D1565784

The International Review of Child Neurology

CHILDREN WITH BRAIN DYSFUNCTION
Neurology, Cognition, Language, and Behavior

The International Review of Child Neurology

The International Review of Child Neurology

Children with Brain Dysfunction
Neurology, Cognition, Language, and Behavior

Isabelle Rapin, M.D.

Saul R. Korey Department of Neurology
Department of Pediatrics and
Rose F. Kennedy Center for Research in
Mental Retardation and Human Development
Albert Einstein College of Medicine
Bronx, New York

Raven Press ■ New York

Raven Press, 1140 Avenue of the Americas, New York, New York 10036

85-2421

Made in the United States of America

Great care has been taken to maintain the accuracy of the information contained in the volume. However, Raven Press cannot be held responsible for errors or for any consequences arising from the use of the information contained herein.

Library of Congress Cataloging in Publication Data
Main entry under title:

Children with brain dysfunction.
    (The International review of child
neurology)
    Includes bibliographical references and
index.
    1. Brain-damaged children. 2. Cognitive
disorders in children. 3. Neuropsychology.
I. Rapin, Isabelle. II. Series. [DNLM:
1. Brain diseases--Infancy and childhood.
WS 340 R218c]
RJ496.B7C47 1982   618.92′8   82-11196
ISBN 0-89004-844-4

Second printing, June 1983

This book is dedicated to the memory of
René Rapin and Saul R. Korey

Foreword

The International Child Neurology Association was founded in 1973 for the purpose of improving the quality of care of children with neurological disorders. It is an association of child neurologists and members of allied professions from all parts of the world dedicated to promoting clinical excellence and scientific research in the field of child neurology. The Association provides, at an international level, an outlet for the interchange of professional opinions for the benefit of the advancement of the neurological sciences in infancy and childhood. It also co-ordinates international meetings, publications, and exchanges in the field of child neurology.

This monograph is the inaugural volume of the International Review of Child Neurology which is the official publication of the International Child Neurology Association. We anticipate that two or three volumes will be published each year and that usually each will be a comprehensive review of a single topic.

We hope to present the best in child neurology wherever that may be found.

John Stobo Prichard

Preface

Despite stunning technical advances such as computerized tomography scanning, frequency spectrum analysis of the electroencephalogram, evoked responses, and others just over the horizon, neurologic diagnosis continues to depend on the clinical evaluation of patients. This is one of the attractions of neurology since this process of diagnosis ensures continued human contact between patient and physician and avoids diagnosis based solely on the perusal of laboratory data. However, correct neurologic diagnosis requires correct interpretation of physical findings and mental status; this in turn requires some knowledge of the nervous system.

The purpose of this book is to illuminate the phenomenology of neurologic dysfunction in children with up-to-date information on how the brain works. It is not intended as a textbook of physical diagnosis nor one of child neurology. It was originally written with pediatricians in mind since I rub shoulders with them daily in the clinics and on the wards. Medical students, pediatricians-in-training, and neurologists-in-training showed me by their questions what they needed to know as we evaluated neurologically impaired infants and children together. In so doing they highlighted areas where knowledge is available and areas where it is not, and led me to include many references that will supply a convenient entry into the clinical, the neuropsychologic, and the neuroscience literature for those who seek more detailed data on a given topic than is provided here.

As I exchanged views with psychologists, speech pathologists, other therapists, and educators who are concerned, as I am, with the welfare of handicapped children, I came to feel that these non-medical colleagues might welcome a book providing them with a basic neurologic framework for thinking in a more structured way about brain dysfunction in children. Would they be able to read my book? Perhaps, if I included a glossary so that the technical terms dear to the physicians's heart would not remain hermetic to them and to parents struggling to understand the jargon bandied about by professionals.

I emphasize deficits of higher cerebral function such as developmental disorders of language, reading, behavior, and cognition for several reasons. First, they are extremely common and every neurologist who sees children, every pediatician, child psychiatrist, and family physician who takes the time to listen to parents, encounters them more often than he or she might wish and needs to know how to approach them. Second, these disorders have attained increasing prominence since the passage of Public Law 94-142 that mandates the education most appropriate to each handicapped child's particular needs. Rational implementation of the law depends on an inventory of what it is the child cannot do, which in turn entails a sophisticated analysis of the behavioral consequences of the developmental and adventitious disorders of brain function. Third, some adult neurologists, child psychiatrists, other professionals, and even some child neurologists harbor misconceptions about deficits of higher cerebral function in children, such as false impressions about criteria for diagnosing brain damage, about the cause of autistic behavior, the interpretation of IQ scores in the child with focal brain dysfunction, or the specificity of a diagnosis of dyslexia.

Neuroscience and neuropsychology are in the exponential phase of their growth curve. This book attempts to capture enough of this current knowledge to help better the sense of children's neurologic and learning disabilities. It will have attained its goal if it can convey some of the excitement I experience when a new discovery in the basic neurosciences unexpectedly clarifies one of my patient's symptoms or opens up an avenue for rational therapy.

Isabelle Rapin

Acknowledgments

This book grew out of two chapters prepared at the request of my colleague Niels L. Low for Brennemann's (now Kelley's) *Practice of Pediatrics*. The first, published in 1964, had the title *Brain Damage in Children*; the second, published in 1981, *Brain Dysfunction in Children*. I thank Vincent C. Kelley and Harper and Row for allowing me to borrow freely from those chapters for the preparation of this book.

Child neurologists spend their lives evaluating children with all manner of symptoms and signs of brain dysfunction. It was therefore lucky for me that Dr. Low's request forced me into wide reading in this area very early in my career. My research on communication disorders in children, supported for many years by grant NS 2503 from the then National Institute of Neurological Diseases and Stroke, deepened my knowledge. My colleagues Barbara C. Wilson, James J. Wilson, and Steven Mattis opened up for me the growing field of neuropsychology as it applies to children with learning disabilities and language disorders. Fruitful collaboration with Doris A. Allen on the psycholinguistics of developmental language disorders added a whole new dimension to my views. At the same time, conversations and collaboration with a host of colleagues in the departments of Neurology, Neuropathology, and Neuroscience of the Albert Einstein College of Medicine and in the Rose F. Kennedy Center for Research in Mental Retardation and Human Development strengthened my understanding of the biologic underpinnings of brain function and behavior. My gratitude is extended to all of these colleagues and to many others outside of my own institution whom I have not named but from whom I learned a great deal. My readings would never have come to life had I not been continuously evaluating children by myself and with younger colleagues. The children taught me what little I know, and I feel priviledged that their parents trusted me to examine their offspring and were willing to listen to whatever advice I could muster on the basis of what I had seen and heard.

It is said that fools venture where the wise fear to tread. Undertaking the task of writing about an area as wide as I have done was probably foolhardy since no one can know enough to cover such a broad topic adequately in all areas. The manuscript was read by Dominick P. Purpura, Herbert G. Vaughan, Jr., and Doris A. Allen, all of whom made constructive suggestions and pointed out areas of obscurity. I thank them for their helpfulness and encouragement.

My colleague from Canada, John Stobo Prichard, pressed the International Child Neurology Association, to which we have both belonged since its inception, to intensify its scientific and educational mission. He proposed that ICNA put out a series of "state of the art" monographs in order to update the knowledge of those around the world who care for children with neurologic problems. I was thrilled and honored to accept his invitation to publish my book as one of this series.

This book would never have seen the light of day had it not been for the cheerful, competent, and untiring help of Helene Manigault and Florence Newmark who typed the countless revisions it went through. Howard Rubin was kind enough to photograph the figures. Finally and not least, the unselfish forebearance and encouragement of my husband, Harold Oaklander, and of my children Anne Louise, Christine, Stephen, and Peter Oaklander has warmed me and enabled me to bring this task to a close.

Contents

1

Introduction

In children, as in adults, gross damage to the brain produces sensorimotor deficits, seizures, intellectual impairment, or a combination of these symptoms. Plasticity, the capacity for reorganization after an injury, was assumed until fairly recently to be so great in the immature brain that full behavioral recovery was thought to be the rule in young children unless damage was extensive. We have come to appreciate that plasticity is limited, and that recovery without discernible deficit is in fact uncommon. Damage, maldevelopment, or dysfunction of the brain often produces syndromes with subtle or circumscribed manifestations that may not become apparent until school age (169).

Strauss and his colleagues (564,565) were among the first to suggest that behavioral problems and school failure might reflect otherwise silent organic brain dysfunction resulting from known or presumed perinatal insults to the brain. The children they described were distractible, hyperactive, impulsive, and inattentive; their moods and energy levels fluctuated; they were often clumsy. They had trouble learning to read, which Strauss ascribed to deficient visual perception. He stressed that while some of the children were dull intellectually others were not, and that their defective school performance was likely to improve substantially when appropriate educational methods were used.

Physicians asked to evaluate one of these children strove to determine whether the child's difficulty reflected an emotional problem—tacitly assumed to be the result of parental mishandling; whether it was caused by "endogenous" mental retardation, or whether "organic brain damage" or "brain injury" was responsible for what was called "exogenous" mental retardation (344), or whether a more subtle learning deficit was its cause. The diagnosis of "organic brain damage" became popular (33,56,67,97,114,261,327,421,453,622). It absolved parents of guilt for the child's problem, removed the stigma of a diagnosis such as mental deficiency, provided a medical, and thus socially acceptable, explanation for the child's scholastic and social difficulties, and brought with it the hope that a medical solution would be found for the child's problem. Medical criteria for diagnosis were sought, for example, minor abnormalities of the motor examination ("soft signs") and of "organicity" in psychologic test protocols. Stimulant medications like amphetamine (dextroamphetamine-Dexedrine®) (70) and methylphenidate (Ritalin®) were prescribed in the hopes of ameliorating the child's ability to learn by increasing his attention span.

As understanding of brain function has progressed, the expectation of a specific syndrome of minimal brain dysfunction or minimal brain damage (MBD) with relatively constant symptoms seems naive. We have swung back from a view of the brain acting as a whole, where the effects of brain lesions upon higher cortical functions were explained in terms of the mass of damaged tissue rather than its location (238,345), to a much more localizationist view (271,378,604).

This position has received strong support from recent technological advances. Localized electrical potentials (90,161) and focal increases in cerebral blood flow, and hence in metabolism, in persons engaged in complex tasks such as speaking, reading silently or aloud, moving their hands, and thinking have been found in the areas of the cortex where involvement in these activities had been predicted on the basis of neuropsychologic studies of patients with focal brain lesions (346). Computerized transaxial tomography (CT) scanning, a noninvasive method for producing images of the brain, is for the first time making it possible to see, if not microscopic, at least macroscopic brain pathology in infants and children who sustain an acute cerebral insult (1,297). A non-negligible number of children with mild motor deficits, learning disabilities, or seizures have detectable lesions or asymmetries on CT scans. We have started to unravel the chemistry of neurotransmitters, which has helped explain some hitherto mysterious drug effects on behavior (363,597). We have learned that the brain produces peptides that influence both brain activity and endocrine secretion, thus exerting general effects on the body (500). Availability of positron emitting radioisotopes with very short half-lives, combined with the use of CT scanning (positron emission tomography = PET), and nuclear magnetic resonance technology will enable us to trace the location and fate of many compounds metabolized in the brain of living, behaving persons (386,465).

Whatever I can say now concerning the consequences of brain damage for the behavior of children is guaranteed to require extensive revision, amplification, and clarification within the next decade, since we are clearly at the threshold of an explosion of knowledge in the neurosciences (580). My goal in this volume is to put the various syndromes that may result from organic brain dysfunction into the context of what we think we know about the brain. A simplified description of a few key aspects of the organization of the brain is provided in the next chapter as well as a glossary of technical terms at the end of the book for the convenience of readers who are not well versed in neurology or neuroscience.

2

Organization of the Nervous System

GENERAL ORGANIZATION

The main divisions of the nervous system are: (a) the two cerebral hemispheres and diencephalon, including a number of paired subcortical gray masses, notably the thalamus, basal ganglia (corpus striatum and globus pallidus), and hypothalamus; (b) the brain stem, comprising the midbrain (mesencephalon), pons, and medulla; (c) the cerebellum, a very large structure lying dorsally to the brain stem; (d) the spinal cord; and (e) the cranial and spinal peripheral nerves (Figs. 1, A–E). Gray areas of the nervous system like the cerebral and cerebellar cortex, nuclei in subcortical areas, and the core of the spinal cord contain neuronal cell bodies. White areas are made up of nerve fibers or axons insulated by myelin. Axons that travel long distances and have common origins and destinations tend to be grouped into bundles or tracts.

The fundamental building block of the central nervous system is the *neuronal circuit*. Circuits may be relatively simple and consist of a chain of just a few neurons, or highly complex with very many interlinked cells. Inputs to a circuit come from other neuronal circuits or from peripheral receptors. The information traverses a more or less convoluted pathway, often with recursive loops, and is elaborated and modified before emerging as a new input to other circuits or as a command to effector organs like the muscles. Individual circuits may be meshed with other circuits into integrated networks or subsystems capable of sustaining complex functions or behaviors. The simplest circuit contains only two neurons, an input and an output cell. Such circuits are called monosynaptic. The familiar knee jerk is a monosynaptic spinal reflex elicited by tapping the tendon of the quadriceps muscle that responds by contracting; the first order sensory neuron is located in the dorsal root ganglion and the output motor neuron in the anterior horn of the spinal cord.

The organization of the nervous system is both hierarchical and parallel in the sense that local circuits made up of simple or complex chains of neurons are under the influence of many distant circuits and that information is usually directed at

3

several circuits rather than just one. Local circuits exist at all levels of the nervous system, from cortex to spinal cord, and function as modules in more complex circuits. For example, some local circuits in the spinal cord are interconnected with cerebellar circuits, brain stem circuits interact with cerebellar ones; the thalamus is linked to the cortex, the cortex to the brain stem, the cortex to the spinal cord, and so on. There are many complex circuits; a well-known one, concerned with fine motor control, runs between cerebellum, thalamus, cortex, basal ganglia, thalamus, cortex, brain stem, and cerebellum (see pp. 57 and 60). Spinal circuits are modulated by descending influences from the cortex and brain stem. Activity in the cortex is modified directly by information from peripheral receptors, relayed through the spinal cord and thalamus.

Some circuits are semi-independent and highly automatized through self-excitatory and inhibitory local feedback or servoloops. The activity of such circuits may be interrupted, triggered, or altered by activity in distant parts of the nervous system. For instance, walking depends on a stereotyped sequence of motor commands whose detailed programming takes place at brain stem and spinal levels, at least in experimental animals (466,539). Starting to walk is triggered by commands from the brain that probably keeps track only of deviations in these programs. Stumbling on a stone no doubt instantly brings into play higher levels of the nervous system, such as cerebellar, vestibular, and basal ganglia circuits (so as to adapt and alter motor patterns in order to avoid a fall), limbic circuits (falling is dangerous, it provokes anxiety), and cortical circuits (thinking, which goes on while one walks, is interrupted by this emergency).

Connections in the nervous system tend to be reciprocal: particular groups of cells both project to and receive information from other cell groups, directly or through relays. For instance, the spinal cord is reciprocally connected to the sensorimotor cortex. As will be pointed out later, reciprocal input-output circuits to the brain, called long tracts, are discrete and highly organized topologically so that information does not lose its detail or get degraded during transmission.

Other reciprocally connected systems have a completely different organization. For example, the reticular formation of the brain stem is made up of a network of interconnected neurons with radiating dendrites. Through neurons with long axons that branch widely, each of which connects with multitudes of cells, the reticular formation can modulate the activity of the entire brain and spinal cord. Information to the reticular formation from most sensory systems and from discrete cortical areas loses its individuality but has widespread effects on the activity of the brain.

FIG. 1A. Lateral view of a normal adult brain. The spinal cord (with the spinal nerve roots) has been severed from the brain stem. Abbreviations: AG = angular gyrus; CS = central sulcus (fissure of Rolando); IFG = inferior frontal gyrus; IPL = inferior parietal lobule; ITG = inferior temporal gyrus; MFG = middle frontal gyrus; MS = motor strip (ascending frontal gyrus); MTG = middle temporal gyrus; OFL = orbital frontal lobe; PCG = postcentral gyrus; PMA = premotor areas; POS = parieto-occipital sulcus; SF = Sylvian fissure; SFG = superior frontal gyrus; SMG = supramarginal gyrus; STG = superior temporal gyrus. (Reproduced and adapted with permission from Hirano et al., ref. 278a.)

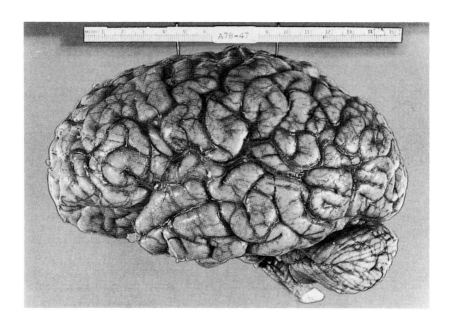

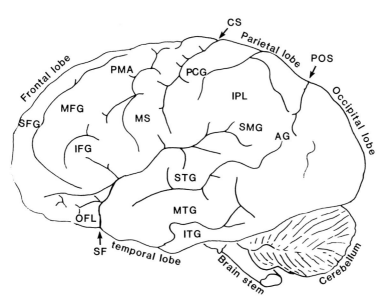

The reticular activating system and so-called nonspecific thalamic nuclei mediate overall behavioral states such as alertness, attention, arousal, and sleep, while the descending reticular formation modulates the tone of the musculature (397).

Reciprocal connections of the brain extend to other body systems through its control of the autonomic nervous system through neurosecretion. Cells in subcortical areas, notably the hypothalamus, secrete peptides that control the pituitary and other endocrine glands (28,281,335). In turn, neurons in many brain areas have been found to have highly specific receptors for cortisol, gonadal steroids, thyroxine, and other hormones (334,354). Differential intrauterine exposure to androgens and estrogens may account in part for personality differences between the sexes (177,256), although the evidence is equivocal at this time (178). Intrauterine and postnatal thyroid deficiency disrupts brain development (25). Observations of this type open the door to exploration of direct effects of various hormones on the brain.

FINE STRUCTURE AND FUNCTION

The central nervous system is made up of synaptically interconnected nerve cells or *neurons*, and of interstitial supportive cells or *glia*. Peripheral nerves consist of the long processes or axons of motor neurons located in the brain stem or spinal cord, and of the long "dendrites" of sensory neurons in cranial nerve and dorsal root ganglia. Supportive cells in peripheral nerves are called Schwann cells. A neuron is a unidirectional polarized cell (Fig. 2) that integrates the bits of information it is continuously receiving from the many neurons to which it is connected. From time to time this information reaches threshold, and the neuron fires and sends out its message to other neurons via its axonal projections. Generally speaking, neurons receive information on their very extensively branched and multiple dendrites and send out information via a single branched axon. Axons are encased in a myelin sheath produced by oligodendroglia in the central nervous system and Schwann cells in peripheral nerves. The neuron's cell body or soma is interposed between dendrites and axon; it contains a nucleus and many organelles responsible for the cell's metabolic machinery. Neurons come in many sizes and shapes, and the geometry of their processes (axons and dendrites) varies in different locations in the nervous system.

Interneuronal communication takes place at *synapses*, which are thin gaps or clefts between specialized areas of the cell membrane (455) (Fig. 3). Typically, presyn-

---

FIG. 1B. Mesial surface of the brain. Midline structures cut to provide this view include the corpus callosum, thalamus, hypothalamus, brain stem, and vermis of the cerebellum. Abbreviations: A = aqueduct of Sylvius; BA = basilar artery; C = cervical cord; CC = corpus callosum; CF = calcarine fissure; CG = cingulate gyrus; CS = central sulcus; F = fornix; M = mesencephalon; MB = mammillary body; ME = medulla; ON = optic nerve; P = pons; PCG = precentral gyrus; PI = pineal gland; POG = postcentral gyrus; POS = parietal occipital sulcus; PS = pituitary stalk; S = septal area; SF = Sylvian fissure; SFG = superior frontal gyrus; SMA = supplementary motor area; SP = septum pellucidum; VM = vermis of cerebellum; III = IIIrd ventricle; IV = IVth ventricle. (Reproduced and adapted with permission from Hirano et al., ref. 278a.)

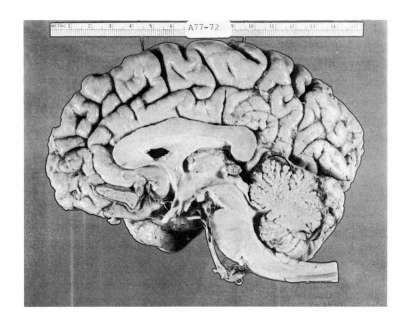

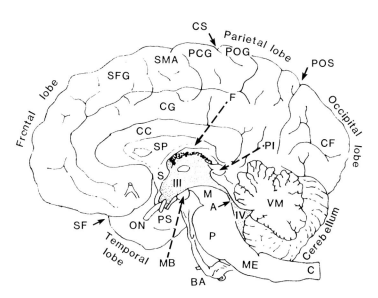

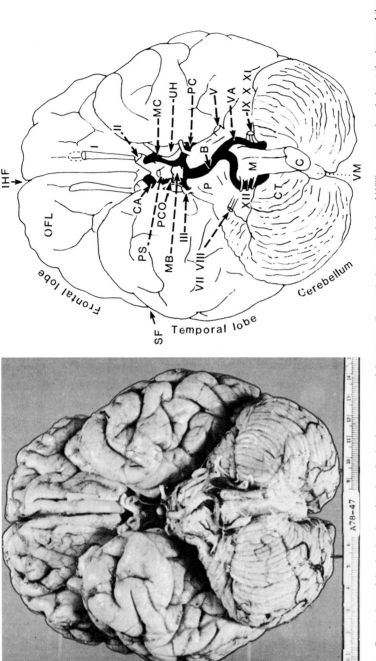

FIG. 1C. Basal view of the brain also showing the brain stem, cranial nerves, diencephalon, and circle of Willis, a vascular circle at the base of the brain shown in black constituted by the anterior communicating artery (not present in this preparation), anterior cerebral, posterior communicating, and posterior cerebral arteries, fed by the basilar and carotid arteries. The middle cerebral arteries are seen to disappear into the depth of the Sylvian fissure. The uncus of the hippocampus of the temporal lobe and the tonsils of the cerebellum are paramedian structures that may herniate through openings of the dura (incisura of the cerebellar tentorium and foramen magnum) in patients with severely increased intracranial pressure. Abbreviations: B = basilar artery; C = cervical cord; CA = carotid artery; CT = cerebellar tonsil; IHF = interhemispheric fissure; M = medulla; MC = middle cerebral artery; MB = mammillary bodies; OFL = orbital frontal lobe; P = pons; PC = posterior cerebral artery; PCO = posterior communicating artery; PS = pituitary stalk; SF = Sylvian fissure; UH = uncus of hippocampus; VM = vermis of cerebellum. Cranial nerves: I = olfactory bulb and tract; II = optic nerve and chiasm; III = oculomotor; V = trigeminal; VII = facial; VIII = auditory and vestibular; IX = glossopharyngeal; X = vagus; XI = spinal accessorius; XII = hypoglossal. (Reproduced and adapted with permission from Hirano et al., ref 278a.)

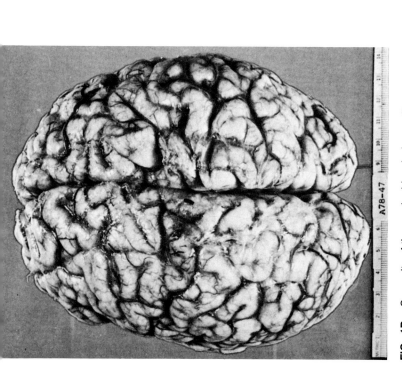
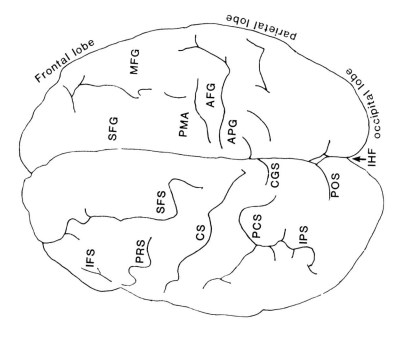

FIG. 1D. Convexity of the cerebral hemispheres. The two hemispheres are normally separated by a fold of the dura called the falx. Note that the left parieto-occipital region is longer and wider than the right, a configuration seen in about 65% of normal right-handed persons that may be related to cerebral dominance for language. Abbreviations: AFG = ascending frontal gyrus (motor strip); CS = central sulcus; CGS = cingulate sulcus; IFS = inferior frontal sulcus; IHF = interhemispheric fissure; IPS = inferior parietal sulcus; MFG = middle frontal gyrus; PCS = postcentral sulcus; PMA = premotor area; POS = parieto-occipital sulcus; PRS = precentral sulcus; SFG = superior frontal gyrus; SFS = superior frontal sulcus. (Reproduced and adapted with permission from Hirano et al., ref. 278a.)

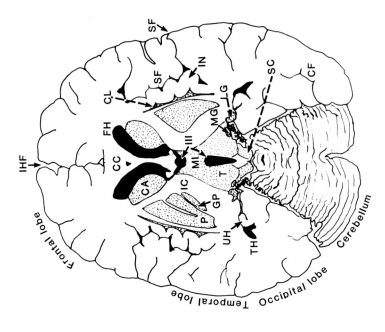

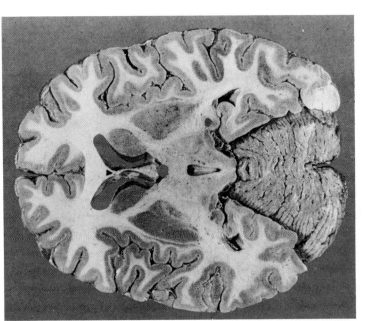

FIG. 1E. Horizontal section of the brain at the level of the superior colliculi. This section is approximately parallel to the plane most commonly used in CT scans and is roughly at the level of the CT scans shown in Figs. 26 and 27. Subcortical gray structures are stippled for clarity. Abbreviations: CA = caudate nucleus; CC = corpus callosum; CF = calcarine fissure; CL = claustrum; FH = frontal horn of lateral ventricle; GP = globus pallidus; IC = internal capsule; IN = insula; IHF = interhemispheric fissure; LG = lateral geniculate body; MG = medial geniculate body; MI = massa intermedia (thalamus); P = putamen; SC = superior colliculus; SF = Sylvian fissure; T = thalamus; TH = temporal horn of lateral ventricle; UH = uncus of hippocampus; III = IIIrd ventricle. (Reproduced and adapted with permission from Hirano et al., ref. 278a.)

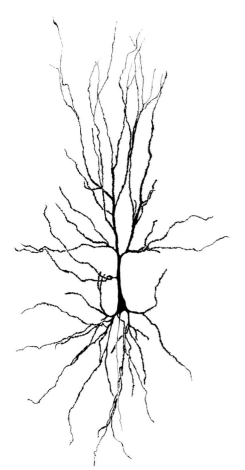

FIG. 2. Pyramidal neuron of the cerebral cortex of a child. Camera lucida drawing of a neuron impregnated with silver salts (Golgi method) and magnified about 300 times. The small dark triangular area is the cell body or soma which contains the nucleus of the cell and its central metabolic machinery. The single thin smooth process emerging from the base of the soma is the proximal portion of the axon which transmits the cell's output; this portion is too short on this micrograph to include recurrent and more distal axon collaterals and axon terminals. All other neuronal processes constitute the elaborate dendritic tree or receptor surface of the cell. Some dendrites fan out from the large apical dendrite which is directed toward the surface of the cortex; others emerge from the basal angles of the soma. The rough surface of dendrites is due to their being studded with thousands upon thousands of spines, specialized areas of receptor membrane upon which the axon terminals of other cells form synapses. Pyramidal neurons of the cerebral cortex of man are among the most complex of nerve cells to have developed in the course of evolution and are assumed to play a key role in sustaining man's cognitive competence. (Courtesy of D. P. Purpura.)

aptic membranes of transmitting neurons are located on axon terminals; postsynaptic membranes of receiving neurons are located on dendrites and cell soma. A single neuron often has thousands of synapses. Synaptic transmission generally takes place through the release of a chemical or neurotransmitter at the presynaptic membrane. The neurotransmitter crosses the synaptic cleft and is bound by specific receptors on the postsynaptic membrane. Excess neurotransmitter is either rapidly destroyed or taken up into the presynaptic terminal. Connections between neurons and muscle cells take place at synapses on the muscle membrane called neuromuscular junctions.

Synaptic inputs generate graded postsynaptic potentials that may be excitatory or inhibitory; the net effect of the many graded potentials a neuron receives and integrates is to either facilitate or inhibit the depolarization or firing of its soma. The action potential or nerve impulse generated in the soma is a large voltage change across the cell membrane that is propagated rapidly along the length of the axon toward the axon terminals where it triggers the release of packets of neurotransmitter. Axodendritic synapses tend to be excitatory and axosomatic ones inhibitory. More recently described axoaxonal and dendrodendritic synapses provide subtle means of communication between adjacent cells; they increase the complexity of the microcircuitry of the cortex and other structures of the nervous system. (455). Some *neurotransmitters* are excitatory, others inhibitory. Acetylcholine, histamine, and glutamate are some of the neurotransmitters that have generally excitatory influences; norepinephrine, dopamine, serotonin, glycine, and gamma aminobutyric acid (GABA) are some of those with predominantly inhibitory effects (363,550) (see Chapter 9). As a general rule, each neuron releases one neurotransmitter, but is in turn sensitive to several excitatory and inhibitory transmitters. Some neurons also release, and are influenced by, neuropeptides that have more prolonged effects than neurotransmitters and are therefore called *neuromodulators* (248,335,474,551). Neurotransmitters exert their effects by binding to receptors and modifying the conformation of channels or pores in postsynaptic membranes. This alters the cell's permeability to small electrically charged molecules or ions. The resulting net flux of ions such as sodium, chloride, potassium, and calcium in and out of the cell alters the potential difference across the cell membrane. Effects of neurotransmitters on synaptic membranes may be rapid and direct, or they may be indirect and mediated by enzymatic alterations in the levels of the cyclic nucleotides, cyclic AMP (adenosine 3' 5', monophosphate) and cyclic GMP (guanosine 3' 5', monophosphate), within neurons. The modulating role of these two cyclic nucleotides on cellular excitability appears to occur, in part, through their opposite effects on intracellular calcium levels (53).

NEOCORTEX

There are two main types of neurons in the cortex, pyramidal cells and nonpyramidal cells, including stellate cells (Fig. 4). Cell bodies of cortical neurons are arranged in horizontal layers whose varying configuration characterizes different areas of the cortex (cortical architectonics) (Fig. 5A and B). Inputs to the cortex from distant cortical areas and from deep nuclear masses such as the thalamus tend to terminate on the dendrites of cells in the upper layers of the cortex. Large pyramidal neurons in the deeper layers of the cortex are mainly output cells with

FIG. 3. Synapses depicted on the dendritic spines and on the shaft of the apical dendrite are excitatory, those on the cell soma are inhibitory. The electron-micrograph to the right of the diagram (provided by C. S. Raine) shows two excitatory synapses on a dendritic shaft cut transversely and magnified 15,000 times. Synaptic vesicles in presynaptic axon terminals store packets of the neurotransmitter particular to that cell. Arrival of an action potential at the axon terminal triggers the release of the neurotransmitter into the synaptic cleft. The neurotransmitter traverses this narrow space and binds to specific receptors on the postsynaptic membrane, which alters the membrane's ionic permeability. This allows fluxes of charged ionic particles across the membrane and results in the generation of excitatory or inhibitory postsynaptic potentials in the receptor cell's dendrites or soma. The action of the neurotransmitter is terminated either by enzymatic degradation in the synaptic cleft or by reuptake into the vesicles of the presynaptic axon terminal. (Reproduced with permission from Iversen, ref. 295a.)

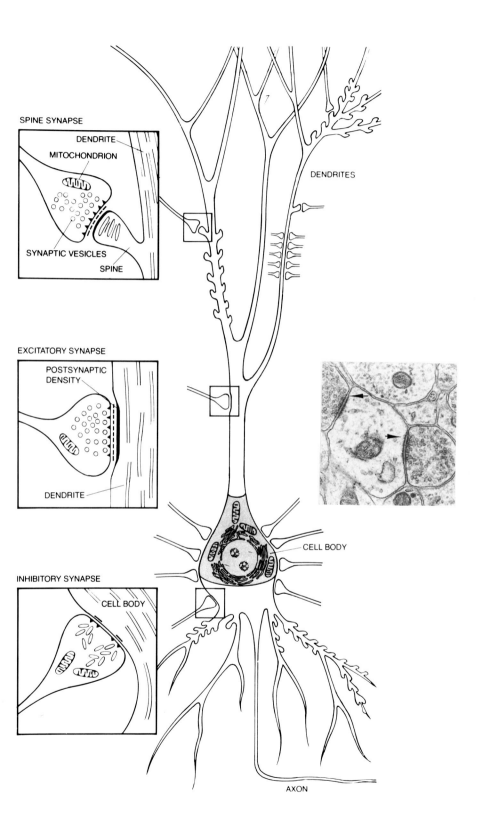

SPINE SYNAPSE

DENDRITE

MITOCHONDRION

SYNAPTIC VESICLES

SPINE

DENDRITES

EXCITATORY SYNAPSE

POSTSYNAPTIC DENSITY

DENDRITE

INHIBITORY SYNAPSE

CELL BODY

CELL BODY

AXON

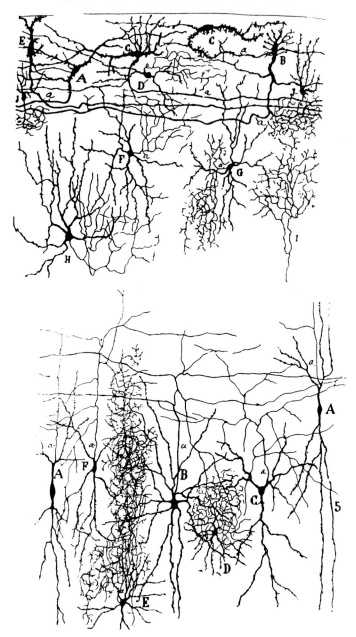

FIG. 4. Variety of neurons in the auditory cortex of a one-month-old child. The cell body, axon *(marked a)*, and entire dendritic tree of each neuron is impregnated with silver (Golgi method), revealing the complex configuration of each cell and some of its interrelationships with other cells. Neurons in the upper part of the figure are mainly intrinsic neurons from the superficial layers of the cortex, those in the lower part mostly pyramidal interneurons from deeper cortical layers. (Reproduced from India ink camera lucida drawings by Ramón y Cajal published in 1902, ref. 483b.)

long axons that transmit at a distance, and short recurrent axons for local communication (176,301). Long axon pathways tend to transmit excitation rapidly and securely to distant and discrete addresses. Through these pathways the cortex is closely coupled with distant cells in subcortical structures (including the spinal cord in the case of the giant pyramidal neurons or Betz cells in the motor cortex), with cells in other areas of the same hemisphere, and with cells in homologous areas of the contralateral hemisphere.

Large pyramidal neurons also communicate locally, through their recurrent axon collaterals, with other pyramidal neurons and with stellate neurons in the immediate vicinity. Small pyramidal neurons in the more superficial layers of the cortex receive inputs from subcortical areas and project mainly within the cortex, including to homologous cortical areas in the contralateral hemisphere (301). Each pyramidal neuron receives thousands of excitatory inputs on the spines of its apical and basilar dendrites. Inhibitory inputs are much less numerous and are located on dendritic shafts and on the cell soma. While the output of pyramidal neurons is excitatory, stellate and other nonpyramidal cells may be either excitatory or inhibitory. The stellate cells, upon which recurrent axon collaterals of pyramidal cells terminate, are mainly inhibitory. Local inhibitory circuits have a stabilizing role; they sharpen messages by the production of surround inhibition and minimize cross-talk or background noise that would interfere with selective transmission. They also prevent uncontrolled excitation from spreading from neuron to neuron within adjacent cortical areas.

In addition to being organized in horizontal layers, neurons of the cortex also have a columnar arrangement. It has been proposed recently that these columns or cores, each of which contains some 110 to 200 cells, respresent the local integrated circuits or modules that are the building blocks of cortical organization (280,432). (Fig. 6).

The cerebral cortex can be divided into the neocortex and archicortex. The archicortex, which is represented by the hippocampus, is phylogenetically older and concerned with processing data arising from internal bodily states. The limbic system, of which the hippocampus is a part, modulates the activity of the neocortex with which it is richly connected. The neocortex occupies the bulk of the surface of the cerebral hemispheres and is concerned with the processing of current data provided by the various senses, with integrating data emanating from the environment with data arising from within the body, and with programming appropriate behaviors based on these external and internal contingencies.

Input-output pathways of the neocortex are relatively discrete and tightly connected, as just stressed. The various sensory systems provide the cortex with integrated and topographically coherent maps of the environment (12). For example, there are specific cells in the sensory cortex of animals that respond to the bending of a single whisker (599). Each spot on the retina projects to specific neurons in the lateral geniculate body of the thalamus and has a sharply defined receptor field in the visual cortex (51). The motor cortex orchestrates the production by the muscles, especially those of the hands and face, of discrete voluntary movements

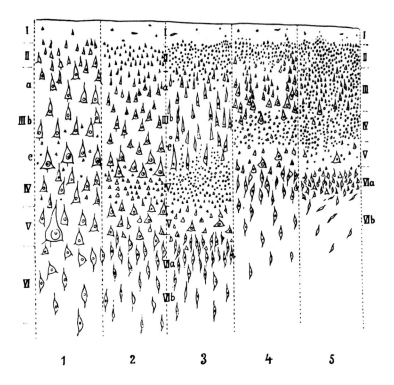

FIG. 5.   Variation in the structure of the neocortex. **(A)** Microscopic anatomy derived from Nissl stains. Neurons tend to be arranged in horizontal layers of alternating large, pyramidal, output neurons and small, granular interneurons. These layers are numbered I to VI going from the surface of the cortex toward the subcortical white matter. Note that the thickness of the cortex and the proportion of large and small cells vary across cortical areas. 1. Agranular cortex, poor in small cells, typical of the motor cortex located in the ascending frontal convolution. The very large cell in layer V is a Betz cell whose axon may project all the way to motor neurons in the spinal cord. 2, 3 and 4. Variations in so-called association cortex which is the most prevalent type of six layered cortex. Small granular or stellate interneurons are most plentiful in layers II and IV and larger pyramidal output cells in layers III, V, and VI. Layer I, the molecular layer, is poor in cells and contains mostly the arborizations of axon terminals upon apical dendrites. 5. Cortex with this configuration is called koniocortex or dusty cortex because it is rich in small interneurons and poor in pyramidal cells. It is typical of sensory projection (input) areas of the cortex. In the visual cortex layer IV, which receives the main visual inputs from the eye, is especially well developed. (Reproduced from von Economo, ref. 176.)

that represent appropriate responses to particular stimuli (466). Lesions in these input-output systems, which encompass sensory and motor areas of the cortex and the tracts leading to and from them, produce relatively specific and predictable sensory and/or motor deficits with limited potential for recovery.

Other areas of the brain, the so-called association areas of the neocortex, participate in complex processing operations. Lesions or stimulation in association cortex do not produce readily detectable effects. For this reason, they are often

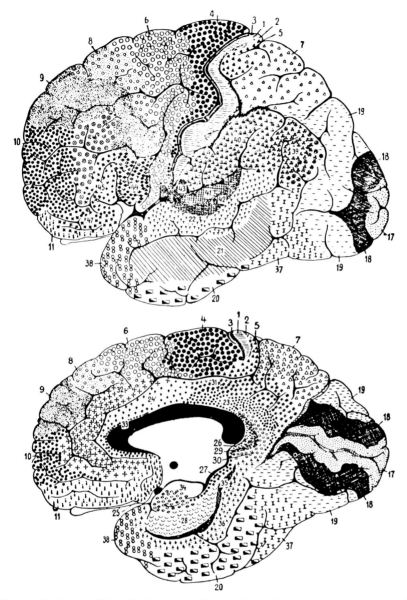

FIG. 5. *Continued.* **(B)** Architectonic map where each symbol corresponds to an area differentiable on the basis of its neuronal configuration and organization studied by silver impregnation. Brodmann (77), who published this map in 1909, inferred that areas of cortex differentiable on morphologic grounds must subserve different functions. His hypothesis has withstood the test of time so well that many cortical areas are still referred to today by the numbers he assigned them on this map; for example, area 17 is the primary visual cortex, areas 18 and 19 secondary or association visual cortex, area 4 the motor cortex, etc.

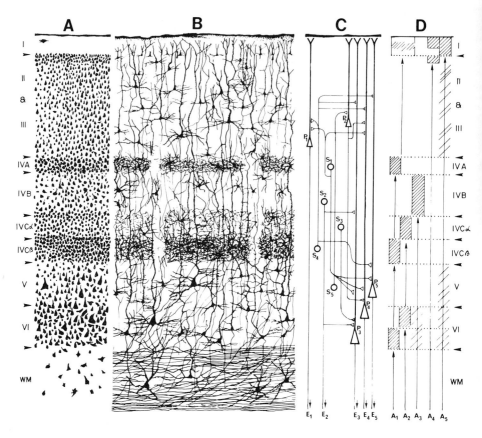

FIG. 6. Laminar and columnar organization of the visual cortex (area 17) and its input-output relationships. This composite diagram of the primary visual cortex of the rhesus monkey integrates observations of several investigators using a variety of techniques. **(A)** Cytoarchitectonic appearance in Nissl preparation which stains cell bodies. Note the subdivisions of layer IV which give the visual cortex a striate appearance visible to the naked eye. **(B)** Cytoarchitectonic appearance in Golgi silver impregnation. The plexus of fibers in layers IV A and IV C are the axonal terminals of the geniculo-cortical afferents terminating on stellate interneurons. An entire vertical column or core, whose width is 350–400μm, is depicted in the center, flanked by two half columns. Each column receives information exclusively from one eye, adjacent columns receiving information from homologous retinal areas of the opposite eye (ocular dominance columns). Cells within a column are heavily interconnected whereas horizontal connections between adjacent columns are sparse. Each column functions as an integrated input-output processing device with very precise topographical connections with other subcortical and cortical areas. **(C)** Simplified diagram of connections within a column and of the cells of origin of its output fibers. S1-5 represents stellate interneurons and their main connection within the column, P = pyramidal neurons. All but P_2 are output cells with targets outside the column: E_1 and E_2 project to other cortical areas—including adjacent visual association cortex, E_3 to the superior colliculus, E_4 and E_5 to different cell groups in the lateral geniculate body. **(D)** Relative position of terminal fields from five major afferent systems: A_1 and A_2 originate from different cell groups in the lateral geniculate body, A_3 from the superior temporal cortex, A_4 from the pulvinar of the thalamus, and A_5 from adjacent visual association cortex (area 18). (Reproduced with permission from Rakic, ref. 483a.)

called silent areas. Association areas are reciprocally and richly connected with multiple cortical and subcortical areas. Some association areas participate in the integration of various inputs and in their evaluation in the context of ongoing cerebral activity and of stored data. Other areas are engaged in choosing among possible courses of action and in programming complex behavioral outputs that are then transmitted to effector systems. Even highly complex activities engage some limited brain systems selectively. For example, lesions in the frontal cortex in adults hinder the ability to wait and choose between behavioral alternatives (378,439,604), while pathology in inferior temporal cortex impairs the memory of complex stimuli (478). Such cognitive operations as making a discrimination that will determine which of two responses to produce have been linked to specific electrical potentials on the scalp of monkeys and humans, some of which are discretely localized (90,161,278).

HEMISPHERIC ASYMMETRY

While it has been known for about a century that activity subsuming language was lateralized to the left hemisphere in most persons, our appreciation that the right hemisphere was specialized for such skills as the ability to recognize melodies, discriminate among complex visual stimuli, and carry out spatial constructional tasks is quite recent. Superficially, the two hemispheres of the brain appear symmetric. Each receives somato-sensory information from the contralateral side of the body, visual information from the contralateral side of space, and more information from the contralateral than from the ipsilateral ear. Each hemisphere controls voluntary movements of the contralateral limbs. Division of labor is not strictly lateralized between the hemispheres since each receives information from, and sends out information to, both sides of the body, and to midline structures like the mouth, neck, and trunk. The neocortex of each hemisphere communicates with lateralized subcortical structures such as the basal ganglia, thalamus, and cerebellum, with cortical and subcortical limbic structures, and with midline subcortical structures like the brain stem and spinal cord.

The importance of communication pathways between the neocortex of the two hemispheres via the corpus callosum and other cerebral commissures is clear. The commissures interconnect homologous areas of the two hemispheres whose activity can thus be integrated. As a result, the environment is perceived as one and activities that depend on harmoniously coordinated movements of both hands can be carried out.

The two sides of the brain have developed some independent and complementary specializations that require separate but integrated programs, and thus interhemispheric transfer of data (164,165,318,431). The best known specialization is, of course, the processing of language in the left hemisphere in right-handed, and in most left-handed persons. The left hemisphere is more efficient than the right for processing serial sensory inputs while the right excels at spatial tasks, pattern recognition, and nonverbal ideation. Experiments in persons whose commissures have been surgically sectioned and in normal individuals in whom care is taken to

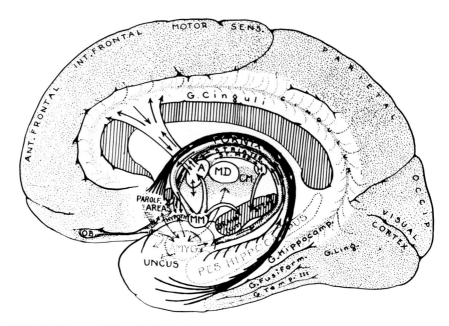

FIG. 7. Diagram of the principal connections of the limbic system, viewed from the mesial aspect of the right cerebral hemisphere. The main directions of connections are indicated by arrows. The cingulate gyrus and hippocampal gyrus were better recognized parts of the limbic cortex than the orbital portion of the frontal lobe at the time the drawing was made. Connections between the brain stem reticular formation and limbic system are not depicted either, notably the major catecholaminergic connections between the mesencephalic portion of the limbic system and its hypothalamic and septal areas (mesolimbic system). Abbreviations: A = anterior nucleus of the thalamus. Amyg = amygdala. CM = center median nucleus of the thalamus. G = gyrus. H = habenula, a small limbic nucleus. Hypoth = hypothalamus. MD = medial dorsal nucleus of the thalamus. MM = mammillary body. The large bundle projecting from the mammillary body to the anterior nucleus of the thalamus is called the mammillo-thalamic tract. OB = olfactory body. Para olf. areas = para olfactory areas, a most important part of which is the septal area which contains a number of olfactory and limbic nuclei, notably the nucleus accumbens septi which is very rich in dopamine. St. Med. = Stria medullaris, which connects the septal area to the habenula. Stria Ter. = Stria terminalis, an efferent pathway from the amygdala to the septal area. (Reproduced with permission from Penfield and Jasper, ref. 459.)

present stimuli to a single hemisphere have highlighted this hemispheric specialization (164,214,216,554,652). It is assumed that in normal persons activity in each of the two hemispheres is continuously integrated via the rich commissural pathways into single solutions that take advantage of the specialization of each. This is no longer the case when the two hemispheres have been disconnected by cutting the commissures. Experiments show that, to a certain extent, each hemisphere of the commissurotomized patient carries on independently, and in some cases, interferes with the activity of its counterpart. Gazzaniga has made a movie showing a commissurotomized patient attempting to reproduce a block pattern: His right hand, commanded by the left hemisphere, interferes with the better performance for such a task of his left hand, commanded by the right hemisphere.

Anatomic asymmetries between the two hemispheres exist and are discernible as early as the second trimester of gestation (223,602,639). In the majority of right-handed persons the superior temporal cortex or planum temporale, an auditory association area, is larger on the left than on the right; the temporo-occipital region is wider on the left, and the frontoparietal wider on the right (206) (see Fig. 1D). It is tempting to correlate this anatomic asymmetry with the specialization of the left hemisphere for verbal processing since hearing is the main channel for language acquisition. Memory for verbal and serial acoustic stimuli is selectively impaired by ablation of the left anterior temporal region while right anterior temporal ablation interferes with memory for visual spatial stimuli (418).

LIMBIC SYSTEM

The limbic cortex, situated in the mesial aspect of the hemispheres, orbital surface of the frontal lobes, and anterior temporal lobes, is richly connected with subcortical limbic structures that include the hypothalamus, amygdala, portions of the thalamus, basal ganglia, and brain stem (Fig. 7). The limbic system is concerned with integrative visceral activities such as feeding, fighting, reproduction, affect, and vigilance; and with the initiation and interpretation of complex species-specific behaviors (295,364,570).

The hippocampus, an archicortical structure of the limbic system, is located in the mesial temporal lobe and plays a crucial role for learning and memory. Learning is obviously essential for survival. It is surely no accident that learning is intimately tied to rewards, as demonstrated by classic conditioning experiments, and to aversive stimuli—avoidance learning. Electrical stimulation of discrete areas in the limbic and hypothalamic systems seems to be perceived by animals as rewarding since they will choose to self-stimulate themselves in these areas. In other discrete areas, stimulation seems to be perceived as unpleasant since the animal will work to avoid such stimulation (450). The limbic system can thus be viewed as the portion of the brain where internal and external stimuli are evaluated in terms of their value to the welfare of the individual (and the species) (364,570).

3

Brain Damage or Dysfunction: General Considerations

DEFINITIONS

Brain dysfunction will be the general term used to refer to the consequences of lesions or damage, maldevelopment, biochemical dysfunction, or altered electrical activity in the brain. The term dysfunction says nothing about the location of pathology in the brain, nothing about severity or type of pathology. The term brain includes the cortex, white matter, subcortical gray matter (thalamus, basal ganglia, amygdala and other nuclei), the brain stem, and the cerebellum.

Mental deficiency means an overall lowering of behavioral competence due to a condition that is static and present from infancy. Mild mental retardation (simple mental deficiency) refers to the condition of high-grade defectives who either represent the extreme lower tail of the normal distribution of intelligence in the population, or those whose retardation probably can be ascribed to an impoverished sociocultural environment. Strictly speaking, mental retardation means delayed cognitive development, mental deficiency, inadequate development. These terms have so much overlap and it is so frequently impossible to determine whether a mildly affected child is mentally "deficient" or mentally "retarded" that the terms tend to be used interchangeably. More severe mental deficiency, whether or not it is accompanied by behavioral problems, is though to represent one of the cardinal symptoms of brain dysfunction. There is overlap between mild and moderate deficiency: Brain damage may result in dull normal intelligence in a child who had potentially high intelligence; the same dysfunction may be responsible for moderate deficiency in a potentially dull child or in one with mild retardation. The relationship between focal brain damage and mental deficiency is discussed in greater detail in Chapter 11.

The terms "behavior disorder" and "emotional disturbance" are often used interchangeably. *Emotional disorder* will be used in the narrow sense of a disorder of affect and emotion, thought to reflect dysfunction in limbic system organization, while *behavior disorder* will be used more broadly to describe any aberrant behavior that is not the direct consequence of a circumscribed defect in brain function such as a deficit in perception or memory. One needs to stress that even circumscribed deficits necessarily have general effects on the child's life experience and thus are likely to produce secondary behavior disorders.

Since the brain is responsible for every aspect of behavior, one could defend the view that all behavioral abnormalities are the result of dysfunction in the brain, since it can be shown that environment shapes the structure and function of the brain (129). Indeed, syndromes with severe behavior abnormalities like schizophrenia, autism, and manic-depressive psychosis are assumed to be the consequence of an as yet unknown structural and/or biochemical defect in the brain which will become manifest if the environment is unfavorable (591). On the other hand, the utility of considering brain function when dealing with the neuroses and the many behavior disorders of childhood that stem from improper rearing practices or disturbed parent-child relationships is doubtful. The wholesale prescription of one drug for a particular symptom, such as methylphenidate (Ritalin®) for hyperkinetic behavior, is just as doubtful.

The consequences of brain damage or dysfunction will vary greatly depending not only on the location and extent of the damage but on characteristics of the child who sustains it. Furthermore, outcome is influenced by the plasticity of the brain, the degree to which it is capable of recovery and of reorganization. Let us now consider these general variables before discussing specific consequences of cerebral pathology.

PLASTICITY AND RECOVERY OF FUNCTION

We saw earlier that lesions affecting the input-output systems of the neocortex are likely to produce predictable deficits with a limited potential for recovery. Lesions in association cortex, in limbic cortex, and in some subcortical areas like the cerebellum and thalamus have less predictable effects or may be silent, either from their onset or after a recovery period. Since it would be ridiculous to suggest that there are parts of the brain that have no function, and since we know that the potential for regeneration after a brain lesion is limited, lack of symptoms must indicate that the brain is capable of performing the same job in several different ways. The anatomic and functional basis for plasticity in brain function is a topic of current research interest (192,558).

Plasticity is assumed to be much greater in early life than in later life. The strongest evidence for this statement is that left-sided lesions are much more likely to produce a permanent aphasia in adults than in young children. But plasticity is limited, even in infancy. As the study of pediatric neuropsychology progresses, we are learning that one can identify rather specific deficits in higher cortical function in young children resembling the classic deficit syndromes of adults with focal brain lesions (628). There is no logical reason to suspect that the child's and the adult's brains are "wired" in substantially different ways.

What are some of the variables that account for recovery from the effects of an acute brain lesion? Early recovery probably reflects the receding of brain swelling and of temporary dysfunction in areas surrounding the lesion. It also reflects recovery from functional synaptic depression (diaschisis) in areas innervated by temporarily incapacitated neurons and from resultant alterations in the balance of the different systems they innervate. Early recovery may also reflect resorption of hemorrhages, improvement in vascular perfusion, and regression of transient metabolic alterations in the vicinity of the lesion.

Late recovery is more difficult to explain. It would seem to reflect reorganization of brain function and, ultimately, perhaps of brain structure. For example, regions of the right hemisphere that under normal circumstances would have limited ability to process language become capable of sustaining it (313). But plasticity is limited and extensive reorganization may be costly (294). Detailed studies of children who recover from an acquired aphasia show that recovery is likely to take place at the expense of other skills that are, presumably, "crowded out" by the right hemisphere's new engagement in linguistic activity (8,264).

What are some of the mechanisms accounting for recovery of function at the cellular level? Two of these are regrowth of axons and synaptic remodeling. To all intents and purposes, neurons, once they are "born," do not divide, so that recovery does not take place by restitution of lost cells.

When a neuron's soma dies, all of the cell's processes also die, whereas the proximal end of an injured axon is capable of regenerating, provided it is attached to its healthy soma (379). Regenerating axons can reoccupy the vacated myelin sheaths left empty by degenerated distal axon segments. Recovery by axonal regrowth is thought to be extremely limited or not to occur within the central nervous system. It takes place regularly, if imperfectly, when peripheral nerves are severed, provided the cut is clean and the cut ends are neatly and tightly sutured together so the axons can find empty myelin sheaths to grow into. It is an extremely slow process since axons grow at the rate of 1 mm per day. Regeneration is often incomplete. Axons regrowing into the "wrong" myelin sheaths will be misdirected and end up innervating muscles previously connected to other motor neurons. For example, aberrant regeneration following damage to the facial nerve may result in involuntary facial movements like winking when smiling, or shedding tears and sweating while eating if autonomic fibers are involved.

Synaptic remodeling reflects the interaction between vacated postsynaptic membranes and adjacent axon terminals. Cells previously innervated by now degenerated axon terminals have denuded postsynaptic areas on their dendrites or cell body. These unoccupied areas seem to attract axon terminals that previously did not end there; these fibers undergo collateral sprouting and slowly reinnervate the denuded neurons (379). The end result of a chronic lesion may thus be the opening of new pathways in the brain. Such aberrant connections may have either beneficial or detrimental functional consequences. We do not know to what extent synaptic remodeling takes place after brain injuries in man. Experiments in fetal monkeys show that significant new pathways, some of them quite large, and judging from their organization, seemingly functional, can develop in the months following a focal hemispheric lesion and, in fact, that proliferating fibers may cross the corpus callosum to find new targets in the other hemisphere (237). (This finding emphasizes, once again, the importance of interhemispheric commissures.)

Another mechanism for recovery of function is more active use of alternate, potentially usable, but until then subsidiary, pathways to produce the movement required to achieve a behavioral goal (192,231,558). Or, an altogether different behavioral strategy may be used; for example, if a monkey's hand is paralyzed it may select another limb or its mouth to grasp a desired object; a child who cannot speak may invent a manual language if he has wants or ideas to convey; a person deficient in visual-spatial skills can verbalize the steps he must follow in order to trace a diagram.

One of the reasons very slowly progressive lesions may be silent for so long is that new behavioral strategies are perfected while old ones are being given up, or new connections made as old ones decay. When the lesion has reached such a large size that compensation is no longer possible, the lesion will rather abruptly make itself known. One of the serious problems in child neurology is to recognize a slowly progressive condition at a time when development is progressing at such a rapid pace that it completely overshadows the consequences of deterioration (485) (see Fig. 23). Slowing of progress is much less obvious than loss of milestones.

CHARACTERISTICS OF THE BRAIN DYSFUNCTION

The term "brain damage" is likely to be a misnomer for many children with organic brain pathology. The term dysfunction appears to be more appropriate and more encompassing, even though it does not have the sanction of tradition. The terms brain damage or brain lesion may continue to be used, provided one appreciates that not all lesions or damage can be seen, even with electron-microscopy.

The location and size of a brain lesion are main determinants of its symptoms. In general, the larger or more diffuse the lesion, the more severe its consequences and the more aspects of behavior will be affected. For example, diffuse or bilateral damage in a child's brain is likely to produce mental deficiency by interfering more or less uniformly with all aspects of behavior and by hindering normal maturation. The correlation between size and severity is by no means simple, however. A relatively small lesion located in a strategic area, for instance the visual cortex, the internal capsule, or the brain stem, will produce highly predictable deficits, while a larger lesion affecting the frontal lobes, the temporal lobes, or the subcortical white matter may go undetected. Furthermore, a large lesion may affect behavior in ways one might not have predicted from a summation of the component deficits it has produced. This supports the notion that in some respects the brain works as a whole in controlling behavior (238,345).

Other characteristics besides size and location of brain lesions are also important determinants of their symptoms: Is the lesion evolving or does it represent the scar of a previously sustained insult? Is it discrete like an infarction, or diffuse like the neuronal drop-out that follows a period of anoxia? Did the damage occur all at once, for instance, following a blow to the brain or an episode of encephalitis, or is it slowly progressive as with low grade hydrocephalus or a neoplasm? In general, acute lesions are much less well tolerated than slowly progressive ones or repeated small insults. Does the lesion obstruct the flow of spinal fluid and raise intracranial pressure? Is it compressing adjacent brain, or destroying it? Is it causing seizures? Does it produce autonomic or endocrine signs by impinging on the hypothalamus?

Alteration of neuronal metabolism and excitability may be just as disruptive to behavior as a structural lesion. Some biochemical lesions, by inactivating a particular neurotransmitter, may have the characteristics of focal pathology since the distribution of many neurotransmitters is discrete and only the pathways where the transmitter is active will be affected. For example, the pharmacologic block of dopamine receptors will mimic pathology in the basal ganglia or limbic system. Of course, some biochemical lesions affect brain structure as well as brain function. For example, sphingolipid storage diseases alter neuronal geometry (482), mucopolysaccharidosis may produce hydrocephalus by infiltrating the leptomeninges, and phenylketonuria (PKU) impairs myelination.

Structural or biochemical lesions occuring during fetal life subvert the genetic programs for development. The result may be a gross alteration in brain organization—a malformation. Later and more subtle alterations may perhaps delay the tempo of development and be responsible for what has been called "maturational lags." For example, lag in head growth and, presumably, in brain growth is frequent among small premature infants during early infancy, with catch-up head growth taking place when the protein-caloric intake of the infant matches his needs (538). Malnutrition after weaning in children growing up in poverty stricken societies also results in a lag in head growth (636). In animals, nutritional lag in brain growth reflects lags in the development of those systems that should have reached their phase of most rapid maturation at the time of deprivation. Is catch-up ever complete after such an insult? Do maturational lags occur because of perinatal insults, and do they account for some cases of dyslexia, of persistant clumsiness or synkinesis (mirror movements) (314,476)? Maturational lags are mentioned frequently in the literature on minimal cerebral dysfunction (MBD) but they are understood poorly and their very existence has been questioned.

Lesions may have negative effects such as paralysis, loss of the ability to perceive complex shapes tactually or visually, or an inability to learn material presented acoustically or visually. They may have irritative effects on surrounding tissue and precipitate focal, complex partial (psychomotor), or generalized seizures. They may release or disinhibit subcortical structures whose disorganized activity may produce a movement disorder or spasticity. Imbalance among particular neurotransmitters may alter mood, raise the threshold for arousal, impair the ability to respond selectively, or be responsible for distractibility and sleep disturbance.

It is important to stress that, depending on their location, lesions that produce identical motor signs, for instance a hemiparesis, may have very different consequences for higher cortical functions. The intelligence of a child with a hemiparesis due to a discrete lesion in the white matter of the brain stem will be entirely normal, while intelligence is likely to be impaired if the hemiparesis resulted from the thrombosis of a cerebral artery producing significant hemispheric damage. Furthermore, the latter is likely to be associated with seizures, while the former is not. Delineating the lesion causing a hemiparesis with a CT scan may therefore be valuable (e.g., see Figs. 26, 27) and help explain differences in symptomatology among children with superficially similar motor signs.

HOST FACTORS

The consequences of brain dysfunction depend, in part, on specific characteristics of the child who is its victim. Age at insult influences outcome at least as much as type and severity of pathology. Organismic characteristics like the innate intelligence and personality of the child, as well as his life circumstances, are other variables to be considered since they too may alter prognosis.

Behavioral development reflects the interface between the genetic programs controlling the organization of the nervous system and the particular environment in which the fetus, infant, and child finds himself. An insult that interferes with these programs during early fetal life will usually bring about more drastic and pervasive modifications in brain organization than damage sustained postnatally. Disruption of normal development by a chromosomal anomaly whose cellular effects are exerted from the time of conception has widespread consequences for behavior. Most major chromosomal anomalies produce severe mental retardation and some are associated with gross brain anomalies, for example, failure of the brain to cleave into two cerebral hemispheres (holoprosencephaly). Genetic disorders like tuberous sclerosis (239) and neurofibromatosis may produce mental deficiency by interfering with cell migration and the orderly organization of the cortex (511). Timing has much to do with the type of pathology since the same anomaly may have a genetic cause in one child and arise from an environmental insult, whereas in another child, an intrauterine infection may be the causative factor. Making an etiologic diagnosis in children with birth defects often requires a number of tests and is by no means always possible.

The brain of the full-term neonate is still very immature, although virtually all neurons have assumed their permanent positions and many have made axonal contact with the distant cells they are genetically destined to innervate. The gross features of the cortex, deep cerebral nuclei, cerebellum, brain stem, and spinal cord, and the major fiber tracts that connect them are present at birth. Postnatal development reflects progressive myelination of these fiber tracts (650), enormous outgrowth of dendrites, and the proliferation and fanning out of axon terminals which will make the myriad and ever more complex neuronal connections that characterize the mature human brain (176,432). Remodeling as a consequence of pathology during fetal life clearly involves different levels of organization than postnatal damage.

Newborns are behaviorally as well as anatomically immature. Damage affecting parts of the brain whose function is not fully developed may be silent until the age when the behavior dependent on the damaged part makes its appearance. Anencephalic and hydranencephalic infants, who are born with essentially no cortical mantle but whose basal ganglia, brain stem, cerebellum, and spinal cord are intact, move their limbs, blink to light, and suck (458). A four-month-old infant with severe congenital micrencephaly learned to smile, regard, and clasp his hands at the same age as normal children; these simple behaviors presumably reflected the activity of his relatively normally developed sensorimotor systems. Pathology, in systems that will sustain behaviors that have not yet emerged, such as fine motor coordination, speech, and cognition, is unlikely to be diagnosed in infancy. This explains, in part, why it may be so difficult to decide, in retrospect, when and how the brain was damaged, and whether a behavorial deficit reflects maldevelopment or an acquired insult (244).

The more subtle dysfunctions that underlie scholastic ineptitude are unlikely to produce stereotyped symptoms. For example, a lesion of the right parietal cortex that, in an adult, would interfere with visual spatial skills might be completely silent for several years, although it might eventually affect the child's ability to learn to read. The same lesion is unlikely to affect the ability to read equally in all children. Some may be able to learn to read if they are taught—or learn on their own—to supplement their less than adequate visual perceptual skills with phonetic analysis of written words and with guesses from contextual cues. An older child, in whom reading has become a highly automatized skill, who sustains the same right parietal lesion may not suffer any reading deficit at all but may draw the face of a clock with all the numbers crowded on the right (132).

Organismic variables like cognitive competence and personality should not be overlooked even though their influence on outcome is likely to be weaker than that of timing, location, and severity of pathology. Dysfunction in a child genetically destined to be highly intelligent will probably have different consequences than the same dysfunction in a child with a less fortunate endowment — whatever the cerebral organization for high intelligence: The first child's IQ may fall within the normal range but he may appear slow compared to his parents and siblings, while the second will seem frankly retarded. In both children, detailed neuropsychologic testing is likely to reveal the uneven levels of performance across abilities that are the hallmark of many brain insults (629).

Those who work to rehabilitate brain-damaged adults know that the patient's personality and mood strongly influence the extent of recovery. Perfectionistic, hypercritical individuals tend to remain depressed and to make less progress than outgoing persons who take a more relaxed view of life. Some children with cerebral palsy will fight to become self-sufficient while others, more passive and shy, will be content to remain dependent on their parents.

One must never lose sight of the fact that biology and environment are inextricably coupled: The circumstances of a child's life, as well as his innate characteristics, contribute to shaping his personality, coping style, and level of competence. Supportive interpersonal relationships, an enriched life experience, and intensive education clearly have favorable effects on a child's ultimate level of functioning

(605). The children of middle-class parents develop earlier and more sophisticated linguistic skills than children growing up in educationally deprived families (60). In musically talented children, the finger dexterity required for virtuoso music performance necessitates both the innate brain organization that underlies the musical talent and extensive practice, started in early childhood. While it is clear that practice, that is learning, must alter the fine structure and function of the human brain, there is no direct evidence on how it does so.

Visual deprivation is known to produce quite specific deficits in visual acuity in children (422), as well as in cats (540), with strabismus or astigmatism (amblyopia) —deficits that are irreversible past a certain age. In monkeys, visual deprivation is associated with anatomic (621) and physiologic (284) alterations in the visual cortex. In fish, an enriched environment alters the structure of dendrites of cortical neurons (129). Rats raised in complex environments and bred for high ability to run mazes were found to have thicker cerebral mantles and more acetylcholinesterase (an enzyme whose concentration accurately reflects that of the neurotransmitter acetylcholine) in their brains than rats that were blinded, reared in simple environments, or bred for poor maze performance (39). It is plausible, therefore, that similar morphologic and functional alterations of the brain take place in man.

This type of experimental evidence seems to have been taken literally by those who propose that very intensive physical and occupational therapy fosters drastic reorganization in the brain of handicapped children (147). There is little reason to suppose that training a child to perform a particular motor act will spill over to other skills (100). It also seems that active, as opposed to passive, experience is required for learning to take place (272). Nonetheless, the experimental evidence does provide some theoretical support for programs of early intervention for children from impoverished environments (Head Start) and for those with handicaps (Public Law 94-142) (454). If preschoolers' IQs can be raised by providing them with a stimulating life experience (286), why not the IQs of children with brain dysfunction? Parents, educators, psychologists, and physicians seem to agree that remedial education, targeted specifically to a child's handicap, is efficacious often enough to mandate its prescription as early as possible for children with known or suspected cerebral or sensory dysfunction. The need for long-term investigation concerning the efficacy of intervention is clear, but the difficulty of rigorous evaluation should not be minimized.

MAJOR AND MINOR BRAIN DYSFUNCTION

The classical signs of gross brain pathology are motor deficits, sensory and perceptual deficits, aphasic disorders, certain rather specific cognitive and behavioral deficits, and seizures. The thesis of this volume is that brain damage or dysfunction tends to affect distinct aspects of behavior differentially. It is true that large acute lesions will lower consciousness or overall brain efficiency, and that diffuse pathology will impair so many aspects of behavior that a label of dementia or mental deficiency, depending on whether the lesion is progressive or static, may be appropriate to describe the person's general ineptitude. Nonetheless, there is so much evidence for specialization of brain structure, brain chemistry, and brain function that one should expect different consequences from different types of lesions. Table 1 attempts to summarize and contrast some of the classic neurologic signs that any physician would readily attribute to gross cerebral pathology with some of the more subtle deficits, often referred to as "soft signs," that have been subsumed under the label of MBD.

The term MBD is often applied to children who show behavioral changes, in particular, learning disabilities, without exhibiting the classic signs of gross brain pathology. Clements (114) gives the following definition: "'Minimal brain dysfunction' refers to children of near average, average, or above average general intelligence with certain learning or behavioral disabilities ranging from mild to

TABLE 1. *Signs of brain dysfunction*

Function affected	Classic neurologic syndromes	Subtle deficits or dysfunction ("Soft signs")
Motor	Spastic diplegia	Toe walking, clumsiness of the hands
	Spastic hemiplegia	Unilateral clumsiness with mild growth arrest
	Pseudobulbar palsy	Excessive drooling, defective articulation of speech
	Choreoathetosis	Prechtl movements of outstretched fingers
	Cerebellar ataxia, tremor	Clumsy gait, impaired fine motor coordination
Sensory	Cortical sensory deficit, astereognosis	Extinction on double simultaneous stimulation
Visual-spatial	Cortical blindness	Visual-spatial deficits, some types of dyslexia
	Homonymous hemianopsia	Visual-spatial deficits, some types of dyslexia
Acoustic	Verbal auditory agnosia	Inefficient processing of acoustic language
Language	Aphasias	Developmental language disability
	Alexias	Some types of dyslexia, dysorthographia
Memory	Amnestic syndromes (e.g., Korsakoff's psychosis, anomias)	Word finding difficulty, deficient memory for acoustic or visual stimuli, problems with sequences, some types of learning disability
Cognition	Severe mental deficiency	Mild mental subnormality; subtest scatter
	Dementia	—
Paroxysmal	Epilepsy (generalized, focal, complex partial or psychomotor, myoclonic)	Minor absences or myoclonus
Attention, arousal	Manic states	Short attention span, hyperkinetic syndromes
	Stupor	Hypokinesis
Affect	Manic depressive psychosis	Labile affect
	Autism	Indifference

severe, which are associated with deviations of function of the central nervous system. These deviations may manifest themselves by various combinations of impairment in perception, conceptualization, language, memory, and control of attention, impulse, or motor function" (p.9).

This definition highlights the lack of specificity of the MBD label. Unfortunately, its very vagueness has blurred awareness of the heterogeneity among children to whom it has been applied. Children with pathologic hyperkinesis or attention deficit disorder (ADD) without learning disability, children with school failure (learning disability) without hyperkinesis (156), children with only clumsiness, and children with combinations of these disorders are often spoken of as though they all suffer from the same condition—MBD. Surely they do not all harbor the same type of brain dysfunction!

While most learning disorders are likely to reflect neocortical dysfunction, disorders of attention may not. Based on experiments performed on rat pups, Shaywitz, et al. (536) have proposed that the restlessness, distractibility, and short attention span of hyperkinetic children may be caused by damage to dopamine systems in the brain or to an inborn error of dopamine metabolism. These symptoms are not specific however. They might reflect the boredom of an intelligent child in a class of slow learners; in a dyslexic sixth grader they might indicate lack of comprehension or be caused by anxiety resulting from the social penalties inflicted by classmates who are competent readers. The time has come to recognize the heterogeneity among children with MBD and ADD and to concentrate on differences rather than similarities.

Explicit in the term MBD is the idea that the child's symptoms are mild. Some workers have argued that the "soft" motor signs of some of the children, like clumsiness, for example, or like the inability to inhibit "mirror movements" in one hand while moving the other hand rapidly, or to keep the fingers quiet while holding the hands outstretched, do not reflect brain damage but immaturity of brain development. Denckla (157) is one of several authors to make the useful distinction between those "soft signs" that, even though they may be very subtle, would be abnormal at any age (she labels them "pastel classic" neurologic syndromes), and those that would be normal if found in a younger child (Table 2). The implication is that "pastel classic" signs must reflect a brain lesion, while the others may not. In the same vein, Kinsbourne (314) argues that many children with learning disabilities (MBD) may be suffering from maturational lags rather than from brain lesions, although elsewhere (315) he argues that maturational lags can also be a consequence of brain damage. Others have suggested that later maturation of boys may explain their greater propensity to suffer from learning disabilities during the early school years. Since maturational lags should have a favorable prognosis and improve with the passage of time, Kinsbourne (315) goes so far as to suggest that benign neglect may be less damaging to the child's self-image than insisting that he learn to read at the same age as his peers. I would suggest that this discussion is specious since specialized educational intervention may be helpful or even crucial, whether MBD reflects "brain damage" or "maturational lag."

TABLE 2. *Examples of "soft signs"*

	"Pastel classic"		"Developmental"
Lateralized	clumsiness weakness hyper- or hypotonia pathologic reflexes mirror movements	Clumsiness or slowness of	gait rapid hand movements tapping (hand or foot) apposing the fingers to the thumb
Asymmetric	associated movements reflexes hopping		Mirror movements (overflow)-bilateral Instability of the fingers with the hands outstretched Difficulty building with blocks Immature holding of a pencil Inability to catch a ball Others

Toe walking
Wide-based gait
Posturing of hands while walking
Tremor of fingers during skilled acts
Dysarthria, drooling, oromotor apraxia, active jaw jerk
Others

Remediability, or lack thereof, cannot be predicted from consideration of the cause (etiology) or mechanism (pathogenesis) of a child's symptoms, unless they are catastrophic or clearly progressive. Rather than focus on etiology and pathogenesis, it is more productive to attempt to isolate and identify the particular deficits of individuals who carry the label of MBD. One can then group children with similar problems into relatively homogeneous subsamples, which will strengthen the analysis of their difficulties. The effectiveness of our management programs will be enhanced if special education is tailor-made to address children's particular difficulty —whatever its cause, and if behavior-modifying drugs with particular pharmacologic effects can be prescribed selectively. While the term MBD may be a useful shorthand label in our present state of ignorance, its very vagueness is treacherous. Hopefully, it is a term that better understanding should render obsolete in the near future.

CONSEQUENCES OF BRAIN DYSFUNCTION FOR COMPLEX BEHAVIORS

In the next two chapters, we shall consider some of the deleterious consequences of brain damage for sensorimotor functions. In some children, sensorimotor dysfunction provides a necessary and sufficient reason for abnormalities of complex behaviors. In others, it is necessary to invoke dysfunction affecting higher order processes like memory, attention, affect, or cognitive competence. The boundaries between sensorimotor deficiencies and higher order deficiencies are admittedly fuzzy. For example, we shall see that deficient decoding of acoustic language has been ascribed by some to the inability to process brief auditory signals (572) rather than to a linguistic deficit impairing the ability to listen in the language "mode" (359), and that reading disability may be a consequence either of visual-perceptual inefficiency or of a language deficit (391).

In addition to deficiencies of motor, visual-spatial, somatospatial, acoustic, and cross-modal processing (57), symptoms of brain dysfunction in children include inadequate ability to learn or remember, attentional deficits, and disorders of mood and drive. The person's verbal skills and problem solving ability and, ultimately, his competence for surviving in his environment may be lowered. In short, his intelligence will suffer. Disorders affecting these so-called higher cortical functions are discussed later in this volume.

4

Disorders of Excitability— Convulsive Disorders

Expression of brain dysfunction is of three types: (1) subtractive deficits responsible for paralysis, sensory loss, or mental deficiency; (2) disorders of excitability producing seizures or paroxysmal loss of function; and (3) imbalance between reciprocally connected neuronal subsystems resulting in positive signs like tremor and other movement disorders. While loss of function is typically thought of as the prime manifestation of brain pathology, seizures are second only to cognitive deficits as far as the frequency of their occurrence during childhood: Seizures are estimated to occur in some 5% of all children (99).

Clinical seizures result from an increase in excitation or a net decrease in one or more of the many inhibitory systems that control neuronal activity in the cerebral cortex. Goal-directed behavior depends on neuronal inhibition as well as on excitation. Inhibitory influences terminate or modulate excitation in single cells; they channel and sharpen the distribution and magnitude of excitation in cell aggregates. Inhibition and excitation are inextricably linked processes at the level of single cells, of local circuits, and of major neuronal systems.

Paroxysmal alterations of excitability are not all in the direction of hyperexcitability (or decreased inhibition), translated behaviorally as tonic-clonic seizures. Pathologic depression is responsible for paroxysmal deficits such as transient weakness, sensory loss, or clouding of consciousness that characterize certain seizure types. Prolonged and diffuse cortical depression results in coma.

Alterations in excitability and inhibition need not all be pathological. Prolonged cyclical changes in the excitability of reciprocally coupled brain stem nuclei underlie the biologic rhythms of arousal and sleep (see p. 101), while variations in excitability of limbic and hypothalamic cell groups are translated as alterations in mood, thirst, and other drives. Regularly phasic behaviors like respiration and walking (539) result from oscillatory excitation-inhibition cycles with a short periodicity in networks of neurons in the medulla and spinal cord.

PATHOPHYSIOLOGY OF SEIZURES

Disorders of neuronal excitability do not become clinically manifest unless sizeable populations of neurons are recruited into a pattern of self-perpetuating hypersynchronous excitation. Rapid recruitment is characteristic of generalized seizures that may start either in the cortex or subcortically but spread through long axons to involve the entire cortex virtually simultaneously. Slow recruitment typifies focal seizures that spread from a small nidus of synchronously discharging neurons to others in the immediate vicinity. It explains the march of clonic movements from the thumb area to the ipsilateral hand, leg, and face that characterizes Jacksonian or focal motor seizures. Strong local inhibitory networks account for the fact that focal cortical seizures often die down without affecting distant brain areas.

The characteristic bursting discharge of an epileptic neuron is caused by a paroxysmal depolarization shift, which has features of a giant excitatory postsynaptic potential (EPSP). The burst of spikes is followed by prolonged after-hyperpolarization. Transition from interictal spikes to the seizure state is accompanied by disappearance of this inhibitory after-hyperpolarization (235). Usually, an epileptic focus is surrounded by an area of inhibition so that the epileptic neurons in the focus rarely have a chance to recruit a sufficient population of normal neurons for a sufficient period of time for their discharge to be translated into clinically apparent symptoms.

The EEG recorded from the scalp is generated by the oscillating excitatory and inhibitory postsynaptic potentials of cortical neurons. Excitatory potentials are depolarizing, inhibitory ones hyperpolarizing. The random spikes that often appear in the interictal EEG of persons with epilepsy (see Fig. 9) result from the transient increase in excitability and summation of EPSPs in a small population of neurons undergoing paroxysmal depolarization shifts. The slow wave that often follows such spikes is the surface reflection of their inhibitory afterhyperpolarization.

During a classic generalized seizure, the EEG mirrors cortical events quite faithfully (Fig. 8). Throughout the tonic phase of the seizure, when the maximally excited cortex is driving brain stem and motor neurons at maximal rates, the EEG consists of an uninterrupted series of spikes. Inhibition reasserts itself during the clonic phase of the seizure with slow waves that interrupt the trains of spikes in the EEG and correspond to pauses between motor jerks. As the seizure runs its course and inhibitory and depressant influences start to predominate, increasingly long periods of flaccidity and longer EEG slow waves separate the clonic jerks and spike discharges until they stop altogether. The patient is then stuporous and the EEG is flat or very slow. Normal rhythms will reassert themselves after a period that may last for no more than a few seconds or that may be very prolonged, depending, in part, on the duration and characteristics of the seizure. When inhibition cannot assert itself, excitability remains unchecked, and the patient experiences continuous seizures or status epilepticus. If status is untreated and extremely prolonged, it may lead to cellular destruction (409) and even to the death of the patient.

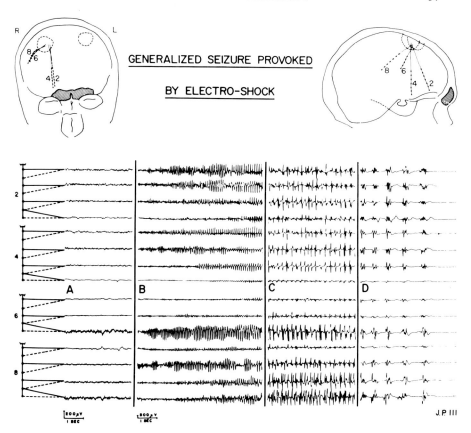

GENERALIZED SEIZURE PROVOKED

BY ELECTRO-SHOCK

FIG. 8. Electroencephalographic pattern of a grand mal seizure produced by electroshock and recorded from multicontact implanted electrodes in an adult schizophrenic patient. Section A: EEG before electroshock. Section B: tonic phase of the seizure which started four seconds after the end of electrical stimulation. Section C: clonic phase of the seizure (interval between B and C: 13 seconds). Section D: end of the clonic phase and start of the postictal coma (interval between C and D: 24 seconds). (Reproduced with permission from Chatrian and Petersen, ref. 105a.)

In generalized seizures such as *absences* where negative effects predominate, a slow wave characteristically follows each EEG spike. The waves reflect strong inhibitory influences responsible for both the interruption in the patient's activity and for the lack of progression to a major generalized seizure despite diffuse involvement of the cortex by the spike-and-wave discharges.

CAUSES OF SEIZURES

Possible precipitants of seizures are legion. It is likely that several factors must coincide in time and act synergistically in order to precipitate a seizure in a susceptible individual, since the occurrence of a clinical seizure is statistically unlikely, even in epileptics in whom seizures occupy but a small portion of life. A drop in seizure threshold may be the consequence of changes in ionic concentration of body fluids. Depolarization may reflect the failure of ionic pumps because of inadequate energy supplies caused by hypoglycemia, anoxia, or other metabolic derangements. Seizures may be triggered by inactivation of inhibitory synapses, or by overstimulation of excitatory ones, caused by alterations in the balance of excitatory and inhibitory neurotransmitters, or by the production of false neurotransmitters that mimic or block the action of natural neurotransmitters. Why some cortical and subcortical lesions are capable of becoming epileptogenic and others are not remains mysterious; and how anatomic lesions foster the epileptic state in neurons adjacent to them is not well understood.

A predominance of inhibition terminates seizures. How these effects come about is not known in detail. Here again, it is likely that multiple mechanisms act synergistically. For example, glial cells may contribute by buffering extracellular ionic concentrations, subcortical inhibitory influences may invade the cortex, and depletion of substrates in discharging neurons interfere with their ability to continue to generate spikes.

In the majority of patients, the cause of recurrent seizures is unknown, and the child is neither mentally retarded nor has other evidence of brain damage. The term *idiopathic epilepsy* denotes a convulsive disorder of undetermined etiology. Strictly speaking, this label should be reserved for patients with recurrent seizures whose only seizure-type is seizures generalized from the onset, since a focal or psychomotor onset or an aura implies that the seizure started in a restricted population of epileptic neurons. In practice, the term idiopathic epilepsy is often used more loosely and applied to any patient who lacks evidence for gross brain pathology and whose seizures have an unknown cause.

That seizures are multidetermined was just stressed. Not only structural and chemical alterations but functional ones can affect seizure threshold. After all, behavior reflects changes in brain state and function. It is not too surprising, therefore, that in some epileptic patients particular emotions like anger or psychic tension may contribute to inducing seizures. These and other emotional states may also be activated by a focal epileptic process and appear as an integral part of complex partial seizures (35,481,624). In a few patients, seizures are triggered by a particular activity such as looking at flashing lights, reading, or listening to music (reflex epilepsy) (144,198,300). The breath-holding spells of infants and toddlers are a particular variant of reflex seizures: The child will have a tonic or tonic-clonic seizure associated with cyanosis, or extreme pallor, and transient asystole precipitated by crying, fright, or pain (392). Most reflex seizures do not respond to anticonvulsant therapy, but may do so to therapies such as desensitization to the offending stimulus (198). Occasional patients can even abort a focal seizure by deliberate behaviors that, presumably, owe their effectiveness to the altering or desynchronizing of brain function they produce; for example, such patients may rub their arm at the start of a Jacksonian seizure, switch their train of thought, or engage in activities like running or singing.

CONSEQUENCES OF SEIZURES

Seizures are usually reversible short-lived events without permanent neurological effects. *Transient postictal deficits (Todd's phenomena)* such as a hemiparesis, homonymous hemianopsia, or aphasia reflect reversible depression of neuronal activity in areas previously preempted by the epileptic process. Todd's phenonema are most common in patients whose epileptic focus reflects a structural brain lesion. Todd's phenomena provide information of localizing value in patients in whom only the generalized phase of the seizure is witnessed. Permanent focal neurologic deficits following seizures are uncommon but do occur. Such deficits, for example an acute infantile hemiplegia, are more likely to be the consequence of an acute lesion responsible for both the seizures and the neurologic deficit rather than a consequence of the seizure itself.

Neuronal metabolism and blood flow increase markedly during seizures. Both can be visualized in persons with a cortical seizure focus by the use of emission computed tomography (PET or positron emission tomography) (336). The metabolic demands of a very prolonged seizure may outstrip available substrates. This results in acidosis and depletion of metabolic fuels in the tissue, in cellular exhaustion or, occasionally, cellular death (608).

A reasonably well-controlled convulsive disorder is usually a benign condition medically, if not socially (607). A chronic convulsive disorder with very frequent seizures has a more ominous outlook. The self-perpetuating character of a chronic epileptic focus may be associated with permanent alterations of postsynaptic membranes and with loss of dendritic spines (areas of dendritic membranes with synaptic specializations, see Fig. 3) (482). One may speculate that loss of spines means deafferentation, and deafferented neurons tend to become hyperexcitable, that is, they respond to smaller and smaller doses of neurotransmitter. A vicious cycle may thus be established. This is one argument for attempting to prevent seizures by the administration of anticonvulsant drugs whose effect is to stabilize neuronal membranes and to decrease the probability of unrestrained firing of epileptic neurons.

Areas that are regularly bombarded by the subclinical epileptic activity of an active seizure focus with which they are synaptically connected may, eventually, be kindled to develop self-sustained independent epileptic activity (403,471). This is especially likely to happen in areas like the hippocampus where excitatory circuits predominate. A mechanism similar to kindling may be responsible for the genesis of a mirror focus in the contralateral temporal lobe of some patients with complex partial seizures (427). Several mechanisms may be at work when a child with a previously localized epileptic focus develops multifocal discharges, such as kindling of new areas of cortex by intermittent subthreshold epileptic activation, cortical damage caused by the anoxia of repeated generalized seizures, and cortical contusions resulting from repeated falls during seizures; rarely, the child may be suffering from a nonrecognized chronic viral infection of the brain (250).

Very prolonged bouts of generalized seizures *(status epilepticus)*, especially if they occur repeatedly and are associated with anoxia, brain swelling, and fever, may produce irreversible damage to the brain (4). Long-lasting seizures associated with fever occurring in infancy, may be one of the causes of incisural sclerosis or scarring of the hippocampus responsible for the later development of psychomotor or complex partial seizures (187). Other seizure types with an ominous outlook for brain development are those that produce frequent massive myoclonic jerks in infants (infantile spasms) and very young children (minor motor seizures) (see p. 43). While in some of the children retardation may reflect the pathology which gave rise to the seizures, in others it is likely that the seizures themselves may have had a deleterious effect on the brain. Purpura (482) has shown apparently progressive changes in dendritic spines in such children. Again, it is not clear whether the dendritic changes are cause or consequence, but they do reflect, at the cellular level, the striking alterations in brain organization that accompany some epileptic syndromes of early childhood and the mental retardation so often associated with them. Futhermore, hypersynchronized populations of epileptic neurons are unavailable to participate in normal brain function. Is it the case that the profound retardation observed in these children reflects, in part, the unavailability of the cortex for encoding inputs from the environment, for processing and storing them, and for programming behavior based on this information?

Chronic epileptic activity may thus interfere with neuronal function and metabolism, with neuronal maturation, with postsynaptic structure and organization, and, at the behavioral level, preclude transiently or permanently a child's ability to interact with his environment, and to learn.

CLASSIFICATION OF SEIZURES BY SEIZURE TYPE

One way to classify seizures is according to clinical and EEG criteria. On that basis, there are two main categories of seizures, those with a focal onset, and those that involve the whole cortex from the start. As stated earlier, seizures in this second category are assumed to arise most often from a subcortical pacemaker in the nonspecific thalamic nuclei or reticular formation that fires the entire cortex through rapidly conducting diffusely projecting pathways. In some cases, generalized seizures are due to a diffuse hyperexcitable state of the cortex. Secondary generalization is presumed to occur either when focal seizure activity in the cortex fires a subcortical pacemaker that in turn fires the entire cortex, or through spread of epileptic activity via interhemispheric commissural pathways (241). The current International Classification of Seizures by seizure type is depicted in Table 3 (123).

The main seizure types in children are (a) generalized (grand mal) tonic-clonic seizures, (b) focal (partial) motor seizures, (c) the so-called psychomotor, temporal lobe, or complex partial seizures, (d) myoclonic seizures—including infantile spasms and minor motor seizures, and (e) absence seizures (staring spells) that may be generalized (true petit mal) or may reflect a complex partial, or psychomotor seizure (365,445).

TABLE 3. *International classification of seizures*[a,b]

I. Partial (focal) seizures
  A. Simple partial seizures (consciousness not impaired)
    1. Motor
    2. Sensory (somatosensory, visual, auditory, olfactory, gustatory, vertiginous)
    3. Autonomic (epigastric discomfort, pallor, flushing, etc.)
    4. Psychic [dysphasic, dysmnesic (déjà vu), cognitive (distortions of time sense, dreamy states), affective, illusions, structured hallucinations]
  B. Complex partial seizures (with impairment of consciousness)
    1. Simple partial onset followed by impairment of consciousness
      a) With simple partial features (I A1–A4) followed by impaired consciousness
      b) With automatisms
    2. With impairment of consciousness at onset
      a) With impairment of consciousness only
      b) With automatisms
  C. Partial seizures evolving to secondarily generalized seizures (tonic-clonic, tonic or clonic)
    1. Simple partial onset
    2. Complex partial onset
    3. Simple partial onset evolving to complex partial seizure evolving to generalized seizure
II. Generalized seizures (convulsive and nonconvulsive)
  A. 1. Absence seizures
      a) Impairment of consciousness only
      b) With mild clonic components
      c) With atonic components
      d) With tonic components
      e) With automatisms
      f) With autonomic components
      g) With a combination of a) through f)
    2. Atypical absence
      a) With changes in tone more pronounced than in II A1
      b) Onset and/or cessation that is not abrupt
  B. Myoclonic seizures (myoclonic jerks, simple or multiple)
  C. Clonic seizures
  D. Tonic seizures
  E. Tonic-clonic seizures
  F. Atonic seizures
III. Unclassified seizures (because of inadequate or incomplete data).

---

[a]The complete document includes ictal and interictal EEG characteristics of each seizure type.
[b]Adapted from the latest proposal for an international classification of epileptic seizures (123).

The clinical manifestations of *focal motor* and of *generalized* or *grand mal seizures* have been described earlier (p. 36). When generalization is secondary, the focal portion of the seizure may be so brief as to pass unnoticed although it may be detectable on the EEG, which shows an interictal focus (Fig. 9) or the focal onset of generalized discharges. Secondary generalization is particulary frequent in epileptic foci of the mesial temporal lobe or hippocampus. The term *aura* or warning denotes that portion of a seizure during which the epileptiform activity is still localized and the patient has not lost consciousness; he is therefore able to describe the subjective experience produced by the focal seizure. Quite often, he may experience auras that are not followed by a major seizure.

Absence seizures are brief lapses of consciousness without loss of posture tone. *Petit mal absences* are characteristically brief (about 10 sec, rarely as long as a minute) episodes of staring and unconsciousness, often accompanied by fluttering of the eyelids, rarely by more complex automatisms (462). They are not preceded by an aura since they are generalized from the onset, and are not followed by postictal drowsiness or confusion. *Psychomotor absences* may be very difficult or impossible to distinguish from petit mal absences without an EEG (14,462). Often, they are more prolonged; loss of consciousness and postictal amnesia are less complete, and they may be associated with complex automatisms, and followed by drowsiness. They are rarely as frequent as petit mal seizures which may occur dozens of times a day. Complex partial seizures are common in childhood; they are often associated with olfactory hallucinations, with autonomic phenomena such as pallor, vomiting, or unpleasant abdominal sensations, and with strong emotional experiences like fear or, less often, anger (596,624). Seizures with paroxysmal laughter (gelastic seizures) often denote a hypothalamic lesion encroaching upon the mesial temporal lobe (213). Complex partial seizures may produce sensory illusions such as the feeling that time is flowing too fast or too slowly, that objects

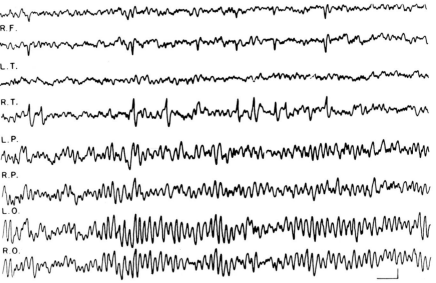

R.F.

L.T.

R.T.

L.P.

R.P.

L.O.

R.O.

FIG. 9. Interictal focal spike discharge in the EEG of a patient with left spastic hemiparesis following birth injury. At 7 years he developed left-sided Jacksonian seizures starting with tingling of the left arm, followed by jerking of the left arm and then the left leg before becoming generalized. The background waking EEG is normal with well-developed alpha at 10 Hz in the parietal (P) and occipital (O) leads. Spikes appear intermittently in the right (R) temporal (T) lead and usually spreads to the right frontal (F) and, at lower voltage, to the left (L) frontal derivations. They are not accompanied by clinical manifestations. Calibration: 500 msc. and 50 μV. (Reproduced with permission from Gibbs and Gibbs, ref. 223a.)

are too large or too small, or unnaturally close or distant; they may evoke memories so that the patient relives a past experience or perceives current events as having happened earlier (déjà vu). Right temporal seizures may be accompanied by formed visual hallucinations, described as being at the movies or the theatre by one patient; left temporal seizures may cause auditory hallucinations such as hearing voices. Many complex partial seizures are associated with automatisms such as walking aimlessly, touching objects, chewing, or speaking unintelligibly (459).

Myoclonic seizures are usually multifocal. They consist of irregular rapid jerks involving a small group of muscles or a single limb, usually without loss of consciousness. Although there are some benign forms of myoclonus, it often denotes underlying structural or metabolic brain pathology. It is characteristic of some genetic progressive brain diseases and of some types of generalized brain damage or maldevelopment. In the majority of children, the etiology of myoclonus is obscure.

In infancy, West's syndrome consists of massive myoclonic jerks of the whole body *(infantile spasms)* associated with a typical EEG pattern called hypsarrythmia consisting of almost continuous high voltage spike-and-wave activity involving the cortex diffusely and asynchronously (Fig. 10). With maturation, this seizure type and EEG pattern evolve to other seizure types or, less often, to recovery (299,388).

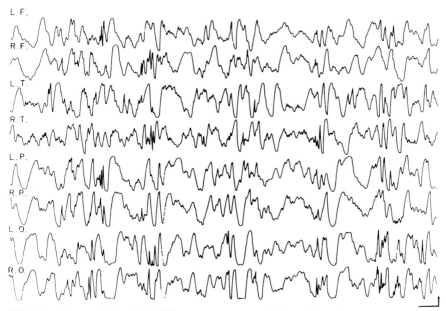

FIG. 10. Hypsarrythmia. This EEG pattern was recorded in an infant who developed infantile spasms (West's syndrome) at age 4½ months. He sustained 2 to 3 attacks per day in which the eyes rolled up, the legs were extended in the air and jerked. Attacks lasted 10-40 seconds and were followed by sleep. Birth and family history noncontributory. The EEG is characterized by irregular high voltage slow activity with frequent spike and polyspike discharges appearing independently in all areas. No normal background rhythms are seen. Calibration: 500 msc. and 50 μV. (Reproduced with permission from Gibbs and Gibbs, ref. 223a.)

The spasms respond poorly to most classic anticonvulsants, better to ACTH or steroids. Unfortunately, infantile spasms are often the prelude to severe mental retardation. In toddlers, a syndrome with similar connotations is manifested by *minor motor seizures* (Lennox-Gastaut syndrome) (108). Children experience brief falls without loss of consciousness as the result of myoclonic jerks. When the jerks are sudden and very frequent the children may appear ataxic (40). The EEG characteristically shows slow (2 cycles/sec) spikes and waves, not to be confused with the 3-cycle-per-sec spike-and-wave pattern of typical petit mal (Fig. 11).

Finally, there are certain extended seizure states that are likely to be misdiagnosed. Prolonged states of foggy consciousness with sluggish behavior and mood changes may coincide with atypical spike-and-wave discharges (233). Abdominal pain and vomiting may accompany these symptoms *(abdominal epilepsy)*. Occasionally, children may be in a state of *absence status* (423). They can walk and are in partial contact with their surroundings. Although they can perform some tasks, their consciousness is clouded, they lack differentiated play and vivaciousness. It is only by specific questioning that one may discover that the child is having staring spells, minor myoclonic jerks, or stereotyped behaviors. Many of these children do not

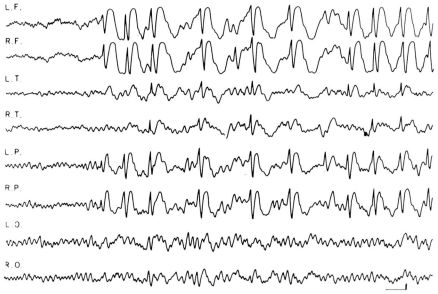

FIG. 11. Slow spike-wave EEG pattern. This EEG was recorded in a mentally retarded adolescent who had one generalized seizure per month starting at age 14 years. No family history of epilepsy. The background waking EEG is normal with alpha activity at 10 Hz in the occipital (O) leads and low voltage fast (beta, 16-20 Hz) activity in the right (R) and left (L) frontal (F) derivations. A run of irregular high voltage slow (approximately 2 Hz) spike-wave activity appears suddenly and synchronously in the frontal and parietal (P) and to a lesser extent in the temporal (T) regions (whose lower voltage is due to placement of reference electrodes on the ears). This pattern is often called petit mal variant (somewhat of a misnomer) and is likely to be seen in toddlers with minor motor seizures (Lennox–Gastaut syndrome). Calibration: 500 msc and 50 μV. (Reproduced with permission from Gibbs and Gibbs, ref. 223a.)

improve dramatically with anticonvulsants unless the EEG, which is crucial to the diagnosis, reveals typical 3-cycle-per-second spike-and-wave absence status.

The syndrome of verbal auditory agnosia or word deafness, discussed on p. 144, may also result from a prolonged seizure state. Bilateral EEG discharges, usually atypical spike-and-wave complexes occuring diffusely or bilaterally over the temporoparietal regions, are common and, some would say, requisite manifestations of this syndrome. The children are not in a state of absence status, although many have a history of seizures or short absences and are mute or nearly so. They tend to have developed a gesture language and usually do not appear autistic or severely retarded although they may have behavior disorders of various types. It is to avoid missing this diagnosis that I recommend obtaining an EEG in all nondeaf nonverbal children.

CLASSIFICATION OF SEIZURES BY ETIOLOGY

Seizures are not a diagnosis but a symptom with many etiologies. They fall into three main etiologic categories, (1) symptomatic seizures, (2) idiopathic seizures, and (3) convulsive disorders with a genetic cause.

Symptomatic Seizures

Acute systemic metabolic derangements, for example, hypoglycemia, hypocalcemia, uremia, anoxia, liver failure, and withdrawal from alcohol or barbiturates may trigger seizures by increasing neuronal excitability in an otherwise normal brain. Chronic seizure disorders may be symptomatic of a genetic-metabolic brain disease like (PKU), various aminoacidurias, the sphingolipidoses, and many others. In storage disorders like Tay-Sachs disease, seizures may be the result of altered cell geometry (482). Commonly, seizures are triggered by focal metabolic alterations in tissue surrounding a brain hemorrhage, contusion, or neoplasm (one needs to stress that neoplasms of the cerebral hemispheres are less frequent in childhood than in middle and late adult life). Seizures may be secondary to bacterial infections of the meninges or parenchyma (cerebritis or brain abscess) or to viral infection of neurons (encephalitis).

Idiopathic Seizures

Chronic convulsive disorders or epilepsy often do not have a detectable cause. Some may reflect an unknown metabolic condition. Others may be caused by a small mesenchymal or glial scar in the cortex, by a developmental malformation such as faulty cell migration or aberrant connectivity, or by some other structural brain anomaly. Neurofibromatosis (von Recklinghausen's disease) and tuberous sclerosis are relatively common dominant genetic traits in which seizures usually reflect aberrant cortical development (239,511).

As stressed earlier, most clinical seizures are probably events with multiple determinants. In patients in whom no etiology can be found for their seizures, genetics may play an accessory role since many studies show that the relatives of epileptics are at a somewhat higher risk of having seizures than unselected persons. This factor may operate even in persons whose seizures are focal and can be presumed to reflect a fortuitous traumatic event: They too are more likely than controls to have a positive family history of seizures (413). A hereditary tendency to neuronal hyperexcitability may act synergistically with adventitious events to explain why some individuals will develop seizures after a brain lesion while others will not.

Convulsive Disorders with a Genetic Etiology

There are several seizure syndromes whose genetic etiology appears well established (413). It is important to be aware of these syndromes since they do not denote brain "damage" and do not require the performance of tests like a CT scan. The best established of these syndromes include (a) true petit mal, (b) benign febrile seizures, (c) benign focal epilepsy of childhood, (d) benign familial neonatal convulsions, and (e) familial photosensitive epilepsy.

True Petit Mal

True petit mal has an autosomal dominant genetic etiology (412). Carriers of the gene do not necessarily have clinical seizures. If they do, the most common seizure type is the classical brief absence described earlier, occurring many times a day, accompanied by the relatively specific EEG pattern of 3 cycles/sec spikes and waves occurring abruptly in all leads in an otherwise normal EEG (Fig. 12). A less common clinical pattern is that of absence seizures associated with occasional grand mal seizures whose initial manifestation is loss of consciousness. Carriers of the gene who do not have clinical seizures often have brief spike-and-wave bursts lasting a second or less in their EEG. One of the characteristics of this gene is that its phenotypic manifestation is age-restricted since clinical seizures are most likely to appear in the early school years and tend to disappear by adolescence (103). Few adults continue to have either absences or generalized seizures, and infants and toddlers virtually never do.

Typical petit mal and grand mal seizures are commonly believed to originate from a pacemaker in the reticular activating system or diffusely projecting thalamic nuclei. They have therefore been called centrencephalic by Penfield and Jasper (459). This theory may not be correct since some patients with otherwise typical absences and EEG discharges have focal spikes in their background EEG (444), and since an excellent model for petit mal seizures has been produced in monkeys by making bilateral focal lesions in the premotor cortex (383). The cerebral commissures, the corpus callosum in particular, also play a role in the genesis of bilateral synchronies (241). This is why commissurotomy is effective in alleviating seizures in some patients with intractable epilepsy (630). Thus, the distinction between primary and secondary bilateral synchronies discussed earlier (p. 40) is not always as sharp as originally believed.

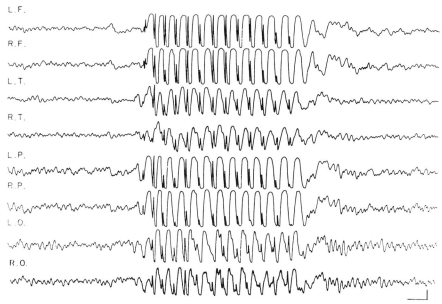

L.F.

R.F.

L.T.

R.T.

L.P.

R.P.

L.O.

R.O.

FIG. 12. Typical petit mal pattern. Onset of absences at age 8 years occurring with a frequency of 4 to 10 per day. No major convulsions. Family history and past medical history noncontributory. Against a normal waking background EEG abrupt onset of regular bilaterally synchronous 3Hz spike and wave discharges with immediate resumption of normal rhythms after 6 seconds. Careful monitoring would show impaired consciousness during the discharge without postictal confusion or drowsiness. Calibration: 500 msc and 50 μV. (Reproduced with permission from Gibbs and Gibbs, ref. 223a.)

Petit mal absences respond to a specific group of anticonvulsants (ethosuximide, trimethadione, and valproic acid); but they may be made worse by the anticonvulsants most likely to be effective against generalized and focal seizures, especially phenytoin. This argues in favor of their having a biochemically distinct pathogenesis. Very recently, Snead and Bearden (547) discovered that the anticonvulsants effective in petit mal were selectively effective against paroxysmal activity produced in rats by the intraventricular injection of leucine enkephalin, while phenobarbital and phenytoin were not. The seizures produced by leucine enkephalin have other resemblances to human petit mal, as do seizures produced in monkeys by gamma-hydroxybutyrate injection. These findings bolster the theory that petit mal is a specific seizure type differing fundamentally from other generalized and focal convulsive disorders.

Benign Febrile Seizures

Benign febrile seizures are also believed to be the reflection of an autosomal dominant genetic trait whose penetrance is incomplete since its manifestation depends on the occurrence of a spike of high fever during the age of greatest susceptibility (352). Benign febrile seizures are most likely to occur between 6 months and 4 years of age. They are rare in older children unless they have had them earlier. Characteristically, benign febrile seizures occur at the height of a rapidly rising temperature spike. They are generalized and brief, lasting only a few minutes. They are not followed by transient or permanent abnormality of the neurologic examination. The EEG is normal during the interictal period. Follow-up studies have shown that such seizures rarely lead to chronic convulsive disorders or epilepsy and that they are not associated with later learning disability or mental deficiency (441). Therefore, if one elicits a history of one or several typical benign febrile seizures in the history of a child with a learning disability, one is not entitled to use the seizure as confirmatory evidence for "brain damage."

Unfortunately, there is a fuzzy boundary between benign febrile seizures and a chronic convulsive disorder whose seizures, initially precipitated by fever, will later occur without fever. There is also an overlap between benign febrile seizures and seizures precipitated by an acute encephalopathy such as the one that accompanies or follows some of the childhood exanthems like roseola and measles, or the encephalopathy of unknown cause that will leave an acute infantile hemiplegia in its wake. As noted earlier, retrospective studies in patients with chronic temporal lobe seizures suggest that in some cases mesial temporal lobe damage (so-called incisural sclerosis) may have been the consequence of a prolonged seizure with fever occurring in infancy (187).

Benign Focal Epilepsy of Childhood

It has recently been appreciated that even seizures with focal characteristics may occasionally have a genetic etiology. Perhaps they reflect a mild genetic aberration of interneuronal connectivity. Benign focal epilepsy of childhood is a dominant genetic syndrome associated with mid temporal-central or Rolandic spikes (61,353). The EEG focus is most likely to be seen during sleep and the seizures, which may be focal or generalized, are also likely to happen during sleep. The seizures typically consist of perioral movements with unilateral jerks of one hand, although more complex psychomotor seizures may occur. This type of seizure tends to be easily controlled with anticonvulsants and to be outgrown by adolesence. This disorder does not have the implication of an acquired or progressive gross structural brain lesion.

Benign Familial Neonatal Convulsions

Another recently recognized dominant genetic disorder is benign familial neonatal convulsions (585). The seizures may be focal or generalized, they are brief, and occur within the first week of life, occasionally within the first days. The children otherwise appear well. The EEG shows paroxysmal features against normal background rhythms. Other laboratory tests are unrevealing. The seizures may be repetitive initially, up to many times in one day, but they are easily controlled with anticonvulsants and are usually outgrown during the first year of life. An occasional patient with this disorder has had a few seizures as an adult. This disorder does not have the serious implications of neonatal seizures caused by anoxia, infection, metabolic disorders, or structural brain anomalies and it is not a prelude to mental deficiency or other neurologic handicaps.

Familial Photosensitive Epilepsy

Still another type of seizure with dominant genetic implications is familial photosensitive epilepsy in which intermittent light stimulation produces a trance-like state, often associated with small myoclonic jerks (300). The EEG of these patients may resemble the EEG of patients with the common type of petit mal or it may contain polyspike-and-wave discharges. Photosensitive patients may suffer generalized seizures, especially if repetitive photic stimulation is prolonged and occurs with a period to which the patient is particularly sensitive. Some children with photosensitivity may experience the altered awareness that accompanies these seizures as pleasureful since they self-induce seizures by waving their fingers in front of their eyes or staring at a flickering television screen (144). Photosensitivity is not always benign since it occurs in some progressive diseases like myoclonus epilepsy of the Lafora type and in some neuronal storage diseases.

EEG AND THERAPEUTIC CONSIDERATIONS

The EEG plays a key role for diagnosis in children with known or suspected seizures. It enables one to distinguish between primary and secondary bilateral synchronies, to differentiate between typical and atypical absences, and to diagnose hypsarrhythmia and absence status. Occasionally, the EEG is also helpful because it suggests that, in that particular child, the seizures are more likely to reflect an active or progressive brain lesion than a static one. Rarely, the EEG is so characteristic that it may suggest a specific diagnosis like subacute sclerosing panencephalitis (SSPE).

The EEG seldom provides evidence concerning brain damage or dysfunction that is germane to the problems of children with attention deficit disorders or learning disabilities. Mildly and diffusely slow EEGs without paroxysmal features rarely have a clinical correlate and are best ignored. Overreading of abnormalities in children's EEGs is, unfortunately, just as common as obtaining an inadequate record (234). Even when the EEG is clearly abnormal and the child has seizures, this does not necessarily signify that the child's learning disability is due to the condition responsible for the seizures and the EEG discharges. This is especially true with the benign seizures of genetic etiology just discussed.

What to make of an abnormal EEG with paroxysmal features in a child who has no clinical seizures and whether to institute anticonvulsant therapy in such a child are difficult questions. For example, should a nonverbal child with autistic behavior and a left temporal spike focus receive carbamazepine or phenytoin? And if an anticonvulsant drug is prescribed, what is the endpoint of therapy, especially if medication produces no change in the child's language deficit? In such doubtful cases, or in the case of a child who has had a single seizure and whose EEG is normal, or of a child with frequent febrile seizures, the physician needs to explain his therapeutic dilemma to the parents since there are no hard and fast rules to guide him.

Seizures are frightening symptoms with inordinately severe social consequences whose management is not always satisfactory. Again, parents need a candid discussion of their child's situation. Many are grateful and helped to understand the therapeutic goals if they are given some written material they can read at their leisure (338).

Unfortunately, all anticonvulsants have possible toxic side effects, even when they are prescribed in doses that keep blood levels within the therapeutic range. The barbiturates, which are otherwise very safe drugs, may worsen some children's attention deficit and hyperkinetic behavior (347). In large doses all anticonvulsants can decrease alertness and interfere with cognitive performance, especially when seizures are very difficult to control and multiple drug combinations are required. In extreme cases, multiple high dose anticonvulsants may even result in a pseudodementia (370). Physicians who prescribe anticonvulsants need to be familiar with their interactions and to learn what drug is most likely to be efficacious for the particular seizure-type and age-group (99,365,445,461). Anticonvulsants are not indicated in children with scholastic problems or with hyperkinetic behavior who do not have seizures.

5

Motor Consequences of Brain Dysfunction

Motor deficit is often the most unequivocal sign of brain damage. As a result, motor dysfunction frequently constitutes the strongest available evidence for brain damage and is invoked to distinguish, among children with learning disability, those with "organic" deficits or "brain damage" from those assumed not to have such problems. The logic of this inference is doubtful on several grounds: While a motor deficit testifies to damage somewhere in the nervous system it may reflect dysfunction in subcortical or spinal systems irrelevant to the child's learning disability. Moreover, neocortical damage or dysfunction does not give rise to motor signs when it spares the sensorimotor cortex. In other words, motor deficits may reflect brain damage outside the cerebral hemispheres; brain damage may occur without motor deficit, and even when motor deficit does reflect brain damage, its relevance to a child's learning disability is likely to be one of guilt by association.

In a very real sense, the only output of the brain is movement, even though movement may be but the vehicle for creative expression: Despite their vividness in the mind of the thinker, unexpressed thoughts remain private and unsubstantial until they are realized through speech, writing, dance, or some other motor behavior. It is not surprising, therefore, that a very large portion of the central nervous system, both cortical and subcortical, is directly or indirectly engaged in motor control, though not necessarily to the exclusion of other integrative activities.

Voluntary or goal-directed movement results from the contraction of muscles activated by motor neurons in the brain stem and spinal cord. These are commanded by pyramidal cells of the motor cortex whose output is modulated by many other systems engaged in programming and controlling skilled movement (466). Motor skill is contingent upon continuous monitoring and adjustment via the multiple external (sensory) and internal feedback loops that signal deviations from the intended movement and that provide the signals for corrective action. Clearly, disorders of movement often reflect pathology outside of the classic motor pathway. Careful analysis of a defective motor performance is required in order to delineate its cause.

Let us start by considering some of the neurologic substrates of movement so as to be able to make sense of the motor symptoms encountered in many children with brain damage or dysfunction.

TYPES OF MOVEMENT

Motor activity is of two main types, sustained or tonic, and transient or phasic. *Tonic muscle contraction* maintains body posture against gravity. Tonic activity is continuously adjusted to compensate for changes in posture as phasic movements alter the distribution of body mass in space. It is never shut off altogether except during some phases of sleep. The maintenance of posture is largely reflex and automatic, and depends on feedback from proprioceptive, visual, and vestibular receptors processed in cerebellar, reticular, extrapyramidal, and spinal loops.

There are many types of *phasic movements*, for example: (a) isolated goal directed gestures, like reaching for an object on sight. These engage motor, premotor, and sensory cortex, together with other cortical and subcortical circuits; (b) series of integrated sequential motor acts culminating in complex activities like speech or figure skating that depend on specific motor learning or practice. They too engage cortical and subcortical loops; (c) sudden isolated movements that compensate for loss of posture or that permit escape from a noxious stimulus. Such acts are largely reflex, they have a short latency, and are organized in shorter loops in spinal or subcortical systems; and (d) highly repetitive or rhythmical motor activities like swallowing or locomotion that are either innate or highly overlearned. As will be seen later, movements of this type depend on cyclical activity in integrated circuits in the spinal cord and brain stem, although triggering and monitoring for dysfunction may engage higher centers, including the cortex. Phasic movements that require prolonged planning and sustained attention are known to engage both neocortical and subcortical systems. Others, for example, laughter, facial expression, and body posture, that mirror a person's mood may originate in the phylogenetically older limbic system.

ORGANIZATION OF THE MOTOR SYSTEM

Final commands for goal-directed discrete voluntary movements of the limbs and face originate in the *motor cortex*. The motor cortex is located on the lateral surface of the frontal lobe and occupies the ascending frontal or precentral gyrus. This gyrus runs parallel to the ascending postcentral gyrus of the parietal lobe from which it is separated by the central or Rolandic fissure (Fig. 1A). The postcentral gyrus receives the primary thalamocortical projections of the somatosensory system. Distinction between these sensory and motor areas of the cortex is not as sharp as may appear at first glance: Both receive inputs from the thalamus and both have descending outputs to subcortical targets in the brain stem and spinal cord. Some investigators prefer to speak of the sensorimotor cortex rather than of the sensory and motor cortical areas.

Another area of the cortex involved with programming motor behavior is located on the mesial aspect of the frontal lobe, just anterior to the mesial extension of the precentral gyrus (see Fig. 1B). This so-called *supplementary motor area* appears to be concerned with automatized repetitive movements like finger tapping and the recitation of overlearned speech sequences, i.e., counting or saying the days of the week (343). It must participate in motor programming since blood flow is said to increase in the supplementary motor area but not in the motor cortex when subjects are asked to picture mentally that they are carrying out a motor sequence without actually executing it with their hands (451).

Areas of the frontal cortex just anterior to the precentral gyrus constitute the *premotor cortex*. The premotor cortex has extensive projections to the sensorimotor cortex, the basal ganglia and, through the pontine nuclei, to the cerebellar cortex. It receives major inputs from the thalamus. The premotor cortex is concerned with motor programming. The frontal eye field, which is a part of the premotor cortex, controls voluntary turning of the eyes toward the opposite side. In the dominant hemisphere, Broca's area can be considered the part of the premotor cortex playing an essential role in speech programming (520).

Each half of the body is represented upside down in the contralateral motor and sensory cortex, with the leg area in its mesial aspect. The motor and sensory representations of the body or homunculi (little men) are similar but not identical (Fig. 13). Areas of the body capable of very complex movements or of refined sensation, like the hand—especially the thumb and index finger—and the lips and tongue have larger areas of representation than body parts such as the proximal portions of the limbs, the neck, and the trunk. Cortical representation of the hand is more strongly lateralized than that of other body parts which receive more equal inputs from both hemispheres. What is represented in the motor cortex is not commands for individual muscles but commands for movement: Stimulation of the surface of the motor cortex produces discrete movements rather than contraction of individual muscles (459), although the latter can be activated by focal intracortical stimulation.

Commands for goal directed motor activity are executed through the activation of a two-neuron system called the *corticospinal* or *pyramidal system*. Neurologists have long referred to the pyramidal neurons giving rise to the corticospinal tract as *"upper motor neurons"*—although, strictly speaking, the only true motor neurons are those that send axons out of the brain stem and spinal cord to skeletal muscles. "Upper motor neurons" are located in layer V of the motor cortex (see Fig. 5A); some of them, notably the giant Betz cells, project directly (monosynaptically) to the motor neurons *("lower motor neurons")* in the anterior horns of the spinal cord and in cranial nerve nuclei of the brain stem, while others project polysynaptically via brain stem and other subcortical relays (466). Each "lower motor neuron" projects onto several hundred muscle fibers in the case of large strong muscles, to fewer muscle fibers in the case of smaller muscles subserving discrete movements of individual fingers and of the face, and to no more than one to a few fibers in the case of the extraocular muscles responsible for moving the eye in the orbit.

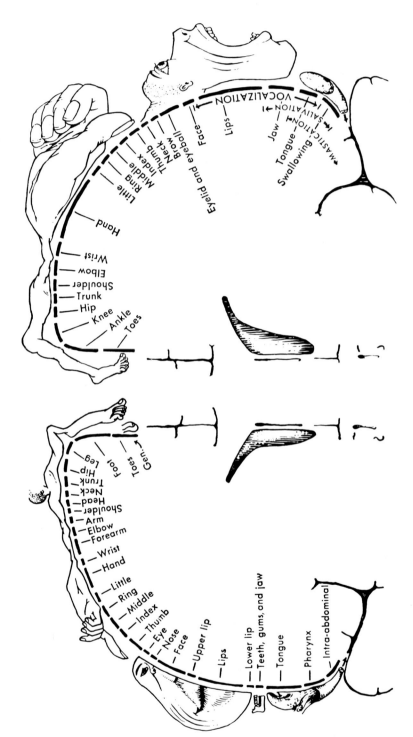

Fig. 13. Representations of the body in the cortex. The homunculus on the left is the somatosensory representation in the postcentral gyrus, the one on the right the motor homunculus represented in the precentral gyrus. Note resemblances and differences. These diagrams were derived from data obtained by electrical stimulation of the cortex of conscious patients who were undergoing surgery for the control of focal epilepsy. (Reproduced with permission from Penfield and Rasmussen, ref. 459a.)

Those muscle fibers innervated by a single lower motor neuron are called a motor unit. The corticospinal executive system is under the control of multiple feedback loops at various neuraxial levels.

Sensorimotor Control at the Segmental Level

Anterior horn cells (alpha motor neurons) receive excitatory inputs not only from the motor cortex and subcortical relays but from primary sensory neurons in the dorsal root ganglia and from sensory interneurons in adjacent areas of the spinal cord. The monosynaptic tendon jerk described on page 3 is the simplest example of a segmental sensorimotor loop. Anterior horn cells are cholinergic cells, i.e., their axon terminals release acetylcholine. They have recurrent axon collaterals that provide them with inhibitory feedback through an interneuron, the Renshaw cell, that releases the inhibitory neurotransmitter glycine.

Anterior horn cells receive information about the length and tension of the muscles they innervate and about the movements of the joints they displace through proprioceptive sensory neurons. There are proprioceptive receptors in skin, bones, joint capsules, muscle tendons, and in specialized (intrafusal) muscle fibers called muscle spindles. Muscle spindles are located in parallel with striated muscle fibers and provide information about muscle length. They receive their motor innervation from small neurons called fusimotor or gamma motor neurons. This so-called gamma loop modulates the activity of the alpha motor neurons in the anterior horns of the cord and plays an essential role in the regulation of muscle tone. Gamma motor neurons, like alpha motor neurons, are under the influence of suprasegmental projection systems.

The influence of proprioceptive information extends beyond the spinal cord; proprioceptive inputs are projected upward to the cerebellum, to the brain stem reticular activating system, and via the thalamus to the sensorimotor cortex. Much proprioceptive information is processed subcortically and does not reach conscious awareness, although recent information suggests an important input of spindle activity to the sensorimotor cortex (399).

Sensorimotor Control at the Cortical Level

Somatosensory information is relayed through the ventroposterolateral thalamus to the primary sensory cortex which is concerned with making fine discriminations about external stimuli and limb movements. In monkeys, inputs from somatosensory modalities like touch, pressure, and joint position are projected to separate representations of the body surface in the postcentral gyrus (see p. 84) (305). The vestibular system provides information about gravity and acceleration of the head, sending such information primarily to brain stem, cerebellar, and spinal cord targets; it also has thalamocortical projections to the parietal lobe (200).

Efficient sensory feedback control calls for the capacity to adapt and correct programs for movement in the light of the movement actually achieved as it is being carried out. This requires a comparison between the sequence of integrated commands to move, reflected by the sequential pattern of firing of the motor neurons, with the proprioceptive feedback provided by the contracting muscles and moving limbs. "Upper motor neurons," like "lower motor neurons," have recurrent axon collaterals (see p. 15). Short axon collaterals project back to cortical neurons in their immediate vicinity (301,432). Longer collaterals provide horizontal intra-cortical connections, through interneurons, to more distant cortical areas and, in particular, to neurons in the sensory cortex. While intracortical loops may account for rapid adjustments in motor programs, modification of firing programs with longer latencies indicates the participation of longer loops to the basal ganglia and cerebellum (79).

Cerebellar Sensorimotor Control Circuits

The cerebellum has phylogenetically old midline structures (vermis), two hemi-spheres, and paired subcortical nuclei. Unlike lesions of the cerebral hemispheres, those of the cerebellar hemispheres give rise to motor deficits in the ipsilateral limbs, whereas vermian lesions tend to produce instability of the neck and trunk.

The cerebellum plays an important role in the timing and control of complex movements requiring integration of feedback information from all the senses with subroutine information provided by various relays of the motor system. It appears particularly concerned with the programming of rapid goal directed *saccadic* or *ballistic* movements that take place too fast to be regulated by peripheral sensory feedback (332). In other words, the cerebellum plays a role in generating self-paced commands for integrated movements to be executed by the sensorimotor cortex (151). Indeed, the major output of the neocerebellum is directed via the thalamus toward the motor cortex, the final orchestrator of goal directed "voluntary" move-ment. Since the cerebellum receives a massive input from the premotor cortex via the fronto-ponto-cerebellar pathway, it is clearly at the focal point of a fronto-cerebellar-frontal loop concerned with motor control (Fig. 14). The ability to pre-program precise sequential movements without requirement for feedback implies previous practice and experience. While the cerebellum no doubt participates in motor learning, its importance for motor memory is still controversial (332).

The cerebellum is informed about what goes on in various relays of the motor system not only through the aforementioned fronto-ponto-cerebellar pathway but through others as well, emanating, in part, from a large relay nucleus in the medulla called the inferior olive. The cerebellum receives sensory information directly from the vestibular system, proprioceptive information via the spinocerebellar tracts, as well as relayed information from oculomotor, visual, and auditory systems. We have a good understanding of the geometry and relationships of these various input fiber systems to the cerebellum with respect to the major output cells of the cerebellar cortex, the Purkinje cells, and with respect to the extremely numerous cerebellar granular cells which are excitatory interneurons, and to other much less numerous inhibitory interneurons of the cerebellar cortex (366) (Fig. 15). The major neuro-transmitters in the cerebellum appear to be amino acids, the main excitatory one being glutamic acid and the main inhibitory one gamma-aminobutyric acid (GABA).

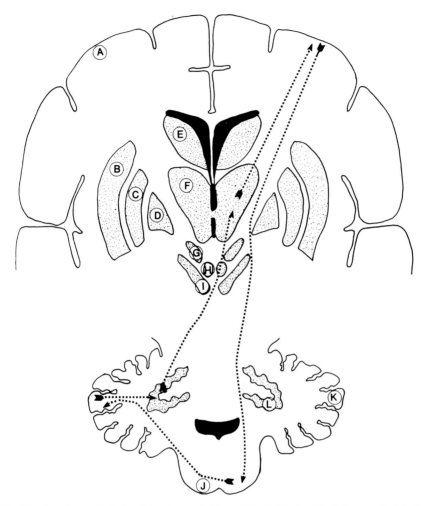

FIG. 14. Fronto-cerebello-frontal motor control loop. This highly simplified diagram depicts the five neuron fronto-ponto-cerebello-dentato-thalamo-cortical pathway. A = premotor cortex; B = outer segment of the putamen; C = inner segment of the putamen; D = globus pallidus; E = head of the caudate nucleus, adjacent to the frontal horn of the lateral ventricle; F = thalamus; G = subthalamic nucleus; H = red nucleus; I = substantia nigra; J = pontine nuclei; K = cerebellar cortex; L = dentate nucleus.

The Purkinje cells of the cerebellar cortex are very large neurons with an extensive dendritic tree. They project to the deep cerebellar nuclei, which they inhibit. These, in turn, are the origin of the main cerebellar excitatory output system which, as was just mentioned, is directed upward toward the ventrolateral thalamus and, ultimately, toward the sensorimotor cortex. Other cerebellar projections are directed toward oculomotor, vestibular, and other brain stem systems.

Basal Ganglia Sensorimotor Control Circuits

The basal ganglia proper are large paired nuclei located deep within each cerebral hemisphere (see Fig. 1E). The *neostriatum* comprises the caudate nucleus and the putamen, divided into an outer and an inner segment, and the paleostriatum, pallidum or globus pallidus (Fig. 16). Two other paired nuclei, the *subthalamic nucleus* and the *substantia nigra*, are usually regarded as belonging to the "basal ganglia" despite their different embryologic origin. The substantia nigra is located in the brain stem and is the source of the dopaminergic nigrostriatal pathway that plays a crucial role in motor control.

Major inputs to the striatum come from the premotor cortex, substantia nigra, raphé nuclei, and from the reticular activating system via the nonspecific thalamic nuclei. The putamen and caudate nuclei receive topographically organized projections from widespread areas of the neocortex, notably the prefrontal cortex (237). Outputs of the neostriatum are directed toward the pallidum and, via GABA and substance P-containing fibers, to the substantia nigra.

The main source of input to the pallidum is the striatum, its main output is directed toward the thalamus. Thus, main outputs of both the neocerebellum and the basal ganglia converge upon the ventrolateral thalamus where they undergo integration and processing before being projected toward the sensorimotor and premotor cortex (466). In short, the basal ganglia are relays in two major loops concerned with motor control, a fronto-strio-pallido-thalamo-frontal loop and a nigro-strio-pallido-nigral loop (see Fig. 16).

The crucial role of the ventrolateral thalamus for motor control is illustrated by beneficial, although usually temporary, effects of stereotaxic thalamic lesions in

---

FIG. 15. Cerebellar cortex **(A)** Low power view of a folium (original magnification 40 ×), prepared by D. S. Houroupian. The surface of the folium, covered by the pial membrane, is at the top. The molecular layer is separated from the granular cell layer by the Purkinje cell layer. The white matter at the center of the folium and part of the granular layer on its other side are seen below. The molecular layer contains the dendrites of Purkinje cells, the parallel fibers (axons) of granular cells, and occasional stellate and basket cells. Most of the nuclei in the granular layer are those of astrocytes. The granular cell layer contains a few Golgi cells whose nuclei are larger and less dark than those of the very numerous granular cells. This section, stained with hematoxylin and eosin, shows cell bodies to much better advantage than cell processes. **(B)** Purkinje cell whose elaborate dendritic tree is deployed in a single plane. a = axon; b = recurrent axon collateral; c and d = space occupied by arborizations of axon terminals of granular and other cells. Camera lucida drawing of a silver stained preparation by Ramón y Cajal (ref. 483c). **(C)** Wiring diagram. The dendrites of the single row of Purkinje cells are arranged in parallel planes deployed transversely along the axis of the folium, while the densely packed parallel fibers of the granule cells are disposed longitudinally. Each parallel fiber makes contact with many Purkinje cells. Inputs to the cerebellum arrive via climbing fibers that twist around the Purkinje cell dendrites and originate in the contralateral olive of the medulla, and via mossy fibers that originate in the spinal cord, vestibular nuclei, reticular formation, and pontine nuclei, and terminate in the granular cell layer. The output cells of the cerebellar cortex are the Purkinje cells. They inhibit the deep cerebellar nuclei, the largest of which is the dentate nucleus. These nuclei project to the thalamus and to brain stem targets. Purkinje, stellate, Golgi, and basket cells are inhibitory. The phenomenally numerous granular cells and the neurons of the deep nuclei are excitatory. (Reproduced with permission from Noback and Demarest, ref. 443a.)

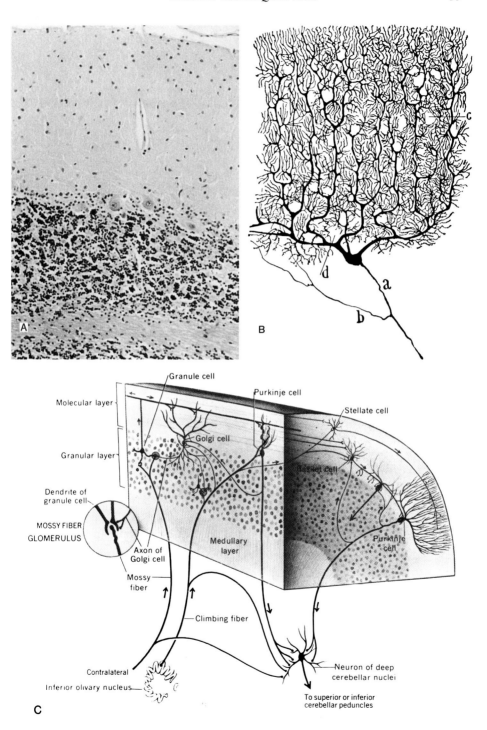

A

B

C

Molecular layer

Granular layer

Granule cell

Purkinje cell

Stellate cell

Golgi cell

Basket cell

Dendrite of
granule cell

MOSSY FIBER
GLOMERULUS

Axon of
Golgi cell

Mossy
fiber

Medullary
layer

Purkinje
cell

Climbing fiber

Contralateral

Inferior olivary nucleus

Neuron of deep
cerebellar nuclei

To superior or inferior
cerebellar peduncles

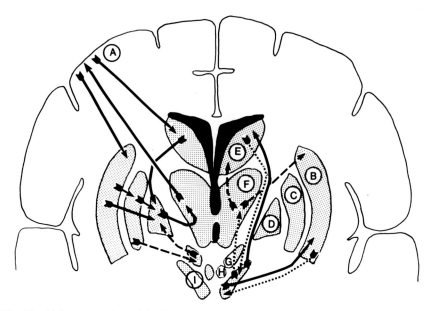

FIG. 16. Major connections of the basal ganglia. The solid black arrows on the left side of the diagram depict the fronto-striato-pallido-thalamo-cortical loop, the dashed arrows on the left main connections of the subthalamic nucleus. On the right side of the diagram the black arrows indicate the dopaminergic nigro-striatal tract and the dotted arrows non-dopaminergic striato-nigral connections. Dashed arrows on the right depict thalamo-striatal and nigro-thalamic fibers. Note that the output of the neocerebellum (dentato-thalamic projections—see Fig. 14) and the output of the basal ganglia (pallido-thalamic and nigro-thalamic projections) overlap and interact in the thalamus. A = premotor cortex; B = outer segment of the putamen; C = inner segment of the putamen; D = globus pallidus; E = head of the caudate nucleus; F = thalamus; G = subthalamic nucleus; H = red nucleus; I = substantia nigra.

patients with movement disorders such as the resting tremor of parkinsonism and the intention tremor of cerebellar pathology (127). (It seems somewhat paradoxical that a second lesion can ameliorate the effect of a first one; perhaps it does so by improving the balance between two systems that should normally be in reciprocal equilibrium.)

Like the cerebellum, the basal ganglia are concerned with motor control and, perhaps, with motor learning (84). Unlike lesions of the cerebellum which have ipsilateral effects, those affecting the basal ganglia produce contralateral motor signs. While cerebellar lesions tend to decrease motor tone, basal ganglia lesions tend to increase motor tone. They also tend to produce a variety of involuntary movements and to interfere with the initiation of movement.

MOTOR PLANNING AND LEARNING

Planning of a "voluntary" motor act requires specification of the goal to be achieved and an evaluation of various potential means for achieving it. It also requires an assessment of the value of the planned activity and of its compatibility with other ongoing activities before the final order to move is put into effect. It is assumed that this aspect of motor control engages the activity of prefrontal and limbic systems. Reactiviation of long-term memories of previously performed actions and their consequences must also play a part in motor planning.

Physiologic studies in animals (466) have shown that neurons in widespread areas, including the cortex and deep nuclei of the cerebellum, the thalamus, striatum, and premotor cortex, discharge as much as 100 msec prior to the inception of a movement. Recordings from the scalp in man have demonstrated "readiness potentials" several hundred msec before the execution of a voluntary finger movement (229). These intervals are considerably longer than the time required for transmitting commands from the sensorimotor cortex to the motor neurons in the spinal cord. It has not been demonstrated yet that activity in one particular location precedes that in others reliably—in other words, we do not know yet where the highest order command for voluntary movement is given (19). In fact, it is likely that the highest commands for movement originate in more than one location, depending on the circumstances of their initiation (432). Disorders of the initiation of movement are common and will be discussed later. They fall into two main categories, akinesia or the inability to initiate movement, and apraxia or the apparent forgetting of how to carry out a particular movement sequence or complex act. The former suggests pathology in the basal ganglia, the latter cortical dysfuntion, usually of the dominant parietal or frontoparietal area.

Motor learning has not been investigated as vigorously as verbal learning but is attracting increasing attention (561). Common experience indicates that motor proficiency usually requires practice, that is, repetition. Learning to ride a bicycle cannot be taught verbally or by imitation; one must experience oneself the proprioceptive, vestibular, and visual feedback provided by riding, and learn by trial and error to utilize it in order to pedal smoothly and stay on the bicycle. Other tasks, for example, learning to knit or play the piano, are greatly facilitated by explicit verbal feedback (telling the student how to move his hands) and by demonstration which provides visual feedback. By so doing, the teacher supplies cognitive strategies that help the student learn to organize the necessary sequence of movements required by the task. This cognitive aspect of motor learning, which corresponds to the cognitive aspects of verbal learning, is now well recognized (561).

We all know that acquiring a new motor skill commandeers our undivided attention. At the start of learning, we monitor individual movements. Even then we are unaware of short-term kinetic memories stored in the motor control circuits at all levels of the nervous system, including the spinal cord. These circuits are called upon to store the vast amounts of ephemeral information that influences, moment to moment, the many subroutines required for maintenance of posture and smooth execution of any planned movement. What we are aware of is the overall goal to be achieved. This goal calls for the retrieval from long-term storage of action plans that constitute our motor memories. As learning progresses and motor skills increase, motor planning embraces longer and longer parts of the sequence of movements required to reach our goal. Individual movements under feedback control become chained and routinized. Conscious attention now encompasses a series of prepro-grammed subroutines that control whole segments of the action, instead of being concerned with the movements themselves. With increasing practice and skill, motor control becomes so strongly hierarchical that only the highest levels of the hierarchy require attention, and a smaller and smaller share of attention at that—so long as all goes well and no error signal is detected.

Execution of skilled movements under visual-kinetic feedback demands that we carry a body-centered map of space in our minds. Kittens (72) and monkeys (273) prevented from seeing their limbs from birth are unable to reach objects in space until after they have been given the opportunity of visually guided reaching; this underlines the importance of integrated visual-proprioceptive feedback for the de-velopment of this map. Feedback from ocular muscles and from neck muscles is also important to the development of the map (561). Since monkeys can learn to perform a skilled act such as grasping a small object between the thumb and index finger after they have been deprived of proprioceptive feedback by deafferentation (cutting all sensory nerves from the limb), a degree of intersensory substitution is possible, with vision compensating in part for the proprioceptive loss (68). For many motor tasks, feedback must be visuokinetic and result from actual perform-ance; passive visual feedback will not do: Kittens carried around in gondolas have diminished capacity for visually guided behavior compared to kittens allowed to walk around and to explore their surroundings (72). Motor learning is quite specific to a particular task: Proficiency at typing hardly enhances piano playing! This should be kept in mind when devising remedial programs for children with brain dysfunction (100).

What is stored in the brain appears to be programs for motor subroutines and action plans for achieving particular goals (561). Programs for activities, rather than programs for movements, must be stored in the cortex since performance keeps at least some of its attributes even when executed with substitute motor neurons and muscles. For example, characteristics of one's handwriting persist whether one is writing on paper or in large letters on a blackboard. Motor learning depends on the integration of the visual-kinesthetic map of space discussed earlier with stored kinesthetic information on how to achieve particular gestures. Corollary discharges provided by commands to move, and fed back locally by recurrent axon collaterals of output cells, may preset sensory systems for the anticipated consequences of voluntary motor acts. Feedback from current movement may thus be compared with stored kinesthetic memories activated by the corollary discharges (577). Motor memory is thus clearly much more complex than the storage of blueprints for carrying out particular gestures.

No one knows where touch typists, dancers, and professional musicians store the programs of mind-boggling complexity they carry in their nervous system. The posterior parietal cortex (inferior parietal lobule, supramarginal gyrus), an associ-ation area that myelinates late and where visual and somatosensory information becomes integrated, plays a crucial role for the execution of learned motor skills. Pathology in this location of the dominant hemisphere is likely to produce an *apraxia* or loss of memory for skilled acts and to preclude the learning of new manual motor skills (268). The dominant hemisphere seems to control skilled movement, not only of the contralateral preferred hand, but also of the ipsilateral, nonpreferred hand via fibers that cross the anterior corpus callosum and project to the contralateral motor cortex. As a result, patients with acquired right hemiplegia due to a left frontoparietal lesion may be clumsy when using their ostensibly normal left hand or may even be quite unable to use their left hand for such an overlearned act as combing their hair.

Very little is known about the recall of motor memories. The hippocampus, especially on the right, clearly plays a role in the retrieval of visual memories and the matching of new visual data with stored spatial maps (74). As will be discussed in Chapter 8, hippocampal activity is essential for verbal and visual learning since bilateral hippocampal ablation results in permanent inablility to remember what was just said or seen. Yet such a patient was able to learn, after many repetitions, to trace a star while watching his performance in a mirror (419), asserting all the while that he had never attempted the task before! Perhaps it is because the networks that participate in motor control are so widespread, and because learning or the gradual shaping of the fine structure and functional properties of these networks takes place over such a long period of time and results in such a hierarchical and distributed organization of motor programs that few deficits affecting motor memory selectively are known to occur.

Control of Walking

Some complex repetitive movement patterns, notably breathing, sucking, swallowing, and stepping, are executed competently from birth (458), and are presumably under tight genetic control. To say that these movements do not require practice or learning may be incorrect, however, since some or all of them are performed *in utero*. These movements appear to be organized in largely autonomous polysynaptic recursive circuits in the brain stem and spinal cord. These circuits do come under at least partial cortical control since we can stop breathing, at least for a few seconds, and can swallow on command. Achievement of other complex motor milestones like sitting, standing, walking, and reaching for an object on sight take time and practice and parallel progress in myelination of the corticospinal tract (650). The ability to stand and walk is innate in many mammals; for example, in horses the foal must be capable of getting up on its feet soon after birth in order to nurse. The nervous system of these animals is more mature and better myelinated at birth than that of man.

In the cat, generators for stepping and for coordination of the two hind limbs reside in automatic cyclically reexcitable circuits in the spinal cord (426,463,539). These circuits do not depend on proprioceptive feedback to maintain their rhythmicity even though the rhythmicity can be altered by proprioceptive feedback. The spinal stepping circuit of the cat can be turned on by dopamine and by stimulation of several defined areas of the brain stem and diencephalon. These so-called locomotor centers, and other areas, including the cerebellum and red nucleus, receive feedback information from the spinal stepping circuits whose activity they modulate. The spinal stepping circuit is also modulated by inputs from the vestibular nuclei, descending reticular activating system, and other brain areas. These supraspinal controls alter gait to fit external circumstances or internally perceived needs and coordinate the movements of the fore- and hindlimbs. The role of the cortex is to trigger these hierarchically organized circuits that control locomotion. Learning to walk is learning to coordinate all of these circuits and the visual, kinesthetic, and vestibular feedback required to maintain the body erect on its small base of support while the rhythmical movements of the legs take place. Further, it is learning how to compensate for tripping, how to run, climb stairs, hop, and skip. It will take 4 to 5 years for children to learn all these alterations of gait competently and to be able to ambulate with minimal need for attention.

Some patients with bilateral frontal damage seem to have forgotten how to walk: They have an *apraxia of gait*. If their deficit is not too severe they can often be made to walk if propelled to take the first step, which probably sets into motion some of the semiautomatic subcortical locomotor circuits just discussed. One can speculate that such patients have lost access to the programs for the initiation of walking. Patients with parkinsonism who suffer from a loss of dopaminergic neurons in the substantia nigra also have trouble starting to walk, but their trouble is best described as akinesia, or inertia. While they appear rooted to the ground when they do get going, their steps are short and shuffling and they tend to walk faster and faster until they are almost running. The loss of dopaminergic input has altered the triggering and the rhythmicity of their locomotor circuits. Differences between apraxia of gait in frontal patients and akinesia in parkinsonian patients illustrate the fact that initiation and execution of walking presumably depend on different programs stored in different parts of the nervous system.

MAJOR TYPES OF MOTOR DEFICITS

Motor disability may affect tone, strength, coordination, and the initiation and planning of motor acts, or consist of the occurrence of abnormal involuntary movements.

Disorders of Muscle Tone

Muscle tone may be pathologically increased. Tone may be increased throughout the range of movement *(rigidity)* or its increase may melt rather suddenly when a muscle undergoes sustained stretch *(spasticity)*. Spasticity denotes dysfunction somewhere along the corticospinal tract while rigidity suggests involvement of basal ganglia circuits. Spasticity may vary dramatically with posture: Spasticity severe enough to prevent ambulation when a child is upright may disappear completely if he is lying supine. The importance for muscle tone of proprioceptive receptors in the neck and of vestibular receptors is demonstrated by changes in tone when the neck is flexed and extended, and by the tonic neck reflex or fencer's position frequently seen in spastic children upon turning the head to one side (automatic extension of the arm and leg ipsilateral to the face and flexion of the contralateral arm and leg). These effects are well-known to physical therapists who attempt to exploit or avoid some of these tonic reflexes when they are training spastic children (64,170).

There are syndromes with greatly increased tone and abnormal postures that indicate that dysfunction has affected the brain stem reticular activating system. Such syndromes are usually associated with impaired consciousness or frank coma. A posture characterized by markedly increased flexor tone in the arms with fisting of the hands and markedly increased extensor tone in the legs suggests diencephalic or upper brain stem dysfunction *(decorticate posture)*. Extensor posture and rigidity of both arms and legs with fisting and pronation of the hands *(decerebrate posture)* points to pontine dysfunction. Evaluation of posture, response to various sensory stimuli, pupil size and reactivity, eye movements, and patterns of breathing provides a means for gauging depth of coma and level of central nervous system dysfunction (473).

When the reciprocal balance between the tone of agonist and antagonist (flexor and extensor) muscles is phasically increased, the child will assume a variety of abnormal postures of the neck, trunk, and limbs called *dystonia*. The severity and extent of dystonia vary greatly as a function of body posture and activity. For example, dystonia so severe as to produce grotesque body posture and to virtually preclude ambulation was observed to decrease strikingly when a child was asked to walk backwards. This observation, incidentally, supports the contention that ordinary locomotion and backward locomotion engage very different brain systems. It is likely that backward locomotion, which is not an overlearned automatized skill like walking, is more dependent on cortical activity and, therefore, is less susceptible to the subcortical dysfunction responsible for dystonia. Dystonia, like many other abnormal postures and movements, disappears during sleep. This is hardly surprising since sleep drastically alters the activity of the brain stem reticular formation and the balance of neurotransmitters in the brain (see p. 101).

Decreased tone, *(hypotonia* or *flaccidity)* occurs as the result of a variety of dysfunctions. It inevitably follows the loss of proprioceptive feedback from muscles since the gamma loop, mentioned earlier, is essential for the maintenance of muscle tone. Muscle tone is also decreased when dysfunction affects the "lower motor neuron" or muscle; hypotonia is then accompanied by weakness and muscle wasting. Hypotonia of peripheral nerve or spinal cord origin is usually associated with loss of tendon jerks.

Loss of vestibular function may result in hypotonia, especially in young children (484). The prevalence and importance of labyrinthine dysfunction in hypotonic hearing children is unknown. Some deaf children with absent vestibular function crawl with a hanging head and have difficulty learning to sit and to stand, although these symptoms disappear as the children mature and they learn to compensate for the lack of this form of sensory input. While it has been suggested that early labyrinthine stimulation hastens the appearance of head control and sitting in normal children (112), to suggest that labyrinthine stimulation has favorable effects in older children with learning disorders is farfetched. Damped labyrinthine function is said to exist in some children with autistic behavior (394). If true, this may explain why some of them enjoy spinning like tops, being carried upside down, or playing roughhouse.

Hypotonia of central origin often points to cerebellar pathology. Hypotonia of cerebellar origin is not associated with weakness but with loss of coordination. There are children with rather diffuse brain damage in whom hyperactive reflexes and other signs of spasticity accompany hypotonia—so-called hypotonic cerebral palsy; the cause of hypotonia in such children is not clear. Children with pathology in the basal ganglia who will later develop athetosis are often hypotonic in infancy. Unilateral hypotonia is rather common in children with infantile hemiplegia with sensory loss; its cause is poorly understood. Generally speaking, hypotonia should suggest derangement in "lower motor neurons," brain stem, or cerebellar circuits rather than dysfunction affecting the cortex. Therefore, one can state rather categorically that hypotonia in a child with school problems is unlikely to be directly related to the cause of the school problem.

Disorders of Strength

Lack of motor strength is called *paralysis* when complete, *paresis* when partial. Lack of strength denotes dysfunction in the corticospinal pathway, "lower motor neuron," neuromuscular junction, or muscles. Lack of movement does not always denote weakness; however, lack of movement may denote markedly increased tone or a severe disorder of body image with neglect (see p. 84).

Pathology in the "lower motor neuron" or muscle is typically associated with wasting and areflexia as well as weakness. Such disorders do not concern us here except to note that *bulbar palsy*, that is, weakness in the muscles of the face and mouth, may preclude normal facial mimic or result in drooling, a nasal voice, and slurred speech. Since such symptoms arise from pathology in the brain stem or cranial nerves, they are not relevant to the disorders of higher cerebral function.

Pathology affecting the "upper motor neuron" is associated with spasticity and hyperactive stretch reflexes. Spasticity reflects increased muscle contraction because brain stem and spinal circuits have lost suprasegmental inhibitory controls. There is no muscle wasting or loss of strength of individual muscle fibers yet the patient is weak, in the sense that he cannot voluntarily move individual fingers or open his fisted hand. Unilateral pathology affecting the corticospinal tract will usually spare, to a greater or lesser degree, the upper part of the face, proximal portions of the limbs, and muscles of the trunk since these muscles receive their innervation from the motor cortex of both hemispheres, directly or through subcortical relays. As a result, persons with a hemiparesis can usually walk and perform some gross movements with their paralyzed arm. (The reasonably functional gait of hemiparetic patients is another argument for the spinal and subcortical programming of locomotion in man as well as in cats.)

What is impaired in corticospinal dysfunction is the ability to translate programs for goal directed and complex motor activities into patterns of motor commands to the lower motor neurons. Where deficits are mild, it is often difficult to decide whether clumsiness of the hand and fingers denotes a corticospinal deficit, impairment of coordination because of pathology in subcortical control circuits, or even an apraxia or disorder of programming. It may also be difficult to determine where, along the corticospinal tract, from motor cortex to brain stem or spinal cord, the pathology may be located. The pattern of muscles affected and signs of dysfunction in other systems are of help for localization.

Disorders of Coordination

We just saw that weakness and disorders of muscle tone may, if mild, masquerade as disorders of coordination. Impaired coordination usually denotes pathology in cerebellar and basal ganglia circuits, although it may reflect loss of proprioceptive input, mild spasticity, mild weakness, or even apraxia.

Lack of sensory feedback precludes smooth motor performance. The three main sensory control systems for movement are vision, proprioception, and vestibular input. Adequate compensation is possible when one sense is missing but not two. Proprioceptive loss produces *pseudoathetosis* which is the inability to maintain the hands outstretched with the fingers immobile, especially when the eyes are closed. Widespread loss of proprioceptive feedback results in a profound disorder of volitional movement, including an ataxic gait, and inability to stand with the eyes closed (Romberg sign). A lesion of the parietal lobe may render the opposite hand almost useless, in part because of the loss of cortical sensory modalities, in part because of a disturbance of body scheme, and in part because of neglect (see p. 85). Children with an infantile hemiplegia with sensory loss can rarely be trained to use their hand except as a prop, whereas children with the same degree of spasticity and lack of individual finger movement are likely to engage in bimanual activity if sensation of the hand is unaffected.

Lack of coordination without weakness or marked change in tone is the hallmark of dysfunction in cerebellar circuits. Movements toward a goal lack smoothness *(dysmetria)* or may be interrupted by an *intention tremor* that increases in amplitude as the goal is approached or as hand posture must be maintained. Gait and the maintenance of the erect posture are affected when pathology involves the vermis. Cerebellar neoplasms in the vermis often produce *titubation* of the head and trunk.

Coordination will also be impaired with disorders of the basal ganglia. A mild chorea may be mistaken for a cerebellar disturbance, especially if accompanied by hypotonia (chorea mollis), while mild athetosis and dystonia will impede proficiency of the hand. Finally, lack of fine motor coordination may be caused by the inability to plan performance—to an apraxia.

It should be clear by now that "clumsiness" and "incoordination" are very nonspecific complaints that may be the end result of many different motor and even sensory disorders. The lack of correlation between *fine motor coordination* of the limbs and signs of *gross motor dyscoordination* affecting locomotor activities observed in some children has anatomic reality since the latter suggests vestibular-vermian dysfunction or bilaterally increased tone, whereas in the former lack of ocular-somatosensory integration or a deficit in the neocerebellar and basal ganglia control circuits to the neocortex are likely to be at fault.

Disorders of the Initiation and Planning of Motor Performance

The initiation of voluntary movement involves the decision to act and the choice of the action to be carried out, as well as the planning of a complex motor sequence. We just saw that these activities are thought to depend on limbic, hypothalamic, and prefrontal-striatal circuits (140,480). *Perseveration*, the inappropriate repetition of a particular act, is characteristic of patients with prefrontal pathology (378). They have trouble thinking ahead and developing problem-solving strategies. It is as though they are stuck on a solution and cannot shift gears. Tasks such as solving mazes or sorting into categories are used to bring out this type of problem (604).

Hypokinesia and *akinesia*, that is, difficulty initiating movement resulting in a paucity of spontaneous movement and of associated movements, reflect pathology in the basal ganglia, most frequently a loss of dopaminergic input from the substantia nigra to the striatum. They are often associated with rigidity. Kornhuber (332) proposed that akinesia indicates a loss of the ramp-generating mechanisms of the striatum while chorea, athetosis, and ballismus reflect their release. Typically, akinetic patients have no difficulty executing sudden ballistic movements, such as catching a ball, that are thought to depend on cerebellar preprogramming. Akinesia is common in parkinsonism but rare in children unless they have suffered massive brain damage.

Catalepsy is a disorder of movement characterized by the very prolonged maintenance of unusual postures without change in tone; it is associated with a lack of response to environmental stimuli and to the request to move. These trance-like states were originally considered to represent a reluctance to move as a consequence of intrapsychic conflict. Newer evidence suggests that they, too, may be caused by a disorder of neurotransmitter metabolism affecting the basal ganglia. Catalepsy can be produced in experimental animals by the administration of neuroleptics like the phenothiazines and haloperidol that are known to block dopamine receptors in the striatum (197). Injection of amphetamine in animals produces forced locomotion and the development of repetitive stereotyped behaviors, an effect thought to be mediated through the release of dopamine in the basal ganglia (311). Recently, Bloom and associates (62) produced a cataleptic state in rats by the injection into the ventricles of the neuropeptide β-endorphin. These effects could be reversed or prevented by naloxone, a specific opiate antagonist (opiate receptor blocker). This effect of endorphin was tentatively attributed to an inhibition of dopamine release in the striatum. Whether there is a relationship between catalepsy produced by drugs and the catatonia of some schizophrenic states is unknown. The evidence just discussed, as well as other observations, raise the question of a possible role of dopamine and of the basal ganglia in the pathogenesis of the major psychoses (530,549,597,606).

Apraxia is often responsible for motor ineptitude in children (247) as well as in adults with acquired brain lesions (81,218,268). Apraxia is the inability to initiate familiar gestures imitatively (50) or in response to a verbal command in the absence of weakness, sensory loss, change in tone, abnormal movements, lack of comprehension, or unwillingness to cooperate *(ideomotor apraxia)*. In some patients, apraxia is so severe as to interfere with the use of common objects like a key or a comb *(ideational apraxia)*. Such patients usually also have an ideomotor apraxia, and either have a receptive aphasia or they are in a confusional state because of diffuse cerebral pathology (268). In some patients, apraxia seems to result from a disconnection between cortical areas concerned with linguistic processing and those, like the premotor cortex, concerned with motor programming (218,219). In other patients, it may reflect an inability to retrieve or activate stored motor programs. Apraxia usually results from a lesion in the dominant hemisphere, notably in the inferior parietal lobule (supramarginal gyrus), unless it reflects pathology in the anterior portion of the corpus callosum. Apraxia interferes with the learning of new motor skills as well as with the execution of previously learned ones (268,312).

Apraxia of gait, that is, inability to initiate walking, is typically seen in demented patients with bilateral frontal pathology, lesions of the anterior portion of the corpus callosum, or hydrocephalus. It is a prominent sign in some of the neuronal storage disorders such as juvenile cerebromacular degeneration (ceroid lipofuscinosis) where the child may appear rooted to the ground. Mild apraxia of gait may be manifested by inability to jump or hop on one foot. Such symptoms are common in children with MBD where they may reflect an apractic disorder rather than be the signs of pyramidal or cerebellar dysfunction.

Oromotor apraxia, the inability to imitate movements of the lips, tongue, and mandible, occurs frequently in children with expressive language disorders and in those with dysarthria (191,330,402,494). It is often associated with pseudobulbar palsy and plays a contributory role in the children's articulation deficit. Oromotor apraxia is rarely severe enough to provide a convincing explanation for complete inability to produce articulated speech.

While the ideomotor apraxias are usually the result of acquired posterior brain lesions in the dominant hemisphere, *constructional apraxia*, or difficulty with tasks such as reproducing block patterns or copying drawings, is likely to reflect non-dominant parietal pathology (46). It is often associated with deficits in visual-spatial perception. Dominant parietal lesions may also be associated with constructional apraxia (469), but in this case the patient may have other signs of an ideomotor apraxia or an aphasia. Non-dominant parietal lesions occasionally produce a *dressing apraxia* limited to the left side of the body in adult patients with left-sided neglect (269). Apraxia confined to the left hand in a patient with a right hemiplegia and an expressive aphasia *(limb kinetic apraxia)* has been attributed by Geschwind (219) to involvement of fibers originating on the left, crossing to the premotor cortex on the right via the anterior corpus callosum, and carrying commands for skilled action from the dominant to the nondominant hemisphere.

Abnormal Involuntary Movements: Neuropharmacology

Abnormal involuntary movements and postures are due to the release of subcortical or spinal cord circuits from inhibitory control or from reciprocal excitatory-inhibitory balance. Abnormal movements usually are not generated in the damaged system, they arise from the malfunction of intact systems that have lost a controlling input. There are abnormal movements of many types. The most common ones are listed on Table 4 and are described in later sections. Abnormal movements are often associated with abnormal postures, abnormal reflexes, and other signs of neurologic dysfunction. Most, if not all, abnormal involuntary movements disappear with sleep and are made worse by stress and anxiety. Abnormal movements do not always denote a lesion of the brain: some, like tremor, dystonia, chorea, tics, and others may appear as side effects of drugs (105). It is likely that some noniatrogenic abnormal movements reflect endogenous, possibly genetic, changes in neurotransmitter metabolism rather than structural brain pathology.

Disorders of dopamine metabolism represent the area of greatest progress to date toward clarifying the neurochemistry and neuropharmacology of movement disorders. In most patients, the *resting tremor* of parkinsonism results from a loss of dopaminergic input to the putamen from the substantia nigra (649) (see Fig. 16), while in an occasional child it may reflect lack of sensitivity of striatal neurons to dopamine (436). Replacement therapy with the dopamine precursor *L*-DOPA or with other dopaminergic drugs capable of crossing the blood-brain barrier alleviates,

TABLE 4. *Abnormal involuntary movements by site of pathology[a]*

Corticospinal system
Clonus
Mass reflexes
Cerebellar systems
Intention tremor
Nystagmus
Titubation
Basal ganglia systems
Resting tremor
Chorea
Athetosis
Dystonia
Hemiballismus
Tics
Catalepsy
Brain stem systems
Intention myoclonus
Palatal myoclonus
Opsoclonus

[a]Site of pathology is presumed.

at least for a time, many of the symptoms of parkinsonism (131). Parkinsonian symptoms may also be alleviated somewhat by anticholinergic drugs like trihexy-phenidyl (Artane®) or benztropine (Cogentin®). The efficacy of anticholinergic drugs is attributed to inhibition of cholinergic interneurons in the striatum that have become overactive as a result of having lost their normal dopaminergic inhibitory input.

Drugs like the phenothiazines and haloperidol (Haldol®) that block dopamine postsynaptic receptors, and drugs like reserpine that deplete presynaptic vesicles of dopamine, produce side effects that resemble parkinsonism (105). Contrariwise, drugs like amphetamine and methylphenidate that increase dopamine levels may precipitate tics, motor restlessness, and choreiform movements in susceptible individuals (232). It seems logical to suppose, therefore, that naturally occurring tics, in particular Tourette syndrome (535), may reflect a hypersensitivity state of dopamine receptors, and that Sydenham's (rheumatic) *chorea* results from excessive release of dopamine by presynaptic terminals (435). This theory is bolstered by the observation that the dopamine receptor blocking agent haloperidol is the most effective drug to date for alleviating the symptoms of Tourette syndrome. It is also consonant with the observation that the phenothiazines and haloperidol ameliorate chorea in some patients with Sydenham's chorea, while others may respond to the adminstration of reserpine, a presynaptic dopamine depleting agent (435).

The chorea of Huntington's disease has been attributed to the loss of small striatal interneurons that produce GABA as neurotransmitter. Unfortunately, this observation has not yet resulted in an effective treatment for the chorea of this illness although some choreic patients may derive modest benefit from agents with central cholinergic effects (323). There is no effective drug therapy either for the *intention tremor* of cerebellar disease, whether it is caused by the loss of gabergic Purkinje cells or by pathology in cerebellar inflow or outflow systems. In contrast, *benign essential tremor* often responds well to diazepam (Valium®), a drug whose effect is to enhance central effects of GABA, and to propranolol (Inderal®) which blocks peripheral and central β-adrenergic receptors (651). Alcohol also alleviates benign essential tremor; whether this effect is related to an affinity of alcohol for β receptors is not certain. The tremor of anxiety has been attributed to overactive peripheral adrenergic receptors in the limbs (385). We do not have an adequate understanding as yet of the chemical pathology underlying movement disorders such as choreoathetosis, dystonia, and hemiballismus. *Intention myoclonus*, especially when it was caused by an acute anoxic insult, may respond to the precursor of serotonin, 5-hydroxytryptophan (579).

CLASSIC MOTOR DEFICIT SYNDROMES

Deficit syndromes involving the "lower motor neuron," myoneural junction, and muscle will not be discussed here. Syndromes attributable to sensory deficits and to disorders of the planning and initiation of movement were described in earlier sections.

Corticospinal or Pyramidal Syndromes

Major Dysfunction

Damage to the "upper motor neuron" in the motor cortex or along the pyramidal tract produces rather clear and predictable symptoms. These include spasticity and loss of voluntary motor control especially of the muscles, like those of the hand, that participate in finely coordinated, rapid, nonrepetitive motor acts (76,348).

Lesions affecting "upper motor neurons" release the subcortical systems they normally inhibit, which produces *spasticity*. Tone is increased in antigravity muscles and there is phasic increase in the resistance to stretch. Tendon jerks are exaggerated and pathologic reflexes like the Babinski sign—dorsiflexion of the big toe and fanning of the other toes when the sole of the foot is stimulated—will appear. When spasticity is severe, minor stimulation of the skin almost anywhere on the lower limb may result in a massive involuntary reflex withdrawal of the leg with dorsi-flexion of the foot and big toe, and flexion of the hip and knee—the so-called triple flexion or mass reflex.

In terms of effects on movement, it matters relatively little where the "upper motor neuron" is damaged, except that the pattern of affected muscles and signs of dysfunction in other systems give clues as to location of pathology. Selective damage to "upper motor neurons" on one side of the brain will produce a contralateral weakness with spasticity called *hemiparesis*, or *hemiplegia* when paralysis is severe or complete. For reasons noted earlier, walking, though spastic, virtually always remains possible in hemiplegia. Since control of fine movements of the hands and fingers is heavily dependent on activity in the motor cortex, one can anticipate the predominance of deficits in the hand in lesions of the motor cortex and pyramidal tract. Hemiparesis is usually associated with weakness of the muscles of the lower face (central facial palsy) on the same side as the hemiparesis. (The muscles of the upper face are spared because of their bilateral innervation.) A hemiparesis acquired in early life often retards growth of the affected side of the body. This is especially true if the lesion responsible for the hemiparesis affects the sensory as well as the motor cortex (302). Growth arrest of the leg may be severe enough to produce a scoliosis, or arrest may be so mild that narrower fingernails and slenderer fingers on the affected side are its only telltale signs. When cortical sensory damage is severe, muscle tone may be decreased and ligaments hyperlax; the affected hand may show spooning, i.e., hyperextension of the metacarpophalangeal joints and flexion of distal interphalangeal joints.

Damage high in the convexity of the brain will produce spasticity in both legs with relative sparing of the arms and face, a pattern of deficit called a *diparesis* or *diplegia*. Diplegia is frequent in children, especially in prematures who have sustained acidosis and ischemia during birth. The parasagittal area, which is the site of origin of fibers that control voluntary movements of the legs, may be particularly vulnerable because it is a watershed area between the territories of the anterior, middle, and posterior cerebral arteries (601). Other causes of diparesis are hydrocephalus and the germinal matrix hemorrhages of premature infants (600); spasticity then reflects bilateral damage to the periventricular white matter or the stretching of motor fibers around the dilated frontal horns. Damage to upper motor neurons in the thoracic spinal cord will also produce weakness and spasticity in both legs, called *paraparesis* or *paraplegia*, but segmental signs of damage to sensory systems and to "lower motor neurons" in the anterior horns will indicate that the lesion is located in the spinal cord rather than in the brain. Bilateral hemiplegia or *quadriplegia* can be distinguished from diplegia because motor deficits predominate in the upper limbs in quadriplegia and in the lower limbs in diplegia.

Pseudobulbar palsy is caused by bilateral loss of "upper motor neuron" innervation to the cranial nerve nuclei. Children with pseudobulbar palsy drool and have difficulty swallowing and speaking. They often have a hyperactive gag reflex and jaw jerk, and may have abnormal facial reflexes such as a snout reflex (puckering of the lips to percussion) or forced sucking movements. Pseudobulbar palsy may be associated with an oromotor apraxia (see p. 69) and with uncontrollably labile emotional expression (forced laughter or crying that is out of proportion to the person's affective experience and mood). Pseudobulbar emotional incontinence is more common in adults than in children.

Pseudobulbar palsy must be distinguished from *bulbar palsy* which reflects bilateral dysfunction of the lower motor neuron innervation of the orofacial musculature. Children with bulbar palsy also drool and have trouble sucking and swallowing. Their face is often flat and expressionless. Their weak palate gives them a nasal voice and causes them to regurgitate through the nose. Their gag reflex is absent and they characteristically have fasciculations of the tongue and pooling of secretions in the mouth and pharynx.

Subtle Dysfunction

Subtle damage to "upper motor neurons" may result in a tendency to walk on the toes. This gait reflects imbalance between muscles in the posterior compartment of the leg compared to the weaker anterior muscles. When the Achilles tendon is tight, passive dorsiflexion of the foot beyond 90° is impossible unless the knee is flexed. Toe walking is common in toddlers who are just learning to walk. If persistent, for instance in a child with hydrocephalus or in one with autistic features, toe walking should not be interpreted as a "bad habit" or as an "emotional problem" but should be viewed as evidence for subtle spasticity. (In a boy, it may be the first sign of Duchenne muscular dystrophy.)

A subtle hemiparesis reflects mild lateralized damage. As just mentioned, it may be associated with mild growth arrest. A left-handed child born to a family of right-handed persons who has a slender, slightly clumsy right hand with narrow fingernails is likely to have a structural lesion in his left hemisphere, whether or not it is detectable by CT scan.

Other subtle signs of corticospinal deficit are mirror movements or synkinesis, that is, involuntary movements of the contralateral hand when the child has to produce coordinated movements with the affected hand. Synkinesis can be brought out by asking the child to pat rapidly, to pronate and supinate the hand fast, or to touch each finger successively with his thumb (finger apposition). Mirror movements are normal in preschool children and become inhibited during the early school years. They are most valuable for diagnosis when asymmetrical.

Neuropharmacology

Knowledge concerning the neurochemistry of corticospinal control is inadequate for effective pharmacotherapy to have been developed. Dantrolene (Dantrium®) and baclofen (Lioresal®) may ameliorate spasticity but are less effective when spasticity is due to cerebral pathology than when pathology is in the spinal cord. Dantrolene often increases weakness and therefore is poorly tolerated by most children.

Cerebellar Syndromes

We saw that the cerebellum is a major system for the integration of sensory information from proprioceptive, vestibular, visual, and auditory receptors with interim information from subcortical and prefrontal motor relays, and that it is involved in the programming of ballistic movements through its feed-forward inputs to the ventrolateral thalamus and cortex. Besides reflecting pathology in the cerebellum itself, cerebellar signs may arise from dysfunction in cerebellar afferents, notably the spinocerebellar tracts, or its efferents, particularly the brachium conjunctivum that extends from the deep cerebellar nuclei toward the brain stem and thalamus. Signs of pathology in the midline of the cerebellum (vermis) include inability to maintain a stable posture of the head and trunk, with resulting *titubation*, and an unsteady *ataxic gait*. Chronic lesions in the cerebellar hemispheres are surprisingly often asymptomatic. When they are not, they interfere with smooth performance of voluntary movements of the limbs. Movements toward a goal are decomposed *(dysmetria)* and are often hindered by the occurrence of an *intention tremor* whose amplitude increases as the limb approaches its goal. Tremor of cerebellar origin is characteristically absent at rest, in contrast with the resting tremor due to loss of dopaminergic neurons in the substantia nigra that abates during voluntary movement.

Intention myoclonus consists of sudden irregular jerks that preclude smooth movements. It is precipitated by movement or the thought of movement. Intention myoclonus may be difficult to distinguish from intention tremor. Its origin is controversial. It may originate in the cortex, in pontine reticular nuclei (255), and perhaps in other subcortical regions including the deep cerebellar nuclei.

Another tremor that occurs during voluntary movement, especially when attempting to maintain a static posture, is *benign essential tremor*. This is a familial condition that starts at any time in life, including in early childhood, and that may interfere significantly with the execution of activities, like writing, that require fine motor control. Like all abnormal movements, it increases greatly with emotional stress. It has features in common with cerebellar tremor but can be differentiated by electromyographic criteria. Essential tremor may be the result of a disorder of β-adrenergic receptors either in the limbs or in the brain (651). When severe enough to require treatment, it may be ameliorated significantly by the use of the β-adrenergic blocker propranolol.

Cerebellar dysfunction affects motor tone which is usually decreased because of depressed activity of muscle spindle afferents (225). Inadequate damping at the termination of movement, and loss of normal reciprocal inhibition between agonist and antagonist muscles results in other characteristic signs of cerebellar dysfunction: pendular reflexes, rebound when a sudden tap is applied to an outstretched limb, and bouncing or loss of check when the load on a limb is lifted unexpectedly.

Oculomotor dysmetria and a variety of other disorders of the control of eye movements that are analogous to the deficits in the motor control of the limbs can be demonstrated by asking patients either to track a moving target (pursuit movement), or to look suddenly from one visual target to another (saccadic movement). Some of these signs may be suppressed by the feedback loops provided to the oculomotor system by the visual input from the retina, so that testing in the dark or with the eyes closed may be required to bring out these signs. Their detailed study requires recording the eye movements (oculogram) in order to obtain a graphic record for quantitative analysis (351). *Oculomotor apraxia* is a supranuclear disorder of motor control precluding the voluntary turning of the eyes in a given direction. The children turn their heads briskly and close their eyes in order to alter the direction of gaze, thus calling upon oculovestibular compensatory mechanisms rather than cortical mechanisms in order to achieve their goal (655).

Pathology affecting the flocculonodular lobe of the cerebellum which is concerned with vestibular processing produces readily observable *nystagmus* on lateral gaze. Nystagmus is often absent when pathology is limited to the neocerebellum (cerebellar hemispheres). Other varieties of nystagmus such as vertical, rotatory, and see-saw nystagmus; and the nystagmus in one eye associated with oculomotor paresis that is characteristic of internuclear ophthalmoplegia are usually due to pathology in the brain stem or diencephalon (116). Oculomotor flutter or rapid oscillation of the eye (654), and opsoclonus, intermittent chaotic movements of the eye(s), are other disorders affecting the control of conjugate eye movements that reflect pathology in the connections between the oculomotor nuclei, the cerebellum, and the vestibular system.

Cerebellar pathology may also affect the coordination of the muscles of articulation. It produces a characteristic disruption of the rhythm of speech called *scanning*. Severe pathology interferes significantly with speech intelligibility and with the control of the voice.

Many drugs such as alcohol, the barbiturates, phenytoin (Dilantin®), and other anticonvulsants produce ataxia and nystagmus among their side effects. Yet knowledge concerning the neurochemistry of cerebellar disorders has not progressed to the point where drugs effective in controlling disorders of movement resulting from cerebellar dysfunction have become available. The value of placing a lesion in the ventrolateral nucleus of the thalamus to control ataxia and intention tremor is still under investigation.

Syndromes of Dysfunction in the Basal Ganglia

Pathology in the basal ganglia produces a number of different disorders of motor control, depending on what systems are affected. Loss of dopaminergic neurons in the substantia nigra that innervate small cholinergic neurons in the caudate and putamen produces *akinesia*, *rigidity*, and a *resting tremor*. This syndrome complex is characteristic of Parkinson's disease. We noted earlier that it can be ameliorated for a time by the replacement of deficient dopamine through the administration of its precursor L-DOPA (131). A similar syndrome is seen in children who have been given excessive doses of drugs like chlorpromazine and haloperidol that block dopamine receptors in the striatum. The drug-induced syndrome is readily reversible by the intravenous administration of diphenhydramine (Benadryl®).

Chorea, or sudden, unpredictable, irregular involuntary movements of the limbs and face, appears to reflect pathology in small neurons in the caudate and putamen that are under direct or indirect dopaminergic control. A deficiency of GABA in the caudate may be responsible for chorea (58). The pharmacology of chorea was discussed on page 71. In children, Sydenham's chorea follows an infection with streptococci of the A strain (20). In adults, chorea is likely to be a symptom of Huntington's disease which is inherited as a dominant trait and which produces dementia as well as chorea. When Huntington's disease becomes symptomatic in children, it is more likely to produce rigidity than chorea (384). Benign familial chorea is a dominant genetic disorder that rarely needs treatment and does not lead to severe neurologic deterioration (257).

Among "soft signs" of motor dysfunction, Prechtl (475) pointed out that a school age child's inability to maintain his or her arms and fingers immobile when holding the upper limbs outstretched with the eyes closed may be correlated with excessive jitteriness in the newborn period and with perinatal anoxia. Although the choreiform syndrome may reflect mild pathology in the basal ganglia, there is no proof for this contention.

Ballismus, a unilateral violent flinging of the limbs, results from a lesion in the subthalamic nucleus. It is rarely seen in children and does not respond well to drug therapy.

Dystonia or torsion spasm is a movement disorder that reflects phasic increases in tone that usually predominate in the axial muscles of the neck, trunk, and proximal portions of the limbs. In some children, it may present with an intorsion of the foot (semilunar foot) or with tightness of the hand while writing (writer's cramp). It may be associated with bizarre facial grimacing and interfere significantly with speech and eating. Naturally occurring dystonia is assumed to reflect an imbalance in neurotransmitter metabolism in the basal ganglia, but its neurochemical basis has yet to be elucidated and its pathology is still unknown. Effective drug therapy for dystonia has not been devised although some dystonic children improve with large doses of cholinergic drugs like trihexyphenidyl (Artane®). Dystonia, as well as parkinsonism, may be ameliorated in some patients, at least temporarily, by placing a lesion in the ventrolateral thalamic nuclei that receives inputs from the basal ganglia and cerebellum (127,246). Since extensive bilateral lesions are often required in patients with bilateral symptoms, and since bilateral thalamic lesions may result in serious and permanent interference with speech, this type of surgery is rarely indicated now that effective drug therapy is available for parkinsonism and may become available for dystonia.

Chorea associated with dystonia and rigidity is called *choreoathetosis*. This is a movement disorder consisting of slow writhing movements of the face and limbs, where they predominate in the fingers. In some children, choreoathetosis is associated with diffuse damage to the basal ganglia and thalamus which have a marbled appearance (status marmoratus). Choreoathetosis occurs almost exclusively in children who have sustained perinatal anoxia and/or hyperbilirubinemia. In the case of hyperbilirubinemia (kernicterus), deep cerebellar nuclei and brain stem nuclei, in particular those of the auditory and vestibular systems, are also affected: Children with kernicterus are likely to be deaf as well as athetotic. *Pseudoathetosis*, discussed earlier, is caused by lack of proprioceptive feedback or by impaired cortical sensation in a hand whose fingers cannot be kept immobile if vision is suppressed. Thus far athetosis has not responded well to any medication.

Tics are sudden rapid repetitive movements involving the face or other parts of the body. They are often bizarre since persons with tics, like those with chorea, will often assimilate their involuntary movement into a voluntary movement. A child may transiently have a tic that disappears after a few weeks or months, or his tic may be replaced by another tic, or by multiple tics. A person can almost always inhibit his tic(s) for several minutes or longer but the tic(s) will then reappear, at times in an almost paroxysmal burst. Tics, like all abnormal involuntary movements, are exacerbated by tension and anxiety and disappear in sleep. In *Tourette syndrome* they often are accompanied by vocal tics like snorting, by involuntary cursing (coprolalia), and by other behaviors like compulsive touching or smelling (535). Tics used to be considered nonorganic bad habits but are now believed to reflect overactivity of dopaminergic receptors in the basal ganglia. Tics may respond to the administration of haloperidol, a drug that blocks postsynaptic dopaminergic receptors; they may be precipitated by the administration of methylphenidate and dextroamphetamine which are catecholamine releasing agents (232).

Most abnormal movements, even those that reflect a perinatal insult, rarely appear until after the first year of life. One exception is the choreoathetosis of an X-linked recessive disorder, the Lesch-Nyhan syndrome, that is caused by a deficit in uric acid metabolism (485). The diagnosis of Wilson's disease must be considered in any school age child or adolescent with an acquired movement disorder suggesting pathology in the basal ganglia or cerebellum. Wilson's disease is a disorder of copper metabolism that is both preventable and treatable with drugs and a low copper diet (485). A number of other rare genetic diseases, as well as rheumatic fever (Sydenham's chorea) and carbon monoxide poisoning, affect the basal ganglia.

These and toxic side effects of drugs, discussed earlier, should be excluded before assuming that the cause of a child's problem is a fixed nonprogressive lesion or athetoid cerebral palsy.

CEREBRAL PALSY

Cerebral palsy (CP) is a label frequently offered as a diagnosis to the parents of children with motor deficits (137). In fact CP is no more a diagnosis than MBD. Cerebral palsy simply means that the cause of the child's motor deficit is assumed to be nonprogressive pathology in the brain owing to maldevelopment or to damage incurred during birth or in early life. A diagnosis of CP is inappropriate for children with progressive or potentially progressive conditions such as hydrocephalus, a neoplasm, or a genetic metabolic disease. The lack of specifity of the CP label needs to be stressed and parents must be told that the diagnosis of CP says nothing about the severity or type of motor deficit present. Table 5 lists some of the motor syndromes most likely to be labelled cerebral palsy.

Infantile hemiplegias are often associated with cortical sensory loss on the affected side and, in some cases, with a homonymous hemianopsia for the side of space ipsilateral to the hemiplegia. They may or may not be associated with cognitive deficiency, seizures, and growth arrest.

Ataxic CP is rare (251) and ataxia should arouse suspicion of a metabolic illness, neoplasm, or gross cerebellar anomaly. Spastic quadriplegia and hypotonic CP denote diffuse neurologic damage usually associated with severe mental deficiency. Children with hypotonic CP characteristically have hyperactive tendon stretch reflexes and upgoing toes. The pathogenesis of hypotonic CP is poorly understood and no doubt diverse; whether the hypotonia reflects cerebellar, vestibular, brain stem, or other pathology is not well known (137). Children who develop athetosis are usually hypotonic during the first year of life. Hypotonia with spasticity may denote anterior horn cell disease or a neuropathy associated with corticospinal involvement. Children with upgoing toes and hypotonia need to have nerve conduction velocity and electromyographic (EMG) studies in order to clarify their diagnosis since such combinations of symptoms suggest diffuse genetic metabolic disease as a possibility (485).

TABLE 5. *Types of cerebral palsy*

Spastic	{ hemiplegia diplegia quadriplegia
Athetosis	
Ataxic CP	
Hypotonic CP	
Mixed CP (spasticity + athetosis)	

MINIMAL BRAIN DYSFUNCTION

MBD, like cerebral palsy, is not a diagnosis. It is a vague term that implies that a child's learning disability and clumsiness have a neurologic basis (see p. 31). The distinction between "hard" and "soft" signs of motor dysfunction has been stressed earlier and some of their relationships were listed in Tables 1 and 2. We also saw that it is often difficult, if not impossible, to pinpoint the type of dysfunction responsible for clumsiness and other mild motor deficits, and to decide, in school age children, whether "soft" signs denote pathology or immaturity, or even whether the child's performance departs sufficiently from the norm to be considered unequivocally pathologic. A number of quantitative scales of motor function have been developed to help make this distinction.

TESTS OF MOTOR FUNCTION

Quantitive assessment is often needed to decide, in the individual child, whether motor performance is actually deficient. Infant scales of developement such as the Gesell (327), Brazelton (72), Denver (199), and Bayley scales (34) provide norms for the passing of various early milestones of gross and fine motor control. They can be used to indicate how much a given infant departs from the norm, but are not good predictors of later performance, nor do they provide information of diagnostic usefulness for detecting the cause of the motor deficit. Touwen's neurologic examination scale (587) and the Oseretsky Test of Motor Proficiency (167) extend the infant scales to older children and provide guidelines for detecting deviance in motor development. Berges and Lezine (50) have developed norms for children's ability to imitate gestures which assesses praxis as well as motor skill per se. Denckla (154,155) has attempted to quantify some aspects of the clinical examination of motor function and provides norms for school age children for such tasks as hopping and tapping. Wolff (641) examined the development of the ability to alternate taps between the two hands and has clearly shown the later maturation of boys' ability to coordinate activity of the two hemispheres, presumably reflecting later maturation of interhemispheric commissures in boys than girls. The Purdue Pegboard Test is a very sensitive test of fine motor skill. It is quick and easy to administer and deserves to be widely used as a screening test for mild motor deficiency. Norms are available for the performance of each hand and the ability to coordinate the activity of both hands in children from age two and one-half years to adulthood (209,625). The Purdue Pegboard Test is sensitive to a wide range of motor, sensory, and visual motor deficits, and is a useful screening instrument for lateralized dysfunction and bimanual integration (493).

Office Examination of Motor Function

Every physician will have his or her own approach to the detection of motor deficits suggesting brain dysfunction (464,587), and this approach will differ at different ages. Tasks such as throwing, catching, and bouncing a ball; building with blocks; and drawing, if well performed, indicate good fine motor coordination, eye-hand coordination, and relatively short reaction times, suggesting efficient sensorimotor processing. Having the child walk, run, hop on one foot, and stand with his eyes closed and his arms outstretched usually enables one to detect ataxia, a mild hemiparesis, or spastic diparesis. These are good tests of gross motor co-ordination. Decreased associated movements or abnormal posturing of the arms while walking are especially revealing; they can be accentuated by having the child walk on his heels, on his toes, and on the sides of his feet. A child's inability to hold the fingers quiet with the arms outstretched and the eyes closed has been called the choreiform syndrome of Prechtl (475). While ability to maintain this posture matures with age, marked difficulty should suggest minor damage to the basal ganglia or cerebellum. Ability to inhibit mirror movements, which develops before the age of 10, can be examined during rapid pronation and supination of one hand or while apposing each finger to the thumb, an excellent test of the ability to control the movement of individual fingers and to execute a sequence (118). Oromotor apraxia, the inability to move the tongue up, down, and sideways; to move the jaw from side to side; to purse the lips and click the tongue rapidly, especially if associated with an increased jaw jerk (pseudobulbar palsy), may provide an explanation for drooling or defective speech articulation.

The approach to examining motor function is to screen by having the child perform a few complex motor tasks that are appropriate for his age and that tax gross and fine motor skills. If the child can perform the tasks, more detailed examination is unlikely to reveal a significant abnormality. If he cannot, the clinician's task is to examine more closely each of the skills required for this performance in order to attempt to pinpoint the aspect that is defective and, if possible, its cause. For example, motor performance may be defective because of weakness, paralysis (inability to move voluntarily), change in tone, or incoordination between the contraction of muscles within the limb. It may be interrupted by parasitic movements like tremors, tics, and chorea or by the occurrence of primitive reflexes like the tonic neck reflex. The child may be unable to maintain posture and adapt to changes in posture because of an inability to inhibit mirror movements or synkinesis or to coordinate the activity of the limbs on the two sides of the body. Occasionally, what appears to be a motor problem may in fact reflect sensory or visual loss. Observation of the child while he walks and performs simple and complex movements should precede the manipulations required to test for tone, bulk, strength of individual muscles, and reflexes. Observing a natural movement, especially one the child enjoys and performs spontaneously, often provides much more reliable data than more formal testing since cooperation and motivation cannot be taken for granted in children.

6

Sensory and Perceptual Consequences of Brain Dysfunction

SOMATOSENSORY DEFICITS

The somatosensory system provides data concerning stimuli that impinge on the surface of the body and on the mucous membranes of the alimentary and respiratory tracts, and data on the state of joints, muscles and viscera. It is customary to divide somatosensory information into three types:

1) Nociception or pain that warns that tissue damage is occurring and mandates action to escape it.

2) Proprioception that provides data on the state of the musculoskeletal system relative to gravity, on the position of various body parts relative to each other, on movement, and on tension in the muscles. This system plays a preeminent role for the maintenance of posture and the execution of motor programs.

3) Tactile discrimination and haptic sensation that yield precise data on the nature and location of the external stimuli that impinge on the body and guide their exploration.

Pain

Pain sensation is processed predominantly subcortically, in the spinal cord, brain stem, and thalamus (95,410). Since pain is an imperative stimulus that may have life-saving implications, responses to strong painful stimuli tend to be reflexive, immediate, and stereotyped, like the withdrawal of a burned finger from a hot stove. The luxury of deliberation and choice provided by cortical processing would be counterproductive at such a juncture! Pain pathways are phylogenetically old and multisynaptic, with projections at multiple levels including the reticular formation, limbic system, and other brain stem sites. These projections account for the strong arousal, motivational, and autonomic aspects of pain, and for the aversive affect it evokes. Pain does become conscious, of course, and it is believed that the projections of long pain fibers to the thalamus and second sensory area in the parietal operculum and insula may be responsible, at least in part, for the conscious awareness of pain. Except acutely, cortical lesions rarely abolish pain so that loss of pain sensation should suggest pathology in subcortical areas, most likely in the brain stem, spinal cord, or peripheral nerves. Cerebral lesions are not painful, with the notable exception of some thalamic lesions that cause burning, tingling, disagreeable, or intolerable dysesthetic sensations on the contralateral side of the body. In experimental animals, electrical stimulation in certain regions of the diencephalon and midbrain that contain opiate receptors and in pathways that interdict transmission of pain afferents from the spinal cord can lead to analgesia.

Recent data show that there are specific neurotransmitters concerned with pain and suffering. Substance P, a polypeptide, is located in pain afferents in the spinal cord (201). The enkephalins and endorphins are endogenous polypeptides whose analgesic and euphoric effects counteract both painful and aversive aspects of nociception (7,283). They bind to specific neuronal receptors in the brain stem and diencephalon which are referred to as opiate receptors because they bind exogenous compounds, like opiates, that mimic the analgesic and euphoric properties of endorphins and enkephalins. There are other peptides like bradykinin and neurotensin, and biogenic amines like serotonin, that play a role in pain perception at spinal cord, brain stem, subcortical, and perhaps cortical levels. The neurophysiology and pharmacology of pain perception, its affective concomitants, and its control are lively areas of neuroscience inquiry.

Proprioception

Proprioception is largely unconscious and processed subcortically in segmental circuits in the spinal cord, with longer loops involving the cerebellum, brain stem, basal ganglia (599), and even the cortex (399). Proprioceptive, vestibular, and visual inputs participate in the stabilization and maintenance of posture, and in the control of eye movements during motion of the head and body (230). Proprioceptive information is essential for maintaining the balance of tone in agonist and antagonist muscles during the execution of movements. Parietal lesions impair aspects of proprioception concerned with the feedback control required for skilled motor acts (466).

Haptic Perception

Detailed perception of tactile stimuli as they are explored with the hand (haptic perception), and the identification and localization of a stimulus on the skin depend on the integration of data arising from a multiplicity of different somatosensory receptors (599). Before one can conclude that a child's inability to recognize an object by palpation reflects a cortical sensory deficit, it is necessary to show that elementary sensory modalities are intact. Table 6 lists the somatosensory modalities.

TABLE 6. *Somatosensory modalities*

"Primary" sensory modalities
    Pain, deep pain
    Temperature
    Light touch
    Pressure
    Vibration (flutter)
    Position
    Movement

"Cortical" sensory modalities
    Tactile localization
    Two point discrimination
    Double simultaneous stimulation
    Graphesthesia (palm writing)
    Haptic perception (texture, shape, size, weight)
    Haptic perception-stereognosis (identification of ob-
        ject by palpation)

Primary sensory modalities that are routinely assessed clinically include the ability to appreciate light touch, pinprick, passive movement of joints, deep pain, temperature, and vibration. So-called *cortical sensory modalities* assessed as part of a routine neurologic examination include the ability to identify an object by palpation (stereognosis), the ability to localize a stimulus on the body (tactile localization), the ability to discriminate two stimuli applied to the skin simultaneously and close to one another (two-point discrimination), or simultaneously to two corresponding points on the two sides of the body (tactile extinction). Graphesthesia, the ability to recognize a digit "written" in the palm of the hand while the eyes are closed is an excellent screening test for cortical sensation; it taps visual spatial skills and the ability to integrate them with verbal information. Two-point discrimination, and judging size and shape are relatively easy tests of haptic perception to quantitate in children (626,627).

The left hand is more efficient than the right for recognizing shapes by palpation (111) and for reading braille (274). Exploration with the index finger of either hand elicits electrical activity in the right hemisphere (160). These findings and the greater efficiency of the right hemisphere for visual recognition (356) are some of the elements of the now well-established dominance of the right hemisphere for tasks requiring spatial processing.

Effects of Parietal Dysfunction

The somatosensory cortex located in the postcentral gyrus of the parietal lobe receives inputs from the spinal cord via the thalamus. It also receives inputs from the cerebellum and basal ganglia, and recurrent inputs from the motor cortex via axon collaterals of pyramidal neurons (301). The main outputs of the somatosensory cortex project to sensory association areas participating in sensory perception and intersensory integration, to the motor cortex, and to the thalamus and subcortical sensory relays. One of the roles of subcortical projections of the somatosensory cortex appears to be the inhibition of ascending sensory inputs at thalamic and brain stem relays (599). This accounts, in part, for rapid adaptation to constant tactile inputs: It is undesirable to be aware of the stimulation produced by the seat of one's chair until pressure on the gluteal muscles becomes nociceptive and commands a shift in posture to relieve it. Adaptation to constant or repetitive sensory stimuli is partly a function of adaptation of peripheral receptors selectively responsive to stimulus onset or change.

Parietal lesions usually raise the threshold for tactile stimulation without altogether abolishing touch. They do not affect the sensation of pain, temperature, and vibration but impair complex somatosensory perception on the contralateral side of the body. The sensory homunculus, like the motor homunculus and like the cortical representation of space, is upside down. Projections from regions of highest receptor density like the mouth, thumb, and index finger occupy more space in the postcentral gyrus than regions of lower receptor density like the leg and trunk. Recent evidence suggests that there are multiple representations of the body in the somatosensory homunculus of monkeys, presumably corresponding to different somesthetic modalities, for example, light touch, pressure, or body movement (305).

Large parietal lesions resulting in severe loss of cortical sensation in the opposite hand usually render the hand almost useless. The child will be unable to maintain the posture of the hand since he lacks information concerning its location in space and the relationship of the fingers to one another. The hand will drift if he closes his eyes and the fingers execute irregular movements called pseudoathetosis. The hand may be used as a prop under visual control but even vigorous rehabilitation is unlikely to make it a truly functional limb capable of executing finely coordinated movements. This lack of use probably reflects not only loss of proprioceptive input to the sensorimotor cortex, but also unavailability of visuokinesthetic motor engrams thought to be stored in the parietal lobe (268,433).

Disorders of Body Image

Studies of patients with brain wounds after World War II (533) showed that sensory representation in the two hemispheres is not strictly symmetrical, and that the left hand projects to both sides of the brain, while the right hand projects mainly to the left hemisphere. These asymmetries may, in part, be responsible for the fact that apraxia and difficulty with right-left orientation are much more common after left brain damage than right brain damage, and that *finger agnosia*, the inability to report which finger was touched or to name it, is also a sign of left brain damage. Norms for the development of finger recognition and right-left awareness have been established (45). Right-left confusion is often reported in children with MBD and has rarely been assumed to indicate focal or lateralized dysfunction. It may be worthwhile to re-examine this assumption.

The *Gerstmann syndrome* is classically taken to indicate pathology in the left temporoparietal region (angular gyrus). It consists of finger agnosia, right-left disorientation, acalculia, and agraphia. It is often associated with an anomia or other aphasic disturbance and with constructional apraxia. A developmental Gerstmann syndrome has been described (321), even though Benton (42,45) questions the uniqueness and localizing value of the acquired Gerstmann syndrome.

Parietal lesions may lead to distortions of body awareness more severe than right-left disorientation and finger agnosia: Patients may neglect one side of their body (269). Even though they may report a stimulus applied to the contralateral hand while their eyes are closed, they do not report it when both hands are stimulated together (tactile extinction).

Patients, usually adults but occasionally children, with right posterior lesions, in particular acute ones, may deny that their left limbs belong to them, they may deny that the limbs are paralyzed *(anosognosia)*, or they may fail to clothe the left side of their body (dressing apraxia). They may neglect the left side of space and draw a clock with digits only on the right side of its face (132). These disorders tend to improve with time. Their pathogenesis is not fully understood. The reason why they are so much more frequent with right than left-sided lesions may have to do with the special role of the right hemisphere for spatial awareness or with the previously noted asymmetry of the cortical projections from the two sides of the body.

VISUAL DEFICITS

Visual perceptual deficits such as difficulty discriminating figure from background were stressed as one of the cardinal signs of MBD by Strauss and his colleagues (564) and other early workers who defined the syndrome. The children did not have visual field cuts or other classical signs of pathology in the main visual pathway. Their deficits were perceptual and more subtle and, in the nonlocalizationist climate of that time, were ascribed to general cerebral inefficiency. Today, we tend to attribute them to dysfunction in secondary (inferolateral occipital) and tertiary (inferotemporal) visual areas.

The visual system provides the brain with an extraordinarily efficient and continuously updated map of the world and of the self in the world. Lesions that affect the eye and the retinocalcarine pathway produce loss of vision (51), lesions in the extrastriate cortex produce perceptual deficits (632), those in collicular and tectal pathways produce deficits in the control of eye movements and the scanning of visual space (230).

Vision and Visual Perception

The pattern of loss in the visual field of each eye indicates the probable location of the causative pathology (Fig. 17). Lesions in the retina and optic nerve produce loss of vision in one eye. Lesions arising from the pituitary or the diencephalon that disrupt crossing fibers at the optic chiasm give rise to bitemporal hemianopsias, that is, loss of vision in the temporal half of the visual field of each eye. This type of visual field deficit quite often goes unnoticed since, with binocular vision, there

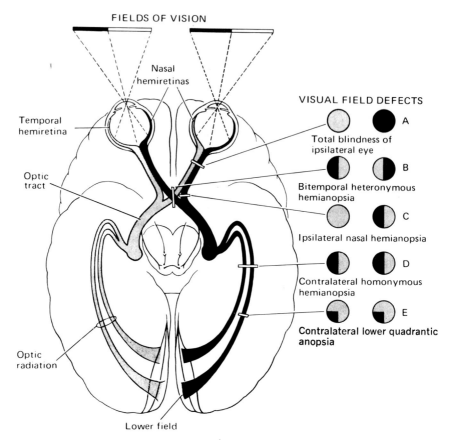

FIG. 17. Diagram of the visual pathways. The key to understanding effects of brain lesions on vision is to recall (1) that because of the lens, images of space are projected upside down, from the retina to the visual cortex, and (2) that thanks to the optic chiasm each half of visual space projects to the contralateral hemisphere. Images originating in the macula project to both occipital poles so that unilateral lesions of the brain typically spare central vision. The diagram indicates the types of visual field defects expected from lesions affecting different levels of the visual pathway. For the reasons already stated, parietal lesions tend to produce contralateral inferior quadrantanopsias and temporal lesions contralateral superior quadrantanopsias. Note that fibers to the tectum and superior colliculus of the midbrain that mediate pupillary light reaction and that control the direction of gaze do not synapse in the lateral geniculate body, which is a thalamic nucleus indicated on the diagram by a knob from which the optic radiations fan out. (Reproduced with permission from Noback and Demarest, ref. 443a.)

is only slight constriction of the visual field. Unilateral lesions in the visual pathway posterior to the optic chiasm produce a homonymous hemianopsia, that is, loss of vision for the contralateral side of space (seen with the nasal half of the contralateral retina and the temporal half of the ipsilateral retina). Homonymous hemianopsia caused by lesions in the optic tract, which are rare, is associated with impairment of the pupillary light reflex when a narrow beam of light is projected onto the blind hemiretina. Lesions in the optic radiations, that travel in the white matter of the posterior hemisphere toward the primary visual cortex in the mesial occipital lobe, and lesions in the visual (calcarine or striate) cortex also produce a homonymous hemianopic defect for the contralateral side of space, but do not involve the pupillary reflex. Temporal lesions affect the upper quadrant, and parietal lesions, the inferior quadrant of the visual field since the lens inverts the image of space on the retina and since visual fibers maintain an orderly relationship throughout their course.

Bilateral lesions in the primary visual cortex result in cortical blindness. These patients characteristically have preserved pupillary light reflexes and conjugate eye movements. They often have persistence of some visually guided behavior, in other words, they are not totally blind. They may not complain of their blindness or may even deny it (Anton syndrome) (159). In young children, sudden cortical blindness resulting from an occipital contusion (245) or basilar artery migraine (80) may produce unexplained agitation and terror as its most obvious symptoms. Chronic cortical blindness may result from previous uncal herniation with posterior cerebral artery infarction (360) or from posterior cortical thinning in hydrocephalus (546).

Cortical representation of visual space depends on the highly topologically organized arrangement of cells throughout the visual system. The crossing of fibers from the nasal half of each retina at the optic chiasm results in information from one half of space projecting from both eyes to the contralateral hemisphere. Columns of cells receiving data from particular points of one retina alternate with columns of cells receiving data from the corresponding points of the other eye (580,621) (see Fig. 6). This arrangement provides for binocular interaction at the cortical level. Thus, each hemisphere processes somatosensory data from the contralateral half of the body, visual data from the contralateral half of space, and commands the muscles in the contralateral side of the body. All these representations are upside-down and spatially congruent with the inverted visual image of the world projected on the retina by the lens (588).

The striate cortex projects to prestriate areas of the occipital lobe where several orderly representations of visual space have been demonstrated in monkeys (632). It is thought that higher order processing of visual attributes like color, shape, and size takes place in prestriate areas, whereas discrimination of brightness, edge, and direction of movement is encoded through the properties of the receptor fields of neurons in the retina, lateral geniculate body, and calcarine cortex. Recognition of visual stimuli calls for a comparison of the pattern produced by a visual stimulus with visual images stored in long-term memory. The inferotemporal cortex and its hippocampal and amygdaloid connections appear to be involved in the ability to recognize a complex visual pattern as familiar (478,616). Integration of data provided by vision, audition, and somatic sensation is thought to take place at the junction of the parietal, temporal, and occipital cortex, one of the last areas of the cortex to mature (650). It comes as no surprise that lesions in this region will interfere with complex tasks requiring visual-spatial perception and may produce visual neglect, as well as somatosensory neglect.

Visual Scanning

Besides this primary geniculocalcarine visual system, a second system controls eye movements and participates in the orientation of the body in space (627). Fibers from the retina project directly to the superior colliculus of the midbrain tectum. This nucleus also receives vestibular, auditory, and somatosensory inputs, as well as fibers from the striate cortex. Its main outputs are toward the pulvinar, a large nucleus in the posterior thalamus, and from there to the prestriate cortex and toward oculomotor, olivary, and other brain stem and cerebellar targets.

The superior colliculus appears to play an important part in active visual exploration, shifting gaze toward a stimulus perceived in the peripheral field in order to bring it into foveal vision. Correlating vestibular data and proprioceptive inputs from extraocular muscles and the muscles of the neck and trunk with inputs from the retina in the superior colliculus makes it possible to distinguish between shifts of the retinal image that result from self-induced head and eye movements from shifts resulting from the movements of a visual target in space (537).

The extrastriate visual system accounts for the preservation of the many aspects of visually guided behavior that survive ablation of the striate cortex in nonprimate species. It also accounts for the fact that cortically blind individuals have conjugate eye movement and orient their eyes toward acoustically perceived targets. How much vision it affords these persons is not clear although it enables many cortically blinded experimental animals, including monkeys, to perceive moving targets and visual patterns (456).

Visual Agnosias

Visual agnosia is the inability to recognize or name an object presented visually while it can be recognized by touch or by its sound. Inability to name an object may reflect an interruption between the visual processing regions of the cortex and the temporoparietal areas of the dominant hemisphere involved in verbal processing (218). This disconnection syndrome differs from the inability to indicate, nonverbally, that an object has been recognized by pointing to another object that matches it, or to a picture of the object, or by mimicking its use (519). Inability to match suggests a large lesion affecting the prestriate cortex and producing a severe deficit in visual perception, while inability to recognize the nature of the use of the object perceived suggests inaccessibility of visual memories because of pathology disconnecting inferotemporal and limbic areas (10). Inability to match colors has been ascribed to a lesion affecting that portion of the visual association cortex involved in color processing (405,457), while color agnosia, the inability to name colors, usually denotes pathology in the parieto-occipital region of the dominant hemisphere that interferes with the retrieval of verbal labels for colors presented visually. Some patients with agnosia for colors can give color names when asked the color of apples or grass or the sky, indicating that access to the repository of color names differs when the stimulus to entry is verbal and visual.

Prosopagnosia or the inability to recognize familiar faces is a deficit in visual perception that has aroused a great deal of interest because it is so surprisingly specific (404). There may be several reasons why faces are processed uniquely. The ability to recognize a person at a glance has always had biologic importance for survival. Very young infants spend more time staring at faces than at any other visual target (252,393). Facial recognition and the reading of facial expression have decisive implications for social interaction. Faces are not readily labelable except by a person's name. Prosopagnosia has been said to reflect bilateral pathology in the inferior occipitotemporal area (404). Since it is often associated with a left upper quadrantic visual field defect, it is the lesion on the right that may be crucial for its occurrence. This is supported by findings in normal persons that indicate that the posterior part of the right hemisphere plays a particularly important role for the discrimination of facial features (356).

Picture identification is more difficult than the visual recognition of three-dimensional objects, and the processing of arbitrary (nonlabelable?) visual patterns more difficult than that of pictures of objects. Difficulty discriminating letters like *b* and *d*, *p* and *q* that differ only by their spatial orientation is very common in children with reading disability (452). The right hemisphere is more efficient than the left for visual spatial processing (164) and the storage of visual memories (418). As stressed earlier, it is also more efficient than the left for somatosensory perception and the awareness of one's body. This is surely no coincidence since both vision and somesthesis are spatial senses. Deficient performance of tasks that require complex visual-spatial processing points toward right, rather than left, posterior hemispheric pathology, even in the absence of left visual field or somatosensory defect.

Differences between the sexes have been observed for the maturation and efficiency of visual-spatial processing, with males tending to outrank females who, in turn, tend to outrank males for tasks requiring verbal fluency (640). These differences may, in some way, be related to the higher prevalence of dyslexia and language disorders in boys than in girls.

Graphomotor Deficits and Constructional Apraxia

Constructional apraxia, or the inability to reproduce a pattern with blocks or match sticks, and impaired ability to copy geometric drawings are considered sensitive indicators of brain damage (46). Tests such as the Bender Gestalt (331) and Beery-Buktenica Developmental Test of Visual Motor Integration (36) are widely used to screen for brain damage. They owe their efficiency to the broad range of skills they call for, and therefore to the wide range of cerebral systems they engage. Successful performance of such a task demands the ability to plan ahead, a function typically impaired by frontal pathology (439,480). It requires adequate visual-spatial perception reflecting integrity of posterior hemispheric function, especially on the right (or nondominant) side, as just discussed. Occasionally, and not nearly as often as those who believe in orthoptic training to cure dyslexia would have us believe, perception of complex visual patterns may be impaired by a disorder of visual scanning and an inability to take in multiple details at a glance (319). Drawing requires skillful use of the right (or dominant) hand, while building with blocks is sensitive to motor dysfunction in either of the hands, and to lack of integration of the motor programs in the two hemispheres through commissural pathways. Constructional apraxia reflecting right posterior pathology tends to be more severe and qualitatively different from constructional apraxia arising from pathology on the left (46,469), a further reflection of interhemispheric asymmetry.

The usefulness of visual-motor tasks to detect brain damage, and the correlation of scores on the Block Design subtest of the Wechsler scale with nonverbal intelligence (604) are no coincidence since both depend on the multiple and complex abilities they sample. Again, it is necessary to break down a task into its component requirements if one is to go further than simply identifying cerebral efficiency or inefficiency, and if one is interested in assessing the particular cerebral systems at fault.

AUDITORY DEFICITS

Audition is a distance receptor that is never turned off. Auditory stimuli are strongly alerting and are a main vehicle for interpersonal communication which, in man, is substantially linguistic. Auditory pathways are both crossed and uncrossed, projecting to both temporal lobes, although the crossed pathway is functionally dominant. Auditory processing takes place at each relay of the central auditory pathway and perception of acoustic stimuli is thus progressively sharpened. Lesions in the brain stem interfere with the ability to localize sound in space and to integrate the inputs from the two ears (259,140). Cortical lesions hinder the ability to discriminate among complex temporal acoustic patterns but not the perception of intensity, frequency, onset, and offset of sounds—that is, they do not produce deafness. Unilateral temporal lobe lesions impair speech discrimination in the contralateral ear, especially when competing messages are presented to the two ears simultaneously (dichotically) or alternately (499).

Peripheral Hearing Loss Versus Pathology in the Central Auditory Pathway

Pathology in the cochlear nuclei has been implicated in the hearing loss of children who suffered from neonatal hyperbilirubinemia and developed kernicterus (172), and that of some children who sustained neonatal anoxia and acidosis (253). Hearing loss in these children characteristically predominates in the high frequencies. Retrocochlear hearing losses, that is, those due to lesions of the auditory nerve and brain stem auditory pathways, interfere more with speech discrimination and with the ability to hear when speech is embedded in noise (for instance, to follow a conversation at a party) than with the ability to detect pure tones at low intensity, that is, with auditory sensitivity (548). Since some hard-of-hearing children learn language less well than one would have expected from the severity of their hearing loss for pure tones, and since the pathologies that damage the cochlea, for instance, hyperbilirubinemia, perinatal anoxia, and meningitis, may also damage the central nervous system, pathology in the central auditory pathway is often invoked, without evidence, to explain this failure. Physiologic tests such as electrocochleography and brain stem auditory evoked potentials can now provide firm evidence to determine how often this postulate of "central" dysfunction is correct.

Early loss of hair cells and spiral ganglion cells, that is, damage to the end organ of hearing, is now known to result in transsynaptic degeneration in the cochlear nucleus and higher auditory relays in experimental animals (610). These anatomic changes have physiologic correlates; for instance, lack of inhibitory interaction at the inferior colliculus has been found in young experimental animals with unilateral conductive losses (115). The central consequences of peripheral hearing loss in man are not yet well known, but may turn out to be significant (518).

A common error is to ascribe to a language deficit what is in fact a peripheral auditory deficit (508). Physicians and other professionals caring for children must be aware that no child is too young to have his hearing tested with physiologic tools that include (a) the recording of the stapedius reflex to loud sound after the mechanical properties of the middle ear have been shown to be normal with tympanometry and impedance measurements (190); and (b) the recording of electrical auditory-evoked responses. With the use of computers it is now possible to record from electrodes pasted on the scalp electrical activity in the cochlea, the auditory nerve, the various levels of the brain stem auditory pathway, and the cortex (190,438,517) (Fig. 18). This approach provides a reliable means for measuring hearing sensitivity and for localizing dysfunction within the auditory pathway even in very young children and in those unable to cooperate because of associated handicaps like mental retardation or autistic behavior. These methods do not provide evidence on the ability of the child to discriminate among complex stimuli or utilize them to program his behavior. Since peripheral hearing loss is the most common and most treatable cause for lack of response to sound and for failure to develop language, it follows that every child with these symptoms must have his hearing tested, regardless of whether or not other handicaps provide a possible explanation for his symptoms.

A common deficit among children with brain damage is unpredictable or inconsistent response to sound. This has been observed most commonly among autistic children who are unusually intolerant of some sounds and appear to experience discomfort even though the sound is not especially loud, while they appear oblivious of other, often more intense sounds. This behavior is poorly understood, but one might speculate that it reflects selective inattention, mediated perhaps by dysfunction in descending inhibitory pathways that bias peripheral receptors and subcortical relays, allowing some stimuli to reach cortical awareness while others are shut out. The existence of such pathways has been demonstrated anatomically (259). Selective gating depending on whether or not the stimulus is relevant to the animal at a particular moment, is reflected by changes of firing rates in subcortical relays. The ability to listen selectively, as in the case of the awakening of a mother by her child's whimper, even though she sleeps through louder traffic noises to which she

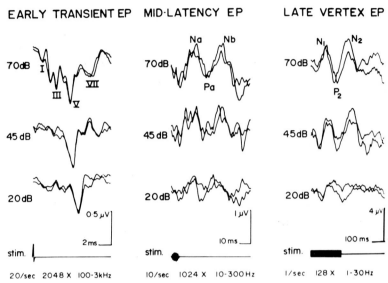

FIG. 18. Some components of the auditory evoked potential. Scalp recordings obtained from a young normal male subject. The early *transient (brain stem) potentials* represent responses to 50 μsec clicks. The most important features for clinical audiometry are wave I, originating in the cochlear nerve, wave V, originating in the vicinity of the inferior colliculus, and the latency difference between waves I and V that measures transit time through the brain stem. Each wave originates in a different subcortical relay of the central auditory pathway. *Mid-latency potentials* that originate in the cortex represent responses to brief 500 Hz tone bursts. The *late vertex* potentials were elicited by 200 msec 500 Hz tones. For all traces an upward deflection indicates negativity of the vertex electrode compared to a mastoid reference. Stimulus repetition rate, number of responses averaged for each tracing, and band-pass of the amplifier filter are indicated below each set of tracings. At the lowest intensity (20dB above threshold of normal hearing) averaging was performed to twice the listed number of stimuli in order to improve the resolution of the wave form. Two replications of each condition are superimposed so as to give some idea of the reproducibility of responses. (Reproduced with permission from Picton, Woods, Baribeau-Braun, and Healey, ref. 468a.)

has become habituated, strongly suggests that similar mechanisms play an important role in auditory processing in man.

Verbal Auditory Agnosia

Total ablation of the auditory cortex bilaterally produces the syndrome of auditory agnosia, that is, inability to recognize the source of a sound and give it meaning, for instance, to recognize a dog's bark or discriminate the ringing of the telephone from that of the doorbell. Complete auditory agnosia is quite rare. A more common syndrome, and one which is often misdiagnosed, is verbal auditory agnosia or word deafness (492,582,647). It is a deficit that seems specific for the decoding of phonology, that is, of the acoustic pattern produced by oral speech. The patient recognizes speech as speech but finds it unintelligible: Adult patients say that speech sounds to them like a foreign language. A child who does not hear or understand speech loses the ability to program speech and rapidly becomes mute.

Verbal auditory agnosia is easiest to diagnose when it is associated with bitemporal epileptic discharges in the EEG, with or without clinical absences, and occurs in a child who previously was able to speak. In some cases, the syndrome may occur so early in life as to preclude all language acquisition. While verbal auditory agnosia is often accompanied by clinical seizures and an abnormal EEG, this is not invariably the case (382). Even if seizures and an abnormal EEG are present, both may recover and disappear with time, suggesting improvement in the underlying pathology. A recent report indicates that in at least one child, this syndrome was the result of a chronic encephalitis (372). One might speculate that some of the mute autistic children who lose their speech in early childhood suffer from similar pathology but that, in them, damage was not limited to the neocortex of the temporal lobes but affected adjacent limbic structures as well.

Verbal auditory agnosia can be viewed as the most peripheral among the disorders of central language processing, since it seems that phonologic decoding precedes the processing of syntax and semantics. It differs from the receptive (Wernicke's) aphasia of adults in that the child remains able to process and use linguistic symbols meaningfully provided they are presented visually. This is a crucial point. While the adult Wernicke's aphasic usually cannot read or write, children with verbal auditory agnosia are capable of acquiring language through the visual modality. This mandates a specialized educational approach for them, based on visual methods of instruction appropriate for deaf children, that rely on the use of sign language associated with oral speech (Total Communication) and on reading.

Other Disorders of Auditory Processing

A variety of auditory processing disorders less severe than verbal auditory agnosia have been described in patients with unilateral temporal lobe pathology, usually adults with brain tumors or infarctions, or following unilateral temporal lobectomy for the relief of epilepsy (499,548). They have occasionally been described in children with congenital aplasia or cystic degeneration of the temporal lobes (340). As was pointed out earlier, the auditory functions of the two temporal lobes are not identical, the left temporal lobe appearing to be specialized for the processing of language and sequential inputs, the right for melodies, environmental sounds, and the prosody of speech (329). These differences have been shown to be present, based on the method of dichotic stimulation, in children as young as 3 years of age (291). Dichotic stimulation consists of presenting two competing messages to both ears simultaneously. The subject is then to report what he has heard. If the stimuli presented to one ear are reported preferentially and more accurately than those presented to the other ear, the hemisphere contralateral to the preferred ear is assumed to be more efficient (dominant) for that particular task. These functional differences are assumed to be the behavioral correlates of the anatomic differences between the auditory association cortex of the two hemispheres (223,602,639).

Patients with unilateral temporal pathology show a stronger ear preference than normal persons (52). They also have difficulty understanding speech presented to the contralateral ear when the speech is degraded by filtering, chopping, or embedding it in noise (548). Patients with left temporal lobe lesions may show a deficit for verbal learning or for learning acoustic sequences even when presented binaurally (418). Asymmetry of auditory evoked responses recorded from electrodes overlying the two hemispheres has been described in patients with unilateral damage (119).

A series of functional tests have been developed to detect disorders of central auditory processing that reflect pathology in the brain stem, thalamus, or cortex (380,499,548). Subtle auditory processing deficits have been found in some children with developmental language disorders (572) and with learning disability.

Adrenoleukodystrophy characteristically affects central auditory processing, presumably by the demyelination it produces in the white matter underlying the temporal cortex. Brain stem gliomas, other leukodystrophies, and, in older patients, the brain stem plaques of multiple sclerosis, may affect earlier stages of auditory processing. The more peripheral the deficit in the central auditory pathway, the more it will resemble deafness rather than verbal auditory agnosia or an aphasia. Brain stem auditory evoked potential tests provide the means for determining whether these disorders reflect unilateral temporal lobe pathology, prolonged conduction velocity in the central auditory pathway, or destruction of auditory brain stem nuclei (438). Their use, together with behavioral tests, will no doubt enhance our still fragmentary understanding of the effects of brain damage on cortical auditory processing.

7

Disorders of Attention and Arousal

The hyperkinetic syndrome or, as it has been labeled in the American Psychiatric Association's recent revision of the Diagnostic and Statistical Manual (DSM III) (171), attention deficit disorder (ADD) with hyperactivity, consists of motor restlessness, short attention span, distractibility, disorganized behavior, impulsivity, and a labile affect, often associated with a sleep disturbance. The hyperkinetic syndrome has received so much attention since it was highlighted in the 1930's (70,109,570) that some consider it virtually pathognomonic of MBD. Rather than viewing it as a possible but by no means invariable sign of brain dysfunction, and its effects as complicating other manifestations of brain dysfunction like learning disability, some have assumed that the hyperkinetic syndrome provides a sufficient cause for learning disability. If true, this would have the attractive corollary that simply administering a pill might mitigate the learning disability since hyperkinesis can be ameliorated in some children by pharmacologic agents such as methylphenidate and amphetamine (29,70,109,552,557). Pharmacologic treatment is cheap and would be much more advantageous than costly interventions such as special education, environmental manipulation, and operant conditioning, the effectiveness of which is difficult to assess. Unfortunately, long-term studies of the effects of stimulants in hyperkinetic children have not documented a better scholastic outcome in children who received them, even though teachers and parents find the medicated child easier to live with and instruct (158,524,542).

ADD can also occur without hyperkinesis, but such children rarely come to medical attention until the structured situation of the classroom exposes their distractibility, since their conduct is acceptable as long as demands for specific behavioral outputs are few. As the name ADD implies, inattentiveness is considered the primary deficit in both variants.

AROUSAL AND SELECTIVE ATTENTION

Attention is a limited capacity system that enables one to select, among the continuous stream of exogenous and endogenous stimuli that bombard the brain, those that are worthy of or demand further processing from those to ignore. Incoming stimuli selected as possibly relevant are collated with ongoing activities in the brain and with memories evoked from long-term storage by these stimuli, in order to decide whether or not the new items require action or storage. Attentional mechanisms also alert the cortex. In some cases, arousal is unselective and affects the entire cortex, but more often it is quite focused and limited to precisely those parts of the brain that will participate most directly in processing the stimuli selected. If one is prepared to see, one will maximize visual detection, possibly at the expense of not perceiving unanticipated weaker signals in another modality. Focused attention is essential for learning since it brings to bear brain processing capacity on salient items selected to the exclusion of others.

Focal or lateralized arousal of the cortex can be detected in the EEG. In alert persons lying with their eyes closed, the dominant EEG rhythm, especially over the posterior part of the head, is in the 8 to 13 Hz or alpha frequency range. When the person opens his eyes, the EEG becomes desynchronized and the alpha activity flattens or disappears (alpha blocking), at least for a period of several seconds. The alpha returns in full force as soon as the eyes are closed again. Galin (208) reports that the integrated whole-band power of the EEG over the left hemisphere decreases during verbal tasks such as speaking, writing, listening, and reading, which he interprets as evidence of selective activation of the left hemisphere during these tasks. The power of the EEG decreases over the right hemisphere during visual-spatial tasks such as block designs or mirror tracking, and during musical tasks such as singing or remembering a melody. The brain electrical activity mapping (BEAM) method (173) displays, in different colors on a diagram of the head, changes in power in various spectral bands of the EEG at various electrode sites as a function of the tasks in which the subject is engaged. Such studies show that changes in activation are not only lateralized but can be very focal and that they occur in the cortical areas that are known to be engaged by the particular tasks. Successive maps over time can be displayed as movies that track these changes in brain activity or in the epileptic discharges of patients with seizures.

Attention, thus, has two facets, selection and arousal. The frontal lobes and limbic circuits participate in selection processes since these require that a value judgement be made as to where to direct attention (228,439). Selection implies the ability to withold an immediate response so that further analysis can take place. Patients with frontal pathology lack selectivity, they tend to act impulsively, and to lack judgement. They also tend to perseverate or repeat what they just said or did, they may repeat what they just heard *(echolalia)* or imitate the examiner's gestures *(echopraxia)*. They are stimulus-bound, they have difficulty shifting their attention from one stimulus to another (378,480).

The focused attention required for selective responsiveness depends not only on prefrontal activity but on descending inputs from association areas to the nonspecific thalamic nuclei (609). The nondominant hemisphere seems to preside over some aspects of attention (270). Geschwind (221) mentions that patients with posterior parietal lesions typically are confused and inattentive. In Chapter 6 we saw that patients with lesions in the right inferior parietal lobule, a multisensory association area, may ignore the left side of space and extinguish stimuli on the left during bilateral simultaneous stimulation, a form of neglect or inattention to the left side of the body. In some cases, this neglect is so severe that the patient may not recognize the left side of his body as belonging to him, fail to clothe it, and may even deny that it is paralyzed. Geschwind (221) ascribes to the right hemisphere the task of scanning both sides of space while the left hemisphere focuses selectively on the right side of space and on the task at hand. Galin (208), and Kinsbourne and Hiscock (317) go so far as to suggest that the two hemispheres may be in competition for attentional mechanisms and that interhemispheric inhibition of competing activities may explain some aspects of cerebral dominance.

Arousal describes a person's degree of responsiveness or alertness. It is mediated, at the physiologic level, by the influence of the brain stem reticular activating system and its thalamic projections on the activity of the cortex (598). Attention fluctuates depending on the time of day and the alertness of the individual. It reaches a minimum but is not completely abolished during sleep since strong stimuli and some low intensity but highly pertinent stimuli like a baby's cry will arouse the sleeper. Fluctuations of arousal during wakefulness depend, in part, on endogenously generated hormonal and autonomic cyclical rhythms (69,304), in part on environmental stimuli, notably light (425), and in part on the relevance of individual events for the person. Pain and novelty are strongly arousing since they mandate investigation to determine relevance, while repeated stimulation is followed by habituation and sometimes even by sleep.

Arousal and attention do not always covary. Children with ADD are typically alert; in fact, they may sleep less than expected, yet they are inattentive or distractible. Perhaps frontal dysfunction is responsible for their symptoms rather than dysfunction in brain stem reticular mechanisms mediating arousal.

States associated with high levels of generalized arousal, such as those produced by anxiety, have deleterious effects on attention by decreasing response selectivity: Inappropriately strong responses such as a jump will occur to low intensity and irrelevant stimuli, for example, the crack of a floor board that would be ignored under other circumstances. The affective tone of stimuli also influences the amount of attention they engage: Neutral stimuli associated, even if rarely, with unpleasant consequences are unlikely to be ignored; habituation tends not to occur and the cortical responses evoked by such stimuli are resistant to extinction (207). In other words, potentially aversive stimuli continue to command attention, in contrast to pleasurable stimuli that pale, at least for a time, if they occur too frequently.

We just saw that the stimuli that impinge on the brain play a dominant role in the maintenance of vigilance. Sensory input projections conveying each modality reach the cortex via two parallel pathways. The first is exemplified by the classical lemniscal pathways that carry detailed environmental information to the brain. Such pathways utilize the modality-specific long tracts from sensory receptors via specific thalamic nuclei to primary sensory receiving areas of the cortex. Relatively few synapses are interposed in these projection pathways from receptors to cortex. The second system mediates arousal (Fig. 19). Most input channels arising in skin,

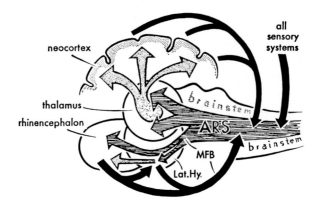

FIG. 19. Reticular activating system. Schematic diagram of the major connections to and from the ascending reticular system (ARS). The ARS is located in the core of the brain stem. Its major projections are (a) to the nonspecific thalamic nuclei, which in turn have diffuse cortical projections, and (b) via the medial forebrain bundle (MFB) of the lateral hypothalamus (Lat. Hy.), to various rhinencephalic structures, notably the septal area, either directly or via lateral hypothalamic relays. The reticular activating system has three major sources of input: (1) from all the sensory systems of the body, (2) from the neocortex, and (3) from the rhinencephalon (including the lateral hypothalamus). (Reproduced with permission from McCleary and Moore, ref. 398a.)

muscles, joints, eyes, ears, tongue, nose, and viscera send collaterals to the reticular activating system of the brain stem (528). This multisynaptic activation pathway, which does not have the modality specificity of the first pathway, carries excitatory impulses from the reticular activating system through the nonspecific thalamic nuclei to widespread areas of the cerebral cortex (562). Thus, behavioral arousal and electrical arousal of the cortex are largely dependent upon the activation of the brain stem reticular formation by sensory inputs.

The cortex sends two types of fibers back to the reticular formation and non-specific thalamic nuclei. Some are excitatory. In the words of Bremer (74), "The cerebral cortex participates actively in its own arousal and in the maintenance of its waking state by the corticofugal impulses which it sends to the brain stem reticular formation" (p. 158). Other corticofugal fibers are inhibitory. Transmission through the modality-specific sensory pathways is rapid because there are few synapses. Through the nonspecific reticular pathway, transmission is slower because of the many synapses interposed. Consequently, there is time for an impulse to reach the cortex through a specific pathway and to relay down to the reticular formation, thus inhibiting the arousal which would have been produced by the stimulus (525). This convergence upon the reticular formation of afferent sensory impulses and corticofugal inhibitory impulses may play a critical role in filtering out irrelevant stimuli, that is, stimuli that do not produce focused arousal of the cortex but are treated as noise.

Selective attention, and habituation or the attenuation of responses to a repetitive stimulus, may both be dependent upon descending inhibitory fibers directed not only to the reticular formation but also to the relay nuclei in the specific sensory pathways and to the sensory receptors themselves. Thus, it is proposed that the brain gates its own inputs selectively at many levels and biases the sensitivity of its receptors, although physiologic evidence for this assumption is still provisional (598).

Complex recursive pathways exist between the reticular formation and many parts of the brain, for example, cortex, limbic system, and hypothalamus, as well as between cortex, thalamus, reticular formation, and classic sensory pathways. The physiologic functions of these feedback pathways have been elucidated to some extent. Their existence permits a tentative explanation for observable behaviors such as selective attention. Focused attention to stimuli and rejection of stimuli as noise vary continuously as the relevance of sensory inputs from outside events is evaluated. If stimuli are considered irrelevant they are filtered out, perhaps at subcortical levels; if not, the sensory channel carrying this information remains open so that more information about the event can reach the cortex. In addition, the brain is aroused by the excitatory effect of the input on the reticular formation; thus, it becomes ready to respond appropriately to the stimulus.

Activity in the classic sensory pathways seems to be stimulus-bound, reflecting the current sensory input more or less accurately. Activity in the nonspecific systems is at least partially determined by prior experience, that is, by previously learned (stored) information. In the cat, when activity in the two systems is concordant, behavior is appropriate to the presented signal; when activity is discordant, behavior is inappropriate (428).

The filtering of sensory inputs is quite selective. In waking man the amplitude of cortical potentials evoked by light flashes increases when the subject is asked to count the flashes; it decreases while he solves a difficult problem in mental arithmetic and recovers after he has finished (278). The amplitude of the visual evoked potential varies as a function of subjective perception of brightness and increases when perception is modified by suggestion (275). While, in general, amplitude of evoked responses is correlated with stimulus intensity, amplitude to occasional unexpectedly weak stimuli (embedded in a train of repetitive clicks) will be higher than amplitude to the louder stimuli of expected intensity. There are even endogenously generated evoked responses to stimuli missing from a rhythmical train occurring at the time the missing stimuli were expected, indicating the arousing effect of the nonoccurrence of an expected event (543) (Fig. 20). Such findings illustrate the active character of perceptual processes and their complex interaction with attentional mechanisms (598).

Attention, then, is a complex system for making choices and for facilitating the processing of selective items. Attention presupposes modulation of incoming stimuli, access to long-term memories, and scanning of current exogenous and endogenous brain processes. Attention determines, and is determined by, the person's state of vigilance and commands his subsequent activities.

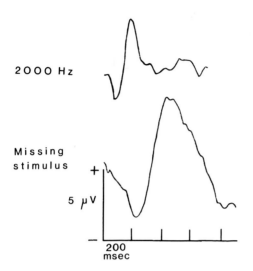

2000 Hz

Missing
stimulus

5 µV

200
msec

FIG. 20. Response evoked by unexpectedly missing stimuli. The top trace is the scalp response evoked by 2000 Hz 50 msec tone bursts delivered at a regular rate of 1/sec. (Grand mean of 4800 presentations to 8 normal subjects.) The bottom trace is a response time-locked to the expected occurrence of stimuli unpredictably missing 10% of the time from this train of tones. (Grand mean of 240 missing stimuli in the same subjects.) The tones evoke a response at the vertex electrode (referred to the tip of the nose) with a negative peak at about 90 msec and a positive peak at about 200 msec, while the missing stimuli evoke a response of greater amplitude (and different distribution over the scalp) with a negativity at about 200 msec and positivity at about 300 msec. (Courtesy R. Simson. See also reference 543.)

CONSCIOUSNESS

A person whose behavior suggests that he is alert and attentive can be assumed to be conscious; one who is asleep or who is unresponsive to even strong and noxious stimuli (coma) is not conscious. (Consciousness of a special sort is present during trance states and perhaps might even be said to be present, for internal stimuli only, during dreaming sleep.) Under everyday circumstances, one tends to infer consciousness in another person from his ability to respond selectively and to communicate verbally or nonverbally. Selectivity implies that a person's responses are not rigidly determined by reflex mechanisms but that the person can choose to respond or not to respond, and that he can choose his particular response. Communication is often the person's answer to a question or his verbal statement about his impressions, wants, or plans, but it might be a gesture or a look. In other words, a person is clearly conscious when he can, figuratively, stand outside of himself in order to make what he experiences as free decisions, and in order to speak about what he perceives is going on in his mind (218,280). We know, and others can infer from our behavior, and EEGs and blood flow studies can show (346), that we are conscious and that our brain is active when we are thinking, even if we neither speak nor move.

Patients who are completely paralyzed as the result of certain brain stem lesions may be in a state called the *locked-in syndrome*. One can determine that such patients are conscious and able to think by asking them to blink or move their eyes in particular directions in response to questions. Their EEGs show that they are alert and that they go through cyclic periods of sleep and arousal. Such patients are sometimes difficult to differentiate from patients in the state of *coma vigil*, who also have their eyes open and move them around but who do not respond to verbal commands through eye blinks or directed eye movements. Most patients in coma vigil have abnormal EEGs. They may or may not go through normal sleep cycles, depending on the location of their lesion (473).

Experiments with split-brain patients have raised interesting new questions about consciousness (214,216,554) (see Fig. 22). Patients who have undergone commissurotomy do not experience any impairment of consciousness or unusual feeling about what is going on in their mind. Under normal circumstances, both hemispheres receive similar or identical stimuli so that the two half-brains are generally focused on similar experiences and tasks. Both hemispheres sleep and are aroused simultaneously by the reticular formation, and as far as can be determined, feelings arising from limbic activity are shared by both sides. It is easy to demonstrate under experimental conditions that the isolated left hemisphere is conscious: It responds to questions, speaks about the tasks it is controlling, and about the subjects's feelings. But what about the mute right hemisphere? The isolated right hemisphere can cause the subject to laugh at a pornographic picture shown in the left visual field which the left hemisphere knows nothing about. The right hemisphere is therefore conscious. But so is the left, since it will cause the patient to confabulate a verbal explanation for a laugh caused by a stimulus it did not experience, a laugh it did not provoke and cannot explain. Consciousness in each of the two hemispheres of split-brain patients is therefore at least partially independent, while the consciousness the patient can speak about is that of the speaking hemisphere. Consciousness in the mute right hemisphere is perhaps analogous to consciousness in a preverbal infant who plays, smiles responsively (communicates), and clearly expresses pleasure and displeasure, but who will be able to remember little or nothing as a child or an adult of what he did and learned as an infant.

VIGILANCE AND SLEEP

Arousal of the brain or its basic excitability state is modulated by the excitatory effects of incoming sensory stimuli on the mesencephalic reticular activating system, and is entrained with circadian rhythmic hormonal fluctuations (69). Norepinephrine has alerting effects on the reticular activating system and on the cortex, as do cholinergic circuits. Sensory deprivation results in drowsiness at first; later it is replaced by endogenously generated sensory activity experienced as hallucinations (656). Destruction of the reticular activating system results in coma, a state of cortical depression during which the organism is incapable of mounting a directed response to sensory stimuli. The EEG correlate of alertness with the eyes open is a low voltage fast EEG, with the appearance of rhythmic alpha waves posteriorly when the eyes are closed. The EEG of coma is usually composed of high voltage slow waves (hypersynchrony) denoting cortical depression.

Sleep is not a homogenous physiologic state. Its two main phases are slow-wave sleep, during which the EEG exhibits high-voltage slow waves; and rapid eye movement (REM), dreaming, or paradoxical sleep during which the EEG exhibits low-voltage fast activity resembling the EEG of wakeful alertness. REM sleep is also characterized by atonia of the muscles and periodic bursts of activity in the extraocular muscles. Alternation between wakefulness, slow-wave sleep, and REM sleep appears to be controlled by cyclical reciprocal interactions between the monaminergic locus coeruleus and raphé nuclei of the brain stem and gigantocellular cholinoceptive neurons in the adjacent pontine reticular formation (397). Raphé neurons are serotonergic, those of the locus coeruleus, noradrenergic. Both nuclei send extensive projections to the cerebral cortex, hippocampus, and other rostral brain areas whose activity they modulate. During the waking state, activity in these monaminergic neurons is high and the pontine reticular neurons are inhibited, while during REM sleep the monaminergic neurons are inhibited and the pontine reticular neurons generate bursts of activity that trigger spikes in the lateral geniculate nucleus of the thalamus and in the occipital cortex (the ponto-geniculo-occipital or PGO spikes characteristic of REM sleep) (152). These reticular neurons also project inhibitory impulses to bulbar reticular neurons that, in turn, inhibit motor neurons in the spinal cord. Slow-wave sleep occurs while neither the reticular neurons nor the monoaminergic neurons are maximally active (397).

Disturbances of the wake-sleep rhythm are frequent in patients with psychoses, illnesses that are associated with alterations in neurotransmitter metabolism, and in hyperkinetic children. Lesions in the raphé nucleus and antiserotonergic drugs abolish slow-wave sleep, at least for a time, while damage to the locus coeruleus and pontine reticular formation abolishes REM sleep. Cholinergic drugs and stimulant drugs like amphetamine have alerting effects and produce insomnia. Drugs that block the effects of monoamines like the phenothiazines and reserpine reduce REM sleep and have sedative effects. Atropine, an anticholinergic drug, also blocks REM sleep. The alerting properties of exogenous sensory stimuli may be mediated in part by their stimulating effects on locus coeruleus and raphé neurons. The alternation of light and dark periods (day and night) entrain cyclical alterations in the concentration of serotonin in the pineal gland through an indirect noradrenergic pathway. The pineal gland has been shown to play a crucial role in the maintenance of circadian rhythms like motor activity and sleep (22). Numerous functions are, in turn, entrained by the wake-sleep cycle, for example, temperature of the body and brain, production of urine, and gastrointestinal motility. The secretion of many hormones occurs in pulses at highly specific times during the cycle, for example, the release of growth hormone which is tied to slow-wave sleep periods (69).

A completely coherent theory of sleep and its control is still lacking. Nonetheless, we have gained some insight into sleep disorders like narcolepsy that appear to affect REM sleep specifically (152) and into the side effects of drugs that alter neurotransmitter metabolism such as the cerebral stimulants and tranquilizers that are used extensively in children with brain dysfunction.

Impaired consciousness usually reflects either a lesion affecting the brain stem reticular activating system, or diffusely depressed cortical activity—by edema or an intoxication, for example (473). It may occasionally reflect diffuse cortical epileptic activity without motor concomitant, such as that seen in infants with infantile spasms (hypsarrhythmia) or with minor motor seizures (Lennox-Gastaut syndrome) who may look awake but are apathetic and "in a shell" in the interval between motor seizures. The cerebral cortex of these children is engaged in epileptic activity. As a result, complex sensorimotor processing is disturbed, although the child may be capable of semiautomatic, presumably largely subcortical, activities like standing and walking (108,233,423).

Pitfalls to be avoided are to mistake coma for deep sleep, or subclinical status epilepticus for a psychiatrically determined impairment of the ability to respond to stimulation, and to mistake for coma the locked-in syndrome seen in patients who are totally paralyzed except for the control of their eye movements. The EEG is obviously extremely useful for making a differential diagnosis in such patients.

THE HYPERKINETIC SYNDROME (ATTENTION DEFICIT DISORDER)

Bradley (70) reported in the 1930's that amphetamine had a "paradoxically" calming effect on hyperkinetic children. Many theories have been advanced to explain the beneficial effects of stimulant drugs in some hyperkinetic children (29,316,552,557). One theory suggests that the children are underaroused. This theory predicts that hyperkinetic children process stimuli inadequately and do not assess the relevance of incoming stimuli efficiently. (This capacity may depend on activity in cholinergic pathways (606) and in the fontal lobes.) Because of inadequate inhibition, the children respond unselectively, are easily distracted, and have a short attention span. This lack of efficiency is also thought to be associated with lack of precision in setting levels of autonomic and affective responsiveness so that the child's reactions are unpredictable, at times too strong, at times too weak. If this state exists in hyperkinetic children who react favorably to stimulant drugs, the effect of the drug is not paradoxical: Increasing cortical arousal, and thus the effectiveness of processing and of subcortical gating of sensory inputs, might explain the calming effect, increased attention span, better focusing, and more appropriate affective responses produced by the stimulant. The hypoarousal theory does not provide a very satisfactory explanation for the hyperkinetic child's sleeping difficulties: Not only does he stay up late at night, he also sleeps restlessly, often fitfully, and awakes early. Allnight EEG recordings with repeated sampling of various hormones and metabolites of biogenic amines will be needed in order to gain better insight into the pathogenesis of these symptoms.

Hyperkinesis, distractibility, and disorganized behavior can be the end result of other mechanisms besides underarousal of the cortex. Hyperarousal is seen in normal persons when they are anxious, or frightened, or given stimulants like caffeine, epinephrine, or amphetamine. Such persons overreact to sensory stimuli, are impulsive—that is, they respond fast and unselectively, without taking the time for due consideration of alternatives, and they do not habituate easily. They have trouble falling asleep. Their levels of autonomic and endocrine responsiveness are increased. Predictably, stimulants are ineffective in children who are anxious and already hyperaroused and such drugs may make them much worse. They are also ineffective in children in whom hyperkinetic behavior reflects the sensory distortions produced by a psychotic process; these would be aggravated by the effects of stimulants on cerebral dopamine systems (549). For clinical reasons, it is therefore important to distinguish hyperactive-impulsive-inattentive children who may respond favorably to stimulant drugs from anxious-hyperkinetic children who may respond to lessening of external pressures, to psychotherapy, and to anxiolytic drugs like the benzodiazepines (12,226). It is also important to distinguish impulsive-inattentive-hyperkinetic children from aggressive-hyperkinetic children who will profit from the imposing of firm behavioral limits and from behavioral modification approaches (339), and these children from psychotic-hyperkinetic children. This latter group may get worse with stimulant drugs while responding favorably to antipsychotic drugs, for example, chlorpromazine (Thorazine®) and thioridazine (Mellaril®) or to drugs such as the butyrophenone haloperidol (Haldol®) (91,194).

Innumerable writings in the past quarter century have espoused the view that hyperkinetic behavior and distractibility are cardinal signs of structural though subtle brain damage, tacitly attributed to some perinatal insult. Recent evidence suggests that a biochemical lesion of an as yet undetermined type caused by chronic exposure to lead at concentrations too low to produce overt signs of poisoning may be still another cause for deficient attention and scholastic achievement in some children (440). Disorders in the balance of neurotransmitters, pathology in the reticular activating system or the thalamus, impaired frontal-limbic activity precluding advance planning (439,480), ineffective inhibitory processes at subcortical relays— any of these might alter arousal mechanisms and preclude selective attention. Even boredom, that can be looked upon as a mild state of sensory deprivation, if it does not lead to sleep may induce self-stimulation or the desire to escape the boring situation, both reflected by fidgetiness. As usual, dysfunction in many different systems may be responsible for an observed symptom. It is important to remember that the hyperkinetic syndrome may reflect a particular temperament (582) and by no means always implies brain damage (106).

Even pathologic hyperactivity is strongly influenced by environmental variables so that pharmacotherapy alone can never be considered adequate management (227). In fact, many pathologically hyperkinetic children will respond so well to environmental manipulation that drugs will not be required. Manipulations may include providing a predictable schedule to be adhered to, insisting that study take place in a quiet environment without competing distractions while providing frequent opportunities for the child to play and move around (564,565), and teaching the child to slow down and speak to himself before responding (408,420). Of course, classic behavior modification approaches are also helpful and are used extensively with such children (210,333,339,618).

8

Disorders of Learning and Memory

In order to adapt to his environment, a person must recognize the stimuli he apprehends, evaluate their significance, and decide upon which of those to act. Each of these operations calls for the processing of new data, registered quasi-automatically in short-term memory, in the light of memories of previous experiences and actions retrieved from long-term storage by the common features they share with the current data. Learning refers to the series of overlapping operations that leads to long-term storage of items in retrievable form. Storage is intimately linked with attentional and affective processes (559): Items in short-term storage that do not achieve sufficient salience to compel further processing are forgotten almost immediately and apparently irretrievably as they are displaced by the stream of new items that take their place (310,369). If fading from short-term stores is due to lack of registration, failure to recall registered items may be the result of either retrieval failure or of failure of consolidation. The probability of storage in retrievable form is enhanced by the significance of the particular items for the individual, by repetition, and by the cognitive organization he or she imposes on the data.

Learning is not limited to the intentional and effortful retention of items or skills deliberately repeated again and again. Learning is a continuous process that operates on all data that reach a threshold of significance. It encompasses the storage of impressions presented to each of the senses, of verbal and nonverbal data and ideas, and the retention of commands for skilled motor acts. We are not sure to what degree sensory, motor, and verbal learning share common brain mechanisms beyond the attention for which they all compete. We shall see that in some ways they are at least partially independent processes (561).

The old adage that intelligence and memory are unrelated is misleading since effective learning is an active cognitive process. We seek new information in order to update what we have already stored. Our ability to hold on to new data depends on our capacity to process them "intelligently" by organizing or chunking inputs into meaningful packages for efficient storage and retrieval (87). We link new information to those previously stored items with which it shares features. If the new item is learned or stored, it will become accessible in turn through this linkage process. The commonalities between new items and stored data, which may be what activates memories and renders them accessible to retrieval, makes them all members of a superordinate class that can be processed as one efficient unit rather than individually. It is this dynamic aspect of memory that provides its power. Learning efficiency varies greatly among individuals. In general, highly intelligent persons have efficient memories; what they store is so well catalogued and cross-indexed that they make rich and unexpected associations in response to new situations. A photographic memory without the ability to make novel associations is useless, witness the occasional severely retarded child with an excellent rote memory (idiot savant) who makes little if any use of what he can parrot (289).

BIOLOGIC BASIS OF LONG-TERM MEMORY

We are still at a loss to understand the biologic basis of learning and of the retention of long-term memories (73,479). Most of the evidence suggests that permanent memories (at least those that are potentially retrievable to consciousness) are stored in the cerebral cortex, although learning, i.e., modification of behavior by past experience, is a general property of neuronal networks that can be shown to take place at all levels of the nervous system, including the spinal cord. It is assumed that permanent memories are coded through structural and/or biochemical changes that somehow modify "educated" cells (3,479) since remote memories survive such "intracerebral holocausts" as major convulsions, electroshock, post-traumatic concussion, and deep anesthesia, all of which profoundly modify cerebral electrical activity. In contrast, it seems likely that sustained electrical activation in particular neuronal networks provides a basis for short-term memory.

Many workers suggest that learning is dependent on the synthesis of macro-molecules like proteins or glycoproteins that either exert their effects at specific synaptic locations or that are biochemically unique, like antibodies, and mark a particular pathway. Some compounds that inhibit protein or RNA synthesis produce amnesia, perhaps by interfering with the consolidation of new memories for long-term storage (3,30,73,504,510). Neurotransmitters play a role in learning. Scopolamine, a cholinergic blocking agent, has been known for years to produce amnesia by impairing both storage and retrieval, while physostigmine, a cholinergic agent with central effects, seems to promote slightly more efficient learning (145,168). Many other agents have as yet poorly understood effects on learning. Perhaps they act through alteration of cholinergic or noradrenergic circuits in the hippocampus, or through their effects on limbic reward systems, or on brain stem alerting pathways. Thus, amphetamine, ACTH, vasopressin, the enkephalins, and various other agents affecting synaptic transmission and membrane permeability have been implicated in altering learning processes (73,335,615). For example, DeWied and Versteeg (162) suggest that in rats extrahypothalamic vasopressin-containing pathways projecting to limbic and midbrain areas may facilitate memory by their interaction with catecholaminergic neurons. These authors indicate that nigrostriatal dopamine may be involved in the retrieval of stored information and norepinephrine in the consolidation of memories. They report that vasopressin was used to good effect in a few patients with posttraumatic amnesia. At this point, we are still too far from understanding the molecular basis of learning to be able to prescribe effective agents to foster learning in our patients.

There is some information about synaptic correlates of learning. Mice deprived of visual experience by being blinded or reared in the dark and, therefore, who have no opportunity for visual learning fail to develop a normal complement of axodendritic synapses in the visual cortex (595). Tectal neurons of fish reared in isolation have less complex dendritic trees and less efficient synapses than those of fish reared in tanks with other fish (129). Whatever the structural or biochemical changes in neurons that accompany learning, they presumably facilitate excitation. In Hebb's terminology (263) the cell becomes part of several cell assemblies and phase sequences, networks of cells that are coactivated even though they may be widely separated in the cortex and particular subcortical structures.

If half of a person's brain is removed he does not lose half of his old memories, nor does he become unable to acquire new ones, that is, to learn. This suggests that memories are stored in possibly nonidentical duplicates in the two hemispheres. Transfer of memories from one hemisphere to the other does not take place when the corpus callosum and other interhemispheric commissures are severed, even though brain stem connections remain intact (214,216,555). Interhemispheric transfer of learning does not occur in rats, even if the commissures are preserved and both hemispheres function normally in between training sessions, when learning is induced in one hemisphere exclusively by temporarily inactivating the other hemisphere during training (521). Memories do not appear to be discretely represented since extensive cortical ablations do not abolish old memories. Pribram (477) proposes that memories may be distributed in the brain much the same as holographic images. A hologram can be reconstructed from any of its parts and is thus highly resistant to damage, a characteristic it shares with long-term memory. Mountcastle (432) indicates how the distributed and resilient organization of the neocortex depends on its modular fine structure, with repeating vertical columns of highly organized interrelated neurons, each of which acts in some ways as an independent integrated unit with well-defined input-output connections (see Fig. 6). Pyramidal neurons in superficial layers II and III of the neocortex provide horizontal intracortical outputs to neighboring and distant columns of the ipsilateral hemisphere and, via the corpus callosum, to discrete addresses in homologous areas of the contralateral hemisphere (301). Larger pyramidal neurons in deeper layers V and VI of the cortex provide vertical outputs to the thalamus and to brain stem and spinal cord targets. Afferents to the cortex originating in the thalamus terminate not only on interneurons in layers IV and on pyramidal neurons in layer III but also on those in layers V and VI, thus providing relatively short loop cortical-subcortical connections; corticocortical afferents terminate mainly in layers II and III which correspond to their locus of origin. As a result of this modular organization of the cortex, only extensive loss of cortical neurons, such as occurs in the late stages of progressive organic dementias of childhood like SSPE or the lipidoses, eventually impairs the maintenance and retrieval of memories for remote events and the performance of overlearned motor skills such as eating and the utterance of stock phrases like greetings.

In contrast to the diffuseness of remote memories, learning—the processes that underlie the storage and retrieval of new memories—seems to depend on focal activity engaging hippocampal-limbic circuits. As will be seen later, lesions affecting the hippocampus bilaterally preclude new learning and produce amnesia. The hippocampus may also participate in retrieval from long-term memory despite the fact that amnesic patients retain access to their remote memories: Patients with temporal lobe seizures often report that during their attacks they relive a particular event in their lives, and Penfield and Jasper (459) were able to elicit complex remote memories by electrical stimulation of the temporal lobe in alert epileptic patients during surgery. Right temporal lobectomy that includes the hippocampus interferes selectively with visual learning, left temporal lobectomy with verbal learning (418). Bilateral temporal lobectomy and hippocampectomy produce permanent inability to learn (anterograde amnesia) (531).

Deciding whether new data should be acted upon now, processed for long-term storage, or allowed to decay because they have fulfilled their use or have been judged irrelevant calls for many complex operations and involves many brain systems including the frontal cortex, the amygdala, and other limbic and subcortical circuits (228,617).

ELECTRICAL CORRELATES OF LEARNING

Electrical recordings from the brains of animals and, with averaging techniques, from the scalp of man during learning tasks have contributed to our knowledge of the neurologic substrates of learning (161). A novel stimulus in a given modality, for example, a sound, produces desynchronization of the EEG over the entire cortex, a change characteristic of alerting. This desynchronization reflects cortical arousal and activation by the reticular formation and is called the *orienting response*. With repetition, desynchronization becomes limited to the auditory cortex; the orienting response has become inhibited and activation is focused, presumably by progressive inhibition or gating of iterative sensory inputs at subcortical relays. After many repetitions, even focal activation disappears, the stimulus is no longer attended to, habituation has occurred. If inhibition becomes generalized the animal may fall asleep.

In man, the amplitude of the brain stem components of average auditory-evoked responses does not decrease with stimulus repetition, in contrast to what happens at the cortex (446). The amplitude of some components of cortical-evoked responses is believed to reflect processes of selective attention, a necessary first step for further processing required for long-term storage; others seem related to retention in short-term memory (101). Evoked responses elicited by expected but missing stimuli were mentioned in Chapter 7 (543). A response produced by a missing stimulus can only be generated endogenously and must reflect data retrieved from storage, together with the alerting effect resulting from thwarted expectancy or from novelty.

Conditioning paradigms provide a means for studying learning and expectancy. As is well known, if a stimulus in one modality, for example, a sound, is regularly preceded by a stimulus in another modality, for example, a light, and if the animal is to respond to the sound to avoid punishment or if he is rewarded after the occurrence of the sound, the warning light will produce preparatory desynchronization in the auditory cortex in anticipation of the sound that has acquired a meaning for the animal through the learning process associated with repetition and with reward or the avoidance of punishment. These changes in the cortical EEG during conditioning are associated with slow waves in the hippocampus, called theta waves, that disappear when conditioning is stable (242). While theta waves parallel the conditioning process and learning, they seem most directly related to focused attentional or search mechanisms and to the inhibition of irrelevant activity in other pathways, all of which are requisites for learning (242,324). Learning is as much or more a matter of inhibition of irrelevant pathways as of closure of specific excitatory pathways (617). The motivational aspects of learning are probably subserved by activity in the hypothalamic-limbic system during conditioning. Thus, interplay of sensory pathways, cortex, reticular formation, and limbic circuits provides the informational, alerting, and motivational components of the learning process (228,428).

In man, reaction time experiments paired with the recording of averaged event-related potentials have shown that a warning stimulus S_1, triggers the appearance of a sustained cortical negativity, called the contingent negative variation, that disappears at S_2, a second stimulus in another modality to which the subject is to respond. This expectancy wave is apparently distinct for the readiness potential that precedes movement and may reflect activation of motor command programs, and from the motor potential of shorter duration whose appearance is restricted to the motor cortex contralateral to the responding hand (229). Expectancy waves and readiness potentials are correlates of conditioning tasks that require a response. These simple tasks are one avenue to the investigation of learning in man.

Learning is selective: Items are stored because of their positive or negative consequences for the individual, whereas the vast majority of neutral items are forgotten. Conditioning and other learning experiments in the laboratory exploit this fact: Reward is used to foster learning and increase the probability that a response will be produced; punishment also fosters learning but decreases the probability that punished responses will be produced and encourages escape; behaviors that are neither rewarded nor punished are produced less and less until they become extinguished. Animal experiments have shown that nigral dopaminergic pathways and noradrenergic pathways of the brain stem and hypothalamus where stimulation produces rewarding effects play an important role in learning (516). Drugs like amphetamine and methylphenidate, widely prescribed to children with learning disabilities, potentiate the effects of these catecholamines. While the drugs are thought to exert their effect by focusing attention and decreasing distractibility, their effects on reward pathways may also be beneficial to learning (29). Operant conditioning paradigms reinforcing desired behaviors and ignoring undesirable ones have been adapted from the laboratory to the classroom, often with notable success (333, 339). In order to be effective, rewards must be individualized for each child. Food reinforcement, which is widely used, is by no means equally rewarding at all times, and is certainly not the most effective reward for every child.

SHORT-TERM STORAGE

Some of the steps involved in learning are (a) registration of the stimulus in a sensory buffer; (b) short-term maintenance while its relevance is appraised and it undergoes processing in the light of material retrieved from long-term stores; (c) acquisition or consolidation; and (d) finally permanent storage in long-term memory (73,184,295,369,479,570). Retrieval is possible at all stages.

Registration of sensory images occurs in a buffer that has a large capacity and is modality-specific (138,369). Its span is very brief: In the absence of rehearsal, visual images decay in less than 1 sec from the iconic store, and auditory ones in less than 4 sec from the echoic store. Subjects can apprehend more than they can report. Averbach and Coriell (21) presented a display of many digits to their subjects. The display was then turned off and after a brief interval, a circle of light appeared in the location previously occupied by one of the digits. The subjects were often able to identify which digit had occupied that space. It is assumed that short-term memory reflects, in part, activity in reverberating circuits, engaging the modality-specific cortical sensory association areas and, presumably, the hippocampus.

Whether there is a short-term memory store distinct from these modality-specific sensory stores is not entirely clear. The "stuff" of short-term verbal memory is auditory or phonologic (125), whether items are presented visually (and presumably labeled by the subjects) or acoustically, although in profoundly deaf children short-term memory appears to operate on visually coded linguistic data. The verbal short-term store enables one, for instance, to wait until the end of an embedded clause to attach meaning to a sentence. In patients undergoing surgery for the control of epilepsy, Ojemann and Mateer (448) were able to identify discrete areas of the left temporoparietal cortex situated at the margins of the perisylvian language area where electrical stimulation interfered with the input or storage phase of short-term verbal memory, and marginal areas in the parietal-prefrontal area where stimulation interfered with retrieval. Ojemann (447) and others (82,188) have shown that the left thalamus participates in verbal and the right thalamus in nonverbal, short-term memory.

Modality-specific short-term storage engages the activity of secondary and tertiary cortical sensory association areas. Ross (512) suggests that memory for nonverbal stimuli presented to visual, acoustic, or tactile channels is impaired selectively by lesions that disconnect cortical sensory association areas for each modality from the structures of the mesial temporal lobe (including the hippocampus) involved in learning.

There is no consensus concerning the stages that intervene between immediate registration and long-term storage. When neurologists speak of short-term memory they are referring to a store that can vary in length from a few seconds to several minutes. They test short-term auditory verbal memory in several ways: (a) they may ask a patient to repeat a string of digits without delay and in the same order they were presented; (b) they may ask the patient to repeat a string of digits in reverse order; or (c) they may ask the patient to repeat, after an interval of minutes, three items he had been warned he would be asked to recall. Neurologists test semantic verbal memory by asking the patient questions about a short-story he has just read or had read to him (27). Note that many of these tasks, ostensibly designed to test short-term verbal memory, are actually tests of learning. They are highly dependent on focused attention, motivation, and cognitive efficiency. The neurologist's tasks do not assess the strategies used by the patient in order to retain the material to be able to repeat it.

When cognitive psychologists speak of short-term verbal memory they are referring to a buffer store of limited capacity that can hold approximately seven items for immediate recall (416). They may ask the subject to repeat a string of items immediately, or after a delay of a few seconds, or after distractor items were presented in order to prevent rehearsal. Items in short-term verbal storage must either be rehearsed or organized semantically (categorized into larger meaningful chunks) in order not to decay and be displaced by new incoming items (87). How individuals organize material they are attempting to learn can be assessed by presenting long lists of words repeatedly and recording the order in which words are remembered on each trial (86). Subjects will automatically cluster words into cognitively advantageous categories. This improves learning efficiency since the subject need only remember the cluster in order to retrieve the items in the cluster.

One of the ways psychologists can distinguish learning from retrieval is by comparing tasks calling for active recall from recognition tasks where all the subject is asked is to state whether an item was presented earlier or not. Neuropsychologists interested in focal brain dysfunction test visual memory in addition to auditory memory by presenting pictures, objects, and nonlabelable nonsense forms for recognition or recall; they may present stimuli to only one of the visual fields in order to compare the efficiency of the two hemispheres. Some of the tests in common use to assess learning efficiency in children can be found in Tables 10 and 11 in Chapter 11.

The term *recent memory* is used by some for tasks that require the recall, after an interval of minutes, of items whose number exceeds the span of short-term memory. These are learning tasks that assess consolidation for long-term storage. The span of the so-called *consolidation* or retention phase of memory extends from a few seconds to perhaps as long as several months following input. Memories in the process of early consolidation are vulnerable to alterations in brain function produced by anesthesia, deep hypothermia, convulsions, and coma, provided these insults occur within 20 to 30 minutes of learning. Interference with consolidation is thought to be responsible for the interval of permanent retrograde amnesia seen in some patients following structural brain insults.

The fact that neurologists and psychologists do not agree fully on the definition of short-term memory highlights the complexities of memory processes which overlap in time: Access to long-term memory occurs immediately upon registration, since perception implies recognition; processing for long-term storage starts as soon as a new item has reached a threshold of relevance. Whether a new item does or does not reach this threshold is determined on occasion by the strength of the stimulus, much more often by what items it has activated in long-term storage, items selected perhaps by the amount of attention the new item has attracted and by the common attributes it shares with stored items (310).

AMNESIA

Amnesia literally means lack of memory. The term amnesia is often used more restrictively to mean inability to learn because of defective storage or consolidation, or to inefficient retrieval of items from permanent storage. Short-term memory is characteristically spared in amnesic patients and impaired in those who are distracted, anxious, confused, or whose state of consciousness is depressed.

Retrograde Amnesia

Retrograde amnesia is a condition that is seen most commonly in patients who have sustained a cerebral concussion. It also occurs after prolonged epileptic seizures and after electroshock. All of these conditions produce profound and prolonged, although reversible, alterations in cortical and brain stem activity. Upon regaining consciousness, patients with retrograde amnesia do not recall events that occurred minutes, hours, or even days prior to their illness. Retrograde amnesia is at its worst immediately after the patient regains consciousness and is said to recede first for items most distant in time, then for more recent ones, although in many patients retrograde amnesia is patchy and does not follow such an orderly course. Eventually, retrograde amnesia shrinks to the point where most patients can recall their past life right up to the time of the accident or shortly before it.

The mechanism of retrograde amnesia is not clear. It seems to interfere with the early states of storage since items in the process of consolidation are most vulnerable, as indicated by the many patients with brain trauma who suffer a permanent loss of memory for items that occurred minutes before the injury. It also seems to affect retrieval, since concussed patients transiently fail to remember items stored for hours, days, or even longer before the injury. It does not seem to interfere with permanent storage, however, since this retrieval failure is reversible, memories regain their accessibility and reemerge intact after recovery. Occasionally, permanent retrograde amnesia may encompass a period of months rather than minutes or hours. This situation was observed following bilateral temporal lobectomy and hippocampectomy in an attempt to control intractable epilepsy (419). The patient, named H.M., to this day remembers nothing of what happened to him for many months before surgery and nothing of what has happened to him since surgery (anterograde amnesia).

Anterograde Amnesia

Anterograde amnesia refers to the inability to learn new material. Learning cannot take place in the absence of interplay between brain stem and cortex, for example, during anesthesia, during sleep, or during the coma caused by brain stem dysfunction. In alert patients, anterograde amnesia may be caused by selective lesions affecting the diencephalon bilaterally, for example, as a result of surgery (531) or of bilateral temporal encephalitis (505). Amnesia may also reflect pathology in the periaqueductal gray matter of the brain stem, mammillary bodies of the posterior hypothalamus, and dorsal medial nuclei of the thalamus (89). Lesions in these locations are characteristic of chronic alcoholic encephalopathy (Korsakoff's syndrome). Patients with anterograde amnesia can maintain items in short-term storage as long as they attend to them; then they forget them, apparently permanently. Skills and information learned weeks to months before the illness are retained intact. Such patients have normal IQs and often intact personalities, but they are disoriented and in need of constant supervision. Some of these patients are inordinately suggestible and can be induced to recount fictitious and highly improbable events to fill in the void of their recent past *(confabulation)*. Anterograde amnesia may be a transient condition if the pathology responsible for its occurrence is transient, for example, if it is caused by a brief period of brain ischemia, or by brain swelling following trauma, or by an acute encephalopathy; loss of memory for items occurring during the period of amnesia is of course permanent. Amnesia is permanent in patients like chronic alcoholics or like H.M., whose damage is irreversible.

Milner and others restudied H.M. 14 years after the operation (419) and even more recently (287,417). They found that the patient had learned nothing since surgery and remembered nothing of intervening events. He thought the date was six months prior to his operation. Surprisingly, he was able to acquire a new visual-manual skill: Although he denied having ever practiced these tasks, he learned after multiple repetitions to trace a star while he looked at its reflection in a mirror, and to trace simple mazes, provided the sequence of lines did not exceed his immediate memory span. He failed to learn more complex mazes. Such observations indicate that bilateral hippocampectomy producing anterograde amnesia for verbal items, facial recognition, visual recognition, and the recall of every day events spares visual-motor learning. Perhaps the sparing ensues from the wide distribution of circuits concerned with motor programming (see Chapter 5), or perhaps, as Cohen and Squire (120) suggest, visual-motor learning belongs to a larger class of skills concerned with the acquisition of rules and procedures, which are spared in amnesia, as opposed to the information that results from the application of these procedures, which is lost.

The evidence cited thus far does not elucidate whether anterograde amnesia should be ascribed to deficient learning (deficient consolidation of memories) or to deficient retrieval (617). Deficient retrieval has been implicated for amnesia in patients with Korsakoff's syndrome (89), and in normal persons when they "forget" (83,86). Recent work in rats (583) and humans (287) may help to clarify this issue: Lesions in the mammillary bodies are reported to impair the formation of new memories without affecting retrieval, while bilateral lesions of the hippocampus may or may not impede the formation of new memories but hinder their retention over time. Evidence for the action of vasopressin on catecholamines also suggests that retention and retrieval may be separable processes (162).

CHILDREN WITH LEARNING DEFICITS

The preceding review of some aspects of the biology of memory and learning highlights the intimate relationships between attention and learning and between affective experience and learning. In young children, learning deficits that resulted from lesions in the mammillohippocampal system would be expected to produce devastating cognitive impairment (220). Perhaps limbic pathology accounts for the severe inability to learn of some autistic children (141,150). Less severe deficits of retention, retrieval, or recognition, especially for sequentially presented stimuli, are encountered in many children with scholastic problems. These deficits may be specific for either the visual or the acoustic-verbal modality (628). Since modality-specific learning deficits are reported in adults after left or right temporal lobectomy (418), it is tempting to suggest that such learning disabled children may have lateralized hemispheric dysfunction. Physiologic correlates of such deficits may become demonstrable through the use of sophisticated techniques such as spectral analysis of the EEG or of evoked responses while the children are engaged in well-defined learning tasks (174). Deficient storage of serial inputs in short-term memory seems to contribute to dyslexia in some children, while in others, anomia or deficient retrieval of verbal labels from long-term stores may be at fault (389).

It is clear that inefficient memory is not always responsible for "learning problems" or school failure. Registration or retrieval processes may not be intrinsically defective, but their inefficiency may be secondary to another problem. Some children's distractibility may preclude the focused attention requisite for learning. The child may be lacking adequate cognitive strategies for organizing new information in the efficient and semantically meaningful ways used by adults (88). He may have a language problem, a perceptual deficit, or he may lack the motivation to learn, not to mention the possibility that his environment may provide him with inadequate opportunity for learning. Often, a combination of factors is responsible for the child's lack of progress. Once again, the teacher who wants to help a particular child needs to have detailed information as to what it is that is keeping him from learning efficiently. There is no educational technique or drill that will meet the needs of all "learning disabled" children.

9

Disorders of Behavior and Affect

Behavior disorders often prompt parents to seek medical advice. Up until recently, environmental determinants of behavior have been emphasized, a trend that can be traced to the Freudian influence on psychiatric thinking. Of late, research in psychopharmacology and neurobiology has turned our attention to the neurologic underpinnings of mood and drive. Of course, environmental and organic theories of behavior should not be viewed as conflicting (180): Emotion is the subjective experience of activity in particular systems in the brain in response to cues arising both from organismic needs and from the effects of environmental stimuli. Drive is the tendency to modify behavior in order to re-establish a desired inner state in the face of internal or external change.

Since behavior is multidetermined, the physician who evaluates a child with so-called emotional problems must consider whether the particular behavioral symptom is a secondary reaction to parental mishandling or to social problems caused by a physical or learning handicap, or whether it is the direct consequence of brain dysfunction or has the characteristics of one of the psychoses. [Today, the psychoses are thought likely to reflect brain dysfunction, with particular biochemical correlates, that alters responses to endogenous or exogenous stimuli, rather than to be reactions to particularly unfavorable environmental circumstances (28,591,597).] In their early work on children with "brain damage", Strauss and his colleagues (564,565) recognized the organic roots of some of the children's abnormal behaviors. Nevertheless, a paradoxical situation persists even today because of the lack of fully validated and accepted diagnostic criteria: Children with identical behavioral aberrations may carry different diagnoses depending on the specialty of the physician their parents happen to consult. Advice for management will vary depending upon whether the child's primary deficit is considered to be brain damage, learning disability, language impairment, mental retardation, attention deficit, emotional disturbance, or autistic behavior. Of course, these diagnoses are not mutually exclusive. The need for better nosologic criteria is obvious.

NEUROLOGIC SUBSTRATES OF DRIVE AND EMOTION

Emotions are intrapersonal experiences associated with approach or avoidance behavior. They are closely interrelated to sensory processes, to the person's state

115

of arousal, and to previous cognitive experiences that enable one to recognize or perceive the nature and significance (value) of a particular stimulus. *Drive or motivation* describes the tendency to translate into action the plans or reactions elaborated in response to these internal and external cues and to their perceived value for the individual (477).

Thus, emotion and drive are strongly related to sensory-perceptual, memory, and arousal processes on the one hand, and to motor, autonomic, and endocrine effector processes on the other. They are at the core of behavior since they enable one to assign priorities to competing stimuli and action programs. This capability is obviously crucial to survival and, not surprisingly, arises from activity in phylogenetically old portions of the brain, the limbic system—especially the amygdala and the hypothalamus (228), areas which we just saw are also concerned with other processes crucial for survival like vigilance and memory. To reiterate what was said earlier, learning enhances fitness and is facilitated if items have clearly pleasureful or aversive consequences and if they promote arousal.

There are many lines of evidence indicating that cortical and subcortical limbic structures play a central role for emotional experience and motivational drive in animals and in man. These are (a) behavioral effects of focal brain lesions, (b) effects of cerebral stimulation, and (c) pharmacologic and neurochemical data combined with histofluorescence microscopy.

Behavioral Correlates of Focal Brain Lesions

Behavioral correlates of focal brain lesions are particularly clear in patients with frontal and temporal pathology. The *frontal lobes*, or more precisely, the prefrontal and orbital regions of the frontal lobes, are connected with the limbic system, neostriatum (basal ganglia), and thalamus, as well as with other areas of the neocortex. They participate in integrating the external and internal data upon which choices among possible actions rest and advanced planning is based (140,439,480). Patients who sustain large frontal lesions, especially bilateral ones, are likely to suffer marked changes in personality: They become passive and apathetic. They are characteristically unmindful of social niceties, boastful but ineffective, distractible, impulsive, perseverative, rigid, uncreative, and they have poor judgement (140,378,480). They are deficient for tasks requiring advance planning and withholding action in order to collect more information and to consider alternatives. These patients do not take into account possible consequences of their actions and do not experience anticipatory anxiety. Attempts have been made to exploit the changes in personality produced by frontal pathology by carrying out frontal lobotomies in chronically hospitalized severely agitated or violent psychotic patients and in patients with severe intractable anxiety or pain (303).

Although we have no definite evidence suggesting that children with attention deficit disorders suffer from frontal lobe dysfunction, or in fact from focal brain dysfunction of any kind, and although the vast majority of children with ADD are neither psychotic nor demented, many of them exhibit behavioral traits that are reminiscent of patients with frontal pathology. It is important to remember, in this context, that the posterior portion of the orbital surface of the frontal lobe is a part of the limbic system.

Patients with *temporal lobe* epilepsy have spurred much of our thinking about affective consequences of brain pathology in man. During the onset (aura) of temporal lobe seizures, patients often experience strong emotions that may be pleasurable (elation, joy, peace) or unpleasant (fear, sadness) (624). They may also experience olfactory and gustatory hallucinations resulting from the activation of limbic areas concerned with these senses. (Note that both taste and smell have strong affective and sexual connotations.) Autonomic symptoms such as flushing or pallor, an abnormal feeling in the pit of the stomach, or vomiting are common and reflect the activation of nearby hypothalamic structures. The patients are likely to have interictal personality problems as well (35): Those with a left-sided epileptic focus are often described as circumstantial, "sticky", and verbose, they may have a thought disorder, a flat affect, or be depressed; those with a right-sided focus tend to be emotionally labile, impulsive, or aggressive.

The amygdala, a large nuclear complex situated within the temporal lobe, is an important relay between olfactory pathways, limbic cortex, hypothalamus, and other limbic areas. The amygdala seems to provide the appropriate affective "bias" to environmental and endogenous stimuli and in so doing to play a role in behavior and in learning or resistance to extinction (228). Repeated stimulation of the amygdala is an effective means for creating chronic epileptic activity in the temporal lobe ("kindling") (471). The amygdala is often involved in temporal lobe seizures which may explain some of their features. Bilateral ablation of the amygdala produces profound changes in social behavior whose type depends on the particular species studied (Klüver-Bucy syndrome) (325). Monkeys seem not to recognize familiar objects and mouth them indiscriminately; they are abnormally tame and hypersexual. In man, bilateral medial amygdalotomy has calming effects in some uncontrollably hyperactive, aggressive brain damaged children (437).

Hemispheric lesions outside the frontal, temporal, and limbic regions may also influence emotional processes. Patients with *right-sided lesions* may be unable to interpret other persons' tone of voice, facial expression, or affect (404). As a result, they may be oblivious to the negative effects of some of their behaviors on others in their environment. They themselves may be inappropriately euphoric or indifferent to the seriousness of their neurologic handicap to the point of denying its existence (anosognosia) (269). Patients with *left-sided lesions*, especially those with an expressive aphasia, tend to be depressed and to experience catastrophic reactions to stress. Patients with fluent aphasia, on the other hand, are often expansive, perhaps because their perceptual and comprehension defects make them unaware of the severity of their deficit. Patients with bilateral subcortical lesions affecting the basal ganglia or frontopontine pathways *(pseudobulbar palsy)* often have a pathologically labile affect and laugh or cry inappropriately at the slightest provocation. These patients report that their inner feelings are dissociated from, and do not match, their uncontrolled emotional expression (593).

Finally, *decortication* in cats is well known to produce the phenomenon of sham rage, unprovoked and uncontrollable raging behavior that reflects disinhibition of hypothalamic and brain stem circuits that mediate aggressive behaviors. Whether temper tantrums in very young children and in some children with brain damage reflect immature or inadequate cortical inhibition of these subcortical limbic structures is plausible but no more than a guess. Uncontrolled aggression is an extremely rare, poorly documented, ictal manifestation of temporal lobe seizures (149,563). Although violent delinquent adolescents are said to be more prone to behaviors suggesting psychomotor epilepsy than less violent ones (470), this does not prove that they are, in fact, epileptic or that epileptics are particularly prone to aggression. Aggressiveness and violence are much more common in males than females, reflecting either direct effects of sex hormones on the brain, or the social consequences of being a male, or both (288). The boundary between temperament and psychopathology is indeed fuzzy.

Behavioral Effects of Electrical Stimulation

Hess (276) was the pioneer who discovered that stimulation of the septum and anterior hypothalamus in cats produces what he called restorative or trophotropic processes of a parasympathetic type such as eating, excretion, penile erection, lowering of blood pressure pulse and respiration, relaxation of muscle tone, decreased responsiveness to environmental stimuli, and even sleep. In contrast, stimulation of the posterior hypothalamus and upper brain stem produces ergotropic somatic and sympathetic responses characteristic of positive action such as the flight or fight reaction characterized by hyperalertness; pupillary dilatation; rise in blood pressure, pulse, and respiratory rates; desynchronization of the EEG; and general excitement of the animal. These effects are now known not only to reflect changes in the autonomic nervous system but also in the pattern of endocrine secretion, controlled by neurosecretory neurons in the hypothalamus.

Electrical stimulation studies have taken on new dimensions, thanks to the discovery by Olds (450,516) that animals will work in order to receive stimulation in certain brain areas. Areas where stimulation seems to be experienced by rats as pleasurable are largely coextensive with the median forebrain bundle of the lateral hypothalamus, a pathway linking the septum, hypothalamus, and mesencephalon. Stimulation need not elicit appetitive or sexual behavior to be rewarding. Other reward areas have been found much more recently in the periaqueductal gray regions of the brain stem which are rich in opiate receptors. The animals will self-stimulate themselves by pressing a bar to deliver shocks to these "reward" areas of their brain in preference to eating. Stimulation of the septal area and periaqueductal gray in man produces euphoria and enables some patients to tolerate the intractable pain of cancer without analgesics (262,283). In contrast, stimulation in some dorsolateral mesencephalic, thalamic, and posterior hypothalamic areas in rats produces avoidance behavior and responses that seem to indicate fear, pain, and rage. The rats seek to discontinue stimulation and will work to avoid it. Highly unpleasant subjective experiences have been reported in man following electrical stimulation in the amygdala and in diencephalic regions immediately adjacent to those producing pleasureful effects (532). They have not been delineated in detail for obvious ethical reasons.

Neurochemical and Neuropharmacologic Correlates of Affect

There has been an explosion of new information concerning the neurochemical basis of mood and emotion (28,363). At least three classes of natural substances are implicated:

1) Catecholaminergic, indolaminergic, cholinergic, and other *neurotransmitters*.

2) *Neuropeptides*, some of which also act as neurotransmitters or as neuromodulators in the brain. These include the enkephalins, hypothalamic-pituitary releasing and inhibiting factors, posterior pituitary hormones, and other peptides, including some released in the gastrointestinal tract and other viscera as well as in the brain (335).

3) *Hormones* such as the adrenal and sex steroids, anterior pituitary hormones, thyroid hormones, and others (Table 7).

All of these substances have been found in the brain although not all are synthesized there. Some of the neurotransmitters and neuropeptides appear to be synthesized in particular neurons and to exert their effects transsynaptically by altering the firing pattern of other neurons they innervate. Others, such as the thyroid and sex hormones, reach the brain from the periphery and act as neuromodulators by attaching to specific neuronal receptors and influencing the cell's activity directly, for example, these hormones alter brain growth and development (25,288,640). Highly specific binding sites for particular hormones, neurotransmitters, and neuropeptides have been demonstrated on the membrane or nucleus of given neurons. It is now clear that the brain affects behavior not only through neurogenic but also through humoral means, and that hormones, in turn, alter brain structure and function, and thus mood and emotion (148).

While systemic administration of a neurotransmitter, its precursor, or its antagonist will have widespread effects on the brain (provided it crosses the blood-brain barrier), it will have much more restricted effects when released by the stimulation of a discrete group of neurons that synthesize it. In other words, the same neurotransmitter has different effects at different sites, depending on which of the several pathways utilizing it is activated. While most neurons characteristically produce but one neurotransmitter, neurons often respond to several neurotransmitters, some of which may be excitatory, others inhibitory. While some neurotransmitters are predominantly excitatory or inhibitory, the effects of others may vary depending on dose and on the neurons upon which they exert their effect.

Much about the brain has been learned through the study of the behavioral, electrophysiologic, and neurochemical effects of drugs empirically found to affect behavior. The major tranquilizers and antipsychotic agents, and the antidepressant, antianxiety, and hallucinogenic drugs derive their influence on mood, drive, and

TABLE 7. Neurohumors[a]

Neurotransmitters	
1. Predominantly excitatory effects Acetylcholine Glutamate Aspartate Substance P Histamine (?)	2. Predominantly inhibitory effects Norepinephrine ⎫ Dopamine ⎬—Catecholamines (Epinephrine) ⎭ Serotonin (5HT) —Indolamine GABA Glycine (cord) Taurine

Neuropeptides	
1. Hypothalamic hypophysiotropic factors Thyrotropin releasing factor (TRF) Gonadotropin releasing hormone (LHRH) Somatostatin (growth hormone-release inhibitory factor) Others?	2. Neurohypophyseal hormones Vasopressin or antidiuretic hormone Oxytocin
3. Adenophypophyseal hormones Thyroid stimulating hormone (TSH) Follicle stimulating hormone (FSH) Luteinizing hormone (LH) Growth hormone ACTH (adrenocorticotropic hormone) Prolactin Melanocyte stimulating hormone (MSH)	4. Brain-gut hormones Cholescystokinin Gastrin Vasoactive intestinal peptide Insulin Glucagon Neurotensin Substance P Others
5. Opioid peptides Endorphins Enkephalins	6. Others Bradykinin Angiotensin Calcitonin Others

[a] A number of peripheral hormones (e.g., sex steroids, cortisol, thyroid hormone, and others) as well as other substances like prostaglandins are believed also to have direct effects on the central nervous system.

behavior from their effects on endogenous neurotransmitter systems (363,597). Various psychotropic drugs may alter neurotransmitter concentration in the brain (a) by competing for access to specific binding sites and blocking them, (b) by mimicking the effects of neurotransmitters, (c) by retarding the degradation of one or more neurotransmitters, (d) by inhibiting their reuptake from the synaptic cleft into presynaptic terminals and thus depleting them, or (e) by releasing them from synaptic terminals. Unraveling of these effects has led to a series of hypotheses, none of which has been substantiated as yet, concerning the pathogenesis of the major psychoses (28,363). It is now believed that alterations in the balance between neurotransmitters, rather than changes in the concentration of a single neurotransmitter, are responsible for particular symptoms (16). Since alteration in one neurotransmitter system produces compensatory changes in others, deciding which change produced by a drug or found in a patient is primary and which is secondary becomes exceedingly difficult. This caveat should alert the reader to the fact that innumerable oversimplistic hypotheses about the neurochemical basis of particular drug effects and behavioral aberrations, for example, hyperkinetic behavior, have been offered. They need to be looked at critically since many are wrong or await further confirmation.

Several techniques have advanced our knowledge of the neural substrates of mood and drive. These include:

(a) Histofluorescence microscopy (185). This method makes it possible to identify neurons that contain a particular neurotransmitter, for example, dopamine, norepinephrine, or serotonin, and to study the distribution of their processes to other brain areas.

(b) Immunocytochemical methods that enable one to visualize the binding of specific antibodies to peptides and other candidate neurotransmitters attached to the surface of individual neuron membranes. This method has extended fluorescence microscopy to many hormones and peptides and to some of the enzymes that control their metabolism (204,281).

(c) Chronic electrical stimulation (sometimes coupled with local drug administration) through indwelling electrodes or cannulas in alert animals whose behavior and EEG can be recorded over extended periods.

(d) Microiontophoretic injections of drugs, hormones, or neurotransmitters with micropipettes into neurons later identified histologically, that enable studies of discrete electrophysiologic, and sometimes behavioral effects.

(e) Microchemical methods to measure minute amounts of neurotransmitters, neuropeptides, hormones, or their metabolites in tissues or body fluids.

EFFECTS OF VARIOUS NEUROTRANSMITTERS AND MODULATORS ON BEHAVIOR

Catecholamines

Areas where electrical stimulation produces rewarding effects tend to be those that are rich in the catecholamines *dopamine* and *norepinephrine*. This is but one line of evidence suggesting that these neurotransmitters play a direct role in the control of mood and affect. Antidepressants like the monamine oxidase inhibitors and tricyclic drugs block the degradation or reuptake of catecholamines, thus increasing their availability. Stimulant drugs like amphetamine release catecholamines and retard their inactivation. Both antidepressants and amphetamine facilitate electrical self-stimulation and reproduce some of its effects. In small doses, amphetamine has alerting and mood elevating effects, but in overdose, it precipitates pathologic behaviors such as motor stereotypies and paranoid ideation, thus mimicking some of the symptoms of the naturally occurring psychoses. The potency of antischizophrenic drugs can be predicted by how strongly they block dopamine receptors and attenuate shock-avoidance behavior, as well as by their effects on prolactin secretion which is under dopaminergic-hypothalamic control. These observations, and better understanding of how the major tranquilizers and antidepressants exert their effects on the brain, have led to speculation, without direct evidence as yet, that the major psychoses, schizophrenia and manic-depressive psychosis, may be the result of disorders of catecholamine (or serotonin) metabolism (28,363,500,530,549): Mania is said to be associated with increased levels of norepinephrine, and the depression that follows it with its decrease, while a popular theory of schizophrenia attributes symptoms to a relative excess of dopamine in critical neuronal circuits.

If rewarding effects are produced by stimulation in some areas rich in catecholamines, they are also produced by stimulating areas rich in opiate (enkephalin) receptors. It is obvious that morphine's effects are not limited to the relief of pain, but owe much to its euphoriant qualities. These characteristics, along with morphine's addictive properties, may be mediated by its effects on central noradrenergic pathways, in particular the locus coeruleus (550). Even in the absence of drugs, euphoria and increased tolerance for pain go together, while depression often accompanies chronic pain. The opiates appear to exert their effects by mimicking those of the endorphins and enkephalins, neuropeptides that also may act as neurotransmitters (606). Moreover, it has been suggested that the endorphins play a role in the pathogenesis of schizophrenia, although this is still a controversial issue (62,514).

Stein (559) proposes that incentive or motivation may be mediated by the action of dopamine in initiating and facilitating pursuit behavior. He also suggests that learning (consolidation of memories) or reinforcement is influenced by norepinephrine and its effects on frontal systems serving to guide response selection via a knowledge of the consequences of the response. Finally, he believes that enkephalin mediates gratification or drive reduction after reward has been experienced, bringing the behavioral episode to a satisfying termination. In short, there is much to suggest that the catecholamines and endorphins may act in concert in mediating pleasurable aspects of experience.

Serotonin, Acetylcholine, and GABA

Areas where stimulation produces aversive effects have not been as clearly related to particular transmitter systems as those mediating rewards, although both acetylcholine and serotonin have been implicated.

Serotonin (5-hydroxytryptamine) is a monoamine whose highest concentration occurs in midline nuclei of the brain stem called the raphé nuclei. Serotonergic neurons project widely to the thalamus, basal ganglia, hippocampus and other limbic areas, and to the neocortex. Important descending serotonergic pathways innervate motor neurons in the spinal cord (28). Serotonin has effects not only on mood but on vigilance, and is responsible for the maintenance of slow-wave sleep (152,304). The major metabolite of serotonin, hydroxyindole acetic acid (5-HIAA) is reported to be decreased in the cerebrospinal fluid (CSF) of about one-third of depressed patients, suggesting that aberrant serotonin metabolism may be relevant to the pathogenesis of depressive symptoms in a particular subgroup of depressed patients.

Since norepinephrine depletion has also been implicated in some forms of depression, and since many of the drugs effective against depression like lithium, the tricyclic antidepressants, and others affect serotonin as well as catecholamine metabolism, it is likely that altered balance between neurotransmitter systems rather than effects on single neurotransmitters needs to be considered. A variety of endocrine changes occur in depression but these are generally considered not to be primary effects (93,354), although the occurrence of depression in menopausal and postpartum women implicates decreased sex steroid levels as one of the potential triggers for depression. Depression is not recognized as often in children as in adults but is probably more prevalent than generally realized (139). Very little is known about its neurochemical basis.

Many potent hallucinogens like lysergic acid diethylamide (LSD) and psilocin resemble serotonin chemically. Their effects have been attributed to suppression of the predominantly inhibitory serotonergic system. Both serotonin depletion and endogenous hallucinogens acting as false neuroregulators have been implicated, without definitive evidence, as a potential cause for the hallucinations of schizophrenic patients (28). Dreaming occurs while the activity of the serotonergic raphé nucleus is inhibited (152,304). Decreased levels of serotonin have been reported in the serum of patients with Down's syndrome and in some with autistic behavior (367), but again, the relevance of these findings to children's behavior is not clear.

The wide distribution of cholinergic synapses in the brain explains the complexity of the effects of *acetylcholine* on motor and sensory processes, learning, and other elaborate behaviors (307,606). Cholinergic pathways in the brain stem reticular formation contribute to the mediation of arousal and, indirectly, by the stimulating effect of acetylcholine on the noradrenergic locus coeruleus of the pons, to the control of paradoxical sleep and dreaming (152,304,397). Acetylcholine also affects the serotonergic raphé nuclei and the periaqueductal enkephalin receptors. In the hypothalamus, it is involved in regulating food and water intake and body temperature, and in controlling the secretion of antidiuretic hormone (vasopressin) and corticotropin (ACTH) releasing factor (CRF). (The identity of CRF remains elusive after 20 years of research.) As we discussed earlier, acetylcholine appears to play a crucial role in learning, presumably through cholinergic pathways to the cortex and limbic system (145,168). Cholinergic blockade impairs the ability to attend selectively to "relevant" stimuli (606). The role of acetylcholine in activating the "punishment system" and in alerting the cortex is another facet of its influence on learning. In rats, it is implicated in some forms of aggression (606). Acetylcholine affects motor control because of its excitatory activity, not only at the neuromuscular junction but also in the basal ganglia and sensorimotor cortex. The modulation of cholinergic pathways at various levels by inhibitory dopaminergic, serotonergic, and other neurotransmitters is complex and not fully understood at this time.

Anxiety, classically associated with adrenergic hypersecretion, appears to respond selectively to the benzodiazepines, a class of drugs that have recently been shown to bind to specific receptors in the brain (573). The drugs interact with receptors for one of the major inhibitory neurotransmitters, *GABA* (gamma aminobutyric acid), to enhance its effects. GABA is widely distributed in the cortex, basal ganglia, cerebellum, spinal cord, and elsewhere in the brain. GABA deficiency in the basal ganglia (striatum) is thought to be involved in the genesis of chorea. The sedative, anticonvulsant, and muscle relaxant properties of the benzodiazepines may be mediated through their activation of the GABA system. The barbiturates may also exert some of their effects by enhancing the inhibitory synaptic activity of GABA (363). The relationship of GABA to other neurotransmitters in the control of mood and vigilance is actively being investigated.

This brief discussion by no means exhausts the list of neurotransmitters that affect behavior. Histamine and numerous other amines and peptides like vasopressin and substance P also seem to act as neurotransmitters or neuromodulators, but their effects on mood and goal directed behavior requires further study (28,335).

Hormones and Peptides

That peripheral hormones like thyroid hormone, cortisol, and the sex hormones influence behavior is well known (93,334,534). The exciting new development of the last decade is that the effects of peripheral hormones have been shown to extend beyond their well-known inhibitory feedback loops to the pituitary and hypothalamus. In fact, it now seems likely that all hormones have nonendocrine functions and influence the activity of extrahypothalamic sites in the brain, and thus behavior, directly.

The secretion of hormones by the anterior pituitary is regulated by neurosecretory peptides produced in hypothalamic neurons (335). The limbic-hypothalamic system thus integrates three major homeostatic systems: behavior, the endocrine system, and the autonomic nervous system. These brain systems exert their effects through classic neurotransmitters as well as through a host of peptides that have been discovered in discrete sites not only in the hypothalamus but in other limbic areas and elsewhere in the brain and spinal cord. Some of these peptides, like gastrin, cholecystokinin, and glucagon, were well known for being secreted by endocrine cells in the gastrointestinal tract, pancreas, and other viscera belonging to the so-called amine precursor uptake and decarboxylation (APUD) system. Some of these peripheral endocrine cells, significantly, have a neural origin since they derive from the embryonic neural crest. The peptides have direct effects on the viscera as well as seeming to act as central neurotransmitter or neuromodulator agents (551). Some, like angiotensin II that subserves drinking, control complex motivated behaviors, whatever the particular acts required to achieve the behavioral goal and reduce the drive.

Some hypothalamic peptides like thyrotropin-releasing factor (TRF) and luteinizing-hormone releasing factor (LRF or LHRH) affect behavior both directly and indirectly: indirectly by stimulating the release of peripheral hormones via their control of the anterior pituitary, directly by acting as neurotransmitters themselves or by modulating the release of a variety of neurotransmitters in limbic and extrahypothalamic sites. For example, TRF antagonizes the sedation produced by barbiturates and other sedatives; it appears to exert this effect by interacting with GABA and acetylcholine (474). Since the action of many peptides is slower and more prolonged than that of neurotransmitters, they may provide sustained modulating effects on entire neuronal networks.

The endorphins and enkephalins, endogenous neuropeptides with opiate-like activities, seem to be derived from the same parent molecule, beta-lipotropin, as the anterior pituitary hormones ACTH, melanocyte stimulating hormone, and others (248,335). As pointed out earlier, they interact with neurotransmitters, and may act as neurotransmitters themselves since they bind to specific "opiate" receptors.

The picture that emerges concerning the role of particular hormones, peptides and neurotransmitters in the control of behavior is complex and admittedly confusing at this time. Where isolated endocrine changes had been thought to be correlated with particular behaviors—for instance increased levels of cortisol with both physical and emotional stress—more recent evidence indicates that stress also affects the secretion of thyroid stimulating hormone, prolactin, growth hormone, vasopressin, luteinizing hormone, and testosterone (534). Endocrine changes associated with depression include decreases in the secretion of growth hormone and prolactin, as well as a blunted response to thyroid releasing factor. Decreased levels of estrogen and progesterone are significantly associated with depression in some women and may help explain the occurrence of depression in the postpartum period and premenstrually; obviously, this hormonal change cannot be invoked in depressed males. Attempts are being made to correlate particular neurotransmitter alterations and particular endocrine changes with particular clinical types of depression such as manic-depressive psychosis, unipolar depression, and agitated depression. Once again, depression is a symptom and not a disease so that heterogeneity in its chemical concomitants is hardly surprising.

It was mentioned earlier that hormones affect brain development as well as behavior (177). This is well known for thyroid hormone where thyroid deficiency starting *in utero* may be responsible for cognitive incompetence (cretinism) in later life (25). The levels of sex steroids to which a fetus is exposed during certain critical periods of gestation may have profound effects not only on sexual behavior in later life but on the organization of the brain (288). In the immature rat, estrogen receptors are found in some areas of the neocortex as well as in the hypothalamus, but the cortical receptors disappear with maturation. Sex steroids affecting the fetus may thus account, in part, for differences in cognitive style and personality between males and females and, perhaps, for some of the differences in the effects of brain dysfunction in each of the sexes (640).

RELEVANCE TO CHILDREN'S BEHAVIOR

The foregoing considerations and the earlier discussions of learning and arousal mechanisms should have made it abundantly clear that endogenous factors in the brain are inextricably interwoven with the consequences of environmental events that impinge upon the individual's life and alter the structure, chemistry, and physiologic state of his brain. The importance of the environment, as contrasted to built-in genetic programs, in forming the personality increases with maturation and with time, yet biologic determinants exert their effects throughout life. Hormones, peptides, and neurotransmitters interact to regulate cyclic physiologic functions such as sleep and wakefulness, to influence complex behaviors like eating, sexual activity, fighting, fleeing, and learning. They also influence the individual's response to the episodic stimuli he experiences which in turn depend on the particular circumstances of the moment. *Mood* seems to represent the background affective set resulting from the sum of these effects, *motivation*, the individual's drive to alter his circumstances, and *emotion* his private experience of his inner state as it varies as a result of these internal and external events (477).

Our knowledge is too scanty at this time to enable us to go beyond educated guesses as to the cerebral underpinnings of the aberrant behaviors we observe in some, but by no means all, children with brain damage or dysfunction. We frequently have difficulty untangling the role of innate traits as an explanation for a child's behavior from the impact of the child's behavior on the family, which in turn will influence the family's behavior toward the child (582). We may also have trouble deciding whether a child's behavior is pathological or simply offensive. We can make the general statement that grossly aberrant behaviors probably reflect the disorder of some cerebral system(s), without necessarily being able to pinpoint the particular pathway or neurohumor responsible. There are cases where we can do so: Lesions of the hypothalamus such as tumors may have prominent signs of endocrine and autonomic dysfunction, sleep disturbances, and a characteristic mood elevation (472); somewhat similar clinical symptoms without a neoplasm are typical of adolescents with anorexia nervosa (374). Since the pathways and neurohumors whose alterations produce behavioral effects are discrete, it is no surprise that brain dysfunction that spares them will not alter mood or behavior. Until our knowledge is much more extensive, our therapies remain limited either to the empirical administration of drugs that might have beneficial effects—but often do not in the individual child—or to environmental manipulations that, hopefully, will enhance learning and reduce misbehavior.

Environmental manipulation might take the form of teaching the child better methods to cope with his environment by circumventing handicaps or avoiding maladaptive behaviors; it might mean fulfilling unmet drives for affection or bolstering feelings of mastery or self-esteem; it might mean reducing anxiety or providing opportunities to vent unexpended anger and frustration. Short of drugs, surgery, or electrical stimulation of the brain, our only tools for altering the brain's chemistry, function, and perhaps, its structure, are to modify a child's experience by altering the circumstances of his life.

The behavior disorders that are encountered most frequently in children with brain dysfunction include deficient attention with or without hyperkinetic behavior, discussed earlier (171,524,618), which is often associated with a labile affect, aggressiveness, temper tantrums, anxiety, and unpredictable mood swings. These behaviors may reflect inadequate or immature inhibitory systems, perhaps associated with a deficit in dopamine metabolism (536,620). On the contrary, the child may show apathy, withdrawal, lack of initiative and of curiosity, suggesting deficient arousal, or, perhaps, frontal lobe dysfunction. Depression may be more common in children than is usually appreciated (139). In some, it may have endogenous roots rather than being the child's understandable reaction to his awareness of the limitations caused by his handicap.

Infantile Autism

The most serious disturbance of emotion occurring in preschool children, especially boys, is without doubt *infantile autism*. Autism is not nearly as rare as the literature would have us believe. Its definition in DSM III (171) specifies that the onset of the illness must occur before 30 months of age. While autistic behavior may already be discernible in infancy, when it is characterized by poor response to mothering and an impoverished behavioral repertoire with stereotyped movements, other parents report that their child caused them no concern until sometime in the second year when developmental progress ceased and behavior and language regressed, without the loss of motor milestones. The fact that this regression often coincided with the birth of a younger sibling has been interpreted by some investigators as evidence that infantile autism is an environmentally determined emotional problem caused by the loss of the parents' undivided love and attention. It seems more likely that, accidentally, this age of onset corresponds to the very common 18- to 30-month time-lapse between the birth of siblings. The current view is that autistic behavior stems from the interaction between a core of behavioral traits arising as a consequence of organic brain dysfunction and each child's social circumstances and temperament. The neurologic basis for autism is not understood (367). The type and severity of the child's symptoms are thought to vary with the extent of brain dysfunction, but they also depend on whether the child is developing in a favorable or unfavorable environment. The etiology of the brain dysfunction varies (see later). In some children, the evidence for cerebral dysfunction may be limited to affective, linguistic, and cognitive deficiencies, while other autistic children show frank evidence of brain damage and some develop seizures (153).

The behavioral signs of autism include a flattened affect with profoundly impaired interpersonal relationships, failure to react normally to pleasurable and painful experiences, rigidity and resistance to change, stereotyped behaviors, and in some children self-mutilation such as head banging or biting. One might ascribe these signs to a severe disorder in limbic reward pathways, catecholamines, endogenous opiate systems, or all three. Autistic children also have signs of neocortical dysfunction. They regularly have a profound communication disorder, discussed in Chapter 10, and cognitive disabilities that are typically less severe for visual-spatial than for acoustic-verbal tasks. As a result, testable autistic children typically have lower verbal than performance IQ scores. Rutter (522) indicates that, at least by school age, the IQ is a good predictor of outcome, and many authors have pointed out that the development of speech, even if echolalic at first, is also an encouraging prognostic sign.

Higher functioning autistic children usually do not have typical signs of brain damage and a few have autistic siblings, indicating the likelihood that genetic factors are involved in some cases. The relationship of autism to the psychoses of later life, in particular schizophrenia, is unknown, although there does not appear to be a higher incidence of adult schizophrenia in the families of autistic children than in the population at large. The two conditions may be etiologically unrelated yet share some common pathogenetic mechanisms since they have some behavioral symptoms in common and since patients in both groups tend to get worse with the administration of amphetamine and methylphenidate (91).

The fragmentary evidence collected thus far does not provide a basis for a coherent hypothesis concerning the cause of autism. The children's usual lack of improvement in response to a variety of psychotropic drugs and environmental manipulations provides no additional clues. It seems quite clear that autism is not the result of a single etiology since tuberous sclerosis (239), hydrocephalus, infantile spasms (hypsarrhythmia) (571), phenylketonuria, congenital blindness caused by retrolental fibroplasia in premature infants (104), congenital deafness due to rubella (107) and to other causes (487), and a variety of brain insults can produce autistic behavior. Some have suggested that in children with the typical story of regression, autism may be the result of an undiagnosed smoldering brain infection of a "slow virus" type that runs its course and leaves the child devastated (250). This is an attractive hypothesis for children with a history of a subacute regression but it is not supported by data at this point. Autistic behavior is likely to be the common expression of a variety of brain dysfunctions, lesions, and maldevelopments that happen to implicate common neurologic targets (141,142,150,260,367). A variety of abnormalities of biogenic amines and other chemical alterations with unknown implications have been reported in autistic children (121,367). While it is possible that a single biochemical abnormality may be responsible for all the signs of autism in some children, in the majority multifocal or multisystem dysfunction appears more plausible (see Chapter 10).

Autism seems to be rarely, if ever, a reaction to purely environmental circumstances, with the possible exception of profound sensory and affective deprivation occurring in early infancy in susceptible children. Yet there is no doubt that environmental manipulation can mitigate some of the child's behavioral aberrations and an unfavorable environment can aggravate his symptoms. This is another example of the complex interaction between environment and the brain in the genesis of behavior (605). Awareness of this complexity should caution physicians not to accept oversimplistic pathophysiologic speculations concerning autism and not to espouse unproven therapies advertised on the basis of flimsy or inaccurate evidence.

There are a number of preschool children who do not fit all the criteria for infantile autism, either because the onset of their illness occurred after 30 months, or because their symptoms are less severe, yet who clearly have thought, affective, and behavior disorders bordering on, or frankly amounting to, a psychosis. Since only behavioral criteria are available for making such a diagnosis, the DSM III (171) has used the expedient of classifying such children under the single noncommittal label, *childhood onset pervasive developmental disorder*. This label embraces conditions we used to call disintegrative psychosis, symbiotic psychosis, early childhood schizophrenia, atypical child, and others. The vagueness of the present label is no doubt deliberate since it was felt unwise to formulate a tight nosologic classification of disorders whose pathogenesis we do not understand and for which we lack firm diagnostic criteria. Some of the children bear strong resemblances to children with infantile autism, and some have a language disorder affecting semantic and pragmatic processing (see Chapter 10). Again, it would appear quite likely that most, if not all of these children, like autistic children, are suffering from a variety of brain dysfunctions that we have yet to define.

10

Disorders of Oral and Written Language

It was pointed out in Chapter 2 that the two cerebral hemispheres are not symmetrical anatomically or functionally, and that the left hemisphere is specialized for language processing in virtually all right-handed persons, and in the majority of left-handed persons (164,165,206,214,216,223,318,418,431,554,602,639). Although this asymmetry is presumably under genetic control and is anatomically discernible long before birth (602), both hemispheres must be capable of sustaining language in early life since there is little if any difference in the language development of children with right and left infantile hemiplegias (15). If such children undergo hemispherectomy at a later age in order to control intractable seizures or severe behavioral disorders, their language is spared whether the damaged hemisphere removed is the right or the left (31). This indicates that if the left hemisphere suffers an extensive injury in early life the right hemisphere is capable of sustaining language (418,496). Such is not the case in adults: Left-sided hemispherectomy for malignant brain tumor in a right-handed man impaired language profoundly, as expected; nevertheless, the patient reacquired some expressive speech and his ability to comprehend language was better than that of some globally aphasic patients with left-sided strokes (85). These observations and those in split-brain patients suggest that both hemispheres have some ability to decode language, but that in most adults the left hemisphere alone has access to the effector pathways for the elaboration of oral speech, possibly because the left hemisphere inhibits the right hemisphere's control of these pathways (317,554).

It is possible to determine which hemisphere is dominant for speech by the Wada test, the intracarotid injection of sodium amobarbital (Amytal®) (603). A contralateral hemiplegia will be produced with either right- or left-sided injection, while interference with language will occur only when the dominant side is injected. The previously discussed method of dichotic stimulation (52,291,329) and studies of cerebral blood flow in conscious patients while they speak, read, and write (343,346) are less invasive methods of assessing cerebral dominance for language.

ACQUIRED APHASIA

Acquired aphasia, impairment of previously normal language, can occur as early as 18 to 24 months of age following an acute lesion of the dominant side. In young children, recovery is often but not invariably rapid and complete (264,645,646). Studies in adult patients who underwent left cortical ablation for the control of seizures following early brain lesions showed that dominance for language had shifted to the right in those patients whose lesions occupied left perisylvian areas, while it had not shifted in patients with lesions outside of the main language area (418,496). A long-standing or congenital lesion such as a low grade glioma or an unruptured arteriovenous anomaly that causes very chronic damage may produce more permanent language deficits than an acute lesion, perhaps because dominance for language is less likely to shift in such cases. In children older than approximately 8 to 12 years and in adults, shift in dominance for language is inefficient so that a massive lesion in the left perisylvian area will almost always result in a permanent language deficit of variable severity. As a group, left-handed and ambidextrous individuals are less likely than right-handed ones to become permanently aphasic following cerebral lesions, but they are more likely to have transient aphasia with right-sided lesions. They seem to have incomplete dominance for speech, that is, both their hemispheres participate in language operations to a greater extent than is the case in right-handed persons (267). As a group, females appear to be less strongly lateralized than males (258,640).

Despite general agreement that the central (frontal-temporal-parietal) region of the left hemisphere is concerned with language (Fig. 21), there is incomplete agreement about the nature and classification of aphasias. No doubt because of variability among individuals in the details of brain organization (449), there are no invariant boundaries of areas in the brain where lesions will produce a particular clinical picture. Overlapping lesions can result in predominantly expressive or predominantly receptive aphasias, although in general, frontal lesions tend to impair speech production and temporal ones its reception. Posterior temporoparietal lesions impair reading, writing, and the ability to calculate (81,215,218,271,378,604). The role for language of the supplementary area in the mesial frontal lobe, located rostrally to the motor cortex controlling leg movements, is not as clear. Cerebral blood flow studies suggest that it is activated during "automatic speech" such as repeating the days of the week or the months of the year (343). The involvement of this region in speech production was first discovered by Penfield and co-workers (459,460) during surgical procedures for the control of epilepsy. They were also among the first to draw attention to the strong connections between the main (posterior) language area of the cortex and the pulvinar of the thalamus (460). The role of the thalamus (82,188,447) and limbic system (503) for linguistic behavior has only recently begun to be appreciated.

Even in right-handed persons, the right hemisphere has some linguistic skills. These have been demonstrated most dramatically in patients who underwent section

S P E E C H   A R E A S

E V I D E N C E   F R O M   S T I M U L A T I O N

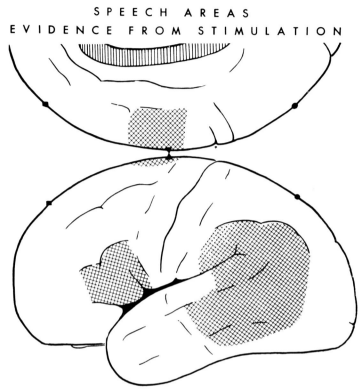

FIG. 21. Language areas of the dominant hemisphere where electrical stimulation of the cortex produces a transient aphasia. These observations were made in awake patients during the course of surgical procedures for the control of epilepsy and were required in order to avoid removing cortex that would result in permanent aphasia. The area located in the third frontal convolution is Broca's area, the larger posterior area encompasses Wernicke's area, the angular and supramarginal gyri, and adjacent temporal and parietal cortex, while the mesial frontal speech area is located just anterior to the leg area of the motor cortex. (Reproduced with permission from Penfield and Roberts, ref. 460.)

of the corpus callosum to control seizures: Words presented tachistoscopically to the right hemisphere can guide the left hand for picking out the correct object among several objects presented out of sight, even though the patient will deny vehemently that he has read anything. The patient is using his disconnected left hemisphere to speak, and the left has no knowledge of what the right is doing (164,165,214,216, 318,431,554) (Fig. 22). The right hemisphere is more efficient than the left for decoding ideograms, and in fact reads by using a whole word approach (652), while only the left hemisphere is capable of phonetic analysis and of generating acoustic-verbal images. These acoustic-verbal images provide the left hemisphere with a superior pathway of access into the lexicon (repository of word meanings) than the visual images accessible to the right hemisphere (355,652). In adults, speech produced under the control of the right hemisphere after an acute lesion to the left is

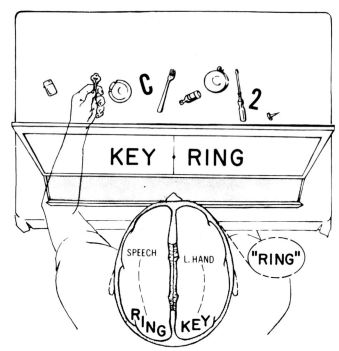

FIG. 22. Performance of split-brain patients. **A.** Each of two words, key and ring, are flashed on the left and right halves of a screen. The commissurotomized subject reports (through his left "speaking" hemisphere) having seen the word "ring." He denies having seen the word "key" and does not recognize that his left hand (hidden behind the screen and commanded by his right "mute" hemisphere) has correctly retrieved and is holding a key in response to the word flashed on the left of the screen. When asked what object he has selected with his left hand he responds "ring." (Reproduced with permission from Sperry, ref. 554.)

limited either to monosyllabic utterances—like the single word produced by Broca's famous patient (424), or to overlearned multisyllabic phrases, often with a highly emotional tone—like curses, or to singing the words of a well-known song. We do not know what mechanisms enable the right hemisphere of young children rendered aphasic by a left-sided lesion to sustain language. There is controversy over whether recovery reflects the reactivation of systems formerly inhibited by the dominant hemisphere or the development of new systems on the right (317,637).

In young children, recovery from acquired aphasia requiring a shift of cerebral dominance is accomplished at the expense of some cognitive ability. The children regain language, but their intellectual progress rarely returns to its premorbid level (8,645). It is as though language is now crowding the access to cortical use of other activities or, perhaps, as though language is permanently preempting previously uncommitted circuits available for temporary operations such as problem-solving or the learning of new skills (371). As a result, some children with right hemiplegia and normal language may have deficits for visual-spatial skills like block designs which ordinarily would suggest right hemispheric pathology.

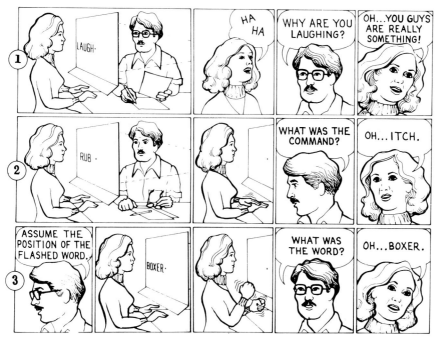

FIG. 22 B. When a series of commands was presented to the left visual field (right hemisphere), of a commissurotomized patient, each evoked a response. Although the left hemisphere did not know what the command was, it attempted to account for the response. When the command was "laugh" or "rub," the left hemisphere instantly "filled in." When the response was less equivocal, the reason generated for the action was quite accurate, as with the word "boxer." (Reproduced with permission from LeDoux, Wilson, and Gazzaniga, ref. 348a.)

Types of Acquired Aphasia

When a brain lesion is sustained after language has developed, it may affect predominantly the ability to decode language ("receptive aphasia") or to encode language ("expressive aphasia") (81,215,218,264,271,378,604).

Receptive Aphasia (Wernicke's Aphasia)

In the adult, receptive or Wernicke's aphasia is usually a fluent aphasia; the patient continues to speak spontaneously even though he has difficulty understanding verbal symbols, regardless of whether they are presented through the auditory channel as speech or through the visual channel as written material. Patients with Wernicke's aphasia are deficient for the semantic (meaning) aspect of linguistic processing. Speech is abnormal, interspersed with jargon or neologisms, perhaps because the patient no longer is able to monitor what he says. Speech is often repetitious and stereotyped although intonation and nonverbal aspects of the communicative interaction, like taking turns to speak, may be well preserved. Geschwind (218) explains adults' retained fluency by the fact that the frontal speech area, through years of practice, does not require much input in order to continue to encode speech. In addition to interfering with comprehension, lesions of the temporoparietal language cortex of children decrease verbal output (8), presumably because speech is not overlearned in children and requires an input to be sustained.

Expressive Aphasia (Broca's Aphasia)

Frontal lesions interfere predominantly with the encoding of language into speech (expressive or Broca's aphasia). Patients may be dysarthric, they speak effortfully and agrammatically. Small words such as prepositions, articles, pronouns, and conjunctions are omitted so that speech takes on a telegraphic quality. It is the phonemic and syntactic aspects of linguistic processing that are most affected, while semantics and the communicative intent of language are largely preserved. Writing is usually interfered with as much as or more than oral speech, and often in much the same way.

Conduction Aphasia

The inability to repeat, conduction aphasia, is typical of patients with subcortical pathology affecting fibers joining the posterior and anterior speech areas (arcuate fasciculus) (218). They typically make many paraphasic errors.

Amnestic Aphasia or Anomia

Amnestic aphasia or anomia, difficulty retrieving the verbal label associated with the visual percept elicited by looking at an object, suggests a posterior temporo-parietal (angular gyrus) lesion. Anomia can also occur with lesions situated else-where in the left hemisphere, including Broca's area, presumably because there are many ways to gain access to the lexicon since words are cross-filed. It is therefore necessary to specify the task precisely (e.g., naming to visual confrontation, or to touch, or when given a verbal cue such as the word's first letter, or providing a missing word in context) in order to define the nature of an anomic patient's deficit (83,265).

Acquired Alexias and Agraphias

Disorders affecting visual language rather than acoustic language are sometimes explained by lesions disconnecting visual processing areas of the cortex from acous-tic and linguistic processing areas, and linguistic areas from premotor areas where the complex fine movements required for writing are programmed and where com-mands are fed to the hand area of the motor cortex (218,265). The importance of interhemispheric pathways for linguistic processing is highlighted by the syndrome of alexia without agraphia: such patients cannot read what they just wrote and cannot copy from a model (222,266). Alexia without agraphia or pure alexia occurs in patients with a left occipital lesion associated with a lesion in the splenium (posterior portion) of the corpus callosum. Verbal symbols seen with the intact right occipital lobe cannot be transmitted to the temporoparietal language area of the left hemisphere for decoding. This difficulty is specific for visually presented words (pure word blindness); hence the patient can write spontaneously or to dictation since under these conditions writing is under the control of auditory association areas concerned with phonetic processing. More common types of alexia, usually with agraphia, are not considered "pure" in that they are associated with an aphasia—and are therefore called dysphasic alexias by Hécaen and Kremin (266). Patients' reading and spelling errors are largely a function of the type of their aphasia.

DEVELOPMENT OF LANGUAGE

A few words about the development of language may be helpful before considering disorders of language acquisition (430). From birth, the infant can focus on certain visual targets and can discriminate among them (306). He soon learns to build meaningful visual percepts and becomes sensitive to recurrent features of his environment (224,468). Tiny infants are capable of discriminating acoustically subtle phonetic cues that provide meaningful linguistic contrasts, for example, the differences between stop consonants like *b* and *p* or *d* and *t* that differ by less than 50 msec in onset of voicing (179,429). These infants rapidly learn to discriminate among other sounds. Later they learn to associate meaningful visual percepts with discriminable auditory ones and to demonstrate this by pointing to objects on verbal command (430).

Language acquisition is not a passive operation based on imitation. The child will not start to repeat the syllables and words he hears until he has learned to segment individual speech sounds and minimum units of meaningful language from the continuous stream of sound that impinges on him. He will not start to produce verbal labels for objects until he can associate a particular, relatively invariant, sound pattern (morpheme) he has learned to reproduce with the visual representation of that environmental referent (object, person, activity) which has acquired visual permanence (293,467). Thus, an executive motor pattern (speech) becomes linked to auditory and visual receptive ones. Later, either the visual image or the auditory one, which have become partially equivalent, will elicit the articulation command pattern, even in the absence of the actual stimulus. As the child's ability to abstract develops, actions, relations, and attributes will be perceived and he will add verbs and adjectives to his vocabulary, and finally relational words such as prepositions and conjunctions (430).

The manner in which the infant acquires the grammar of his language, that is, the rules that govern the meaningful linking of words into sentences, is being studied intensively (63). Behaviorists have offered a model for language acquisition that stresses the reinforcement of correct word chains produced by the child and the extinction of ungrammatical ones which are often misunderstood or corrected by the adults around him. This model may account for some aspects of the perfecting of children's utterances but not for their development: Children's errors indicate that they utter what they know about the language, not what they hear (411). They learn to string words into sentences they have never heard according to the rules of grammar. What the infant is learning is a set of rules for generating basic sentences. He is helped in this task by the manner in which his caretakers simplify their own language to speak to him (430). The acquisition of many of these rules is essentially complete by age 4. It will take the child much longer to perfect his articulatory skills and to learn to produce highly complex sentences. The addition of new words to the vocabulary continues throughout life.

Lenneberg (350), Chomsky (110), and others stress that the brain must have innate, biologic characteristics that favor linguistic processing in order for language acquisition to proceed so smoothly and universally, despite the great complexity of all languages. Lenneberg (350) recorded the time table of language acquisition in children with trisomy 21 (Down's syndrome), and reported that while the tempo was slower, the stages of acquisition were essentially identical to those observed in normal children at a younger age. Improvement in basic language skills reaches an asymptote in adolescence in both normal and trisomic children, a time at which brain maturation is essentially complete. As a result, the language of persons with Down's syndrome and other causes for mental deficiency never equals the sophistication of the normal person's language. Virtual standstill in the acquisition of fundamentally new linguistic skills beyond adolescence may also explain why most adults learning a second language require explicit instruction and virtually never lose their foreign accent, in contrast to the ease and rapidity with which young children can become multilingual.

Language learning requires the availability of language models, since language is a socially derived system of arbitrary symbols people use to transmit information, a system that eventually comes to be used by the individual as a major vehicle for thought (135). The social interaction between child and caretaker has not been subjected to as much formal analysis as children's speech output. The child must learn to listen and take turns and to interpret and produce the signals, both visual (facial expression, gestures) and acoustic (tone of voice, prosody), that govern interpersonal communication (32,404). Failure in these interactional aspects of language learning which seem to depend on nondominant and limbic activities (503,513) may jeopardize language development. Typically they are defective in children whose developmental language disorder is complicated by autistic behavior (141,150,367).

The secondary verbal skills of reading and writing develop at a later date and require formal instruction, in contrast to oral language acquisition which proceeds apparently effortlessly, without special instruction, in every normal child who grows up among speaking persons. Reading and writing call for the child to learn to associate visual linguistic symbols with word-sounds and with the corresponding objects or pictures, and to develop the visuomanual skills necessary for their reproduction. The relationships between acoustic and visual language reception, and articulatory and manual language production, as well as the role of memory in learning these skills, are the subject of many recent studies (215,271,309,652).

Thus, language competence is based upon many complex operations and probably engages a significant portion of the brain's processing capacity, at least during its acquisition. In addition to the specialized perceptual, executive, and memory skills language requires, it is also dependent on more general aspects of brain function such as intelligence, the ability to focus and sustain attention, and the motivation to communicate.

There are relatively few tests of language development with well standardized norms outside of the verbal items of standard intelligence test batteries, such as the Wechsler Preschool and Primary Scale of Intelligence (WPPSI) (613), Stanford-Binet (576), and McCarthy Scales (398). Most language tests such as the Carrow Test for Auditory Comprehension of Language (94), the Peabody Picture Vocabulary Test (175), the Token Test (66,166), the Illinois Test of Psycholinguistic Abilities (322), and the Reynell Scales, developed in Britain and not yet used extensively in this country (502), do not come close to assessing the richness of a child's verbal skills. Recordings on audio, or even better, video tape of the child's language use in an informal play situation provide fruitful and more realistic data to supplement scores on formal tests (11).

DEVELOPMENTAL LANGUAGE DISORDERS (DYSPHASIAS)

Despite progress made in the study of language acquisition and of the disruptions of language resulting from acquired brain lesions, our understanding of language is far from complete. Our understanding of the disorders of language acquisition is even less adequate (376,377,489) in as much as children at the age of language acquisition are difficult to study. Many of the published investigations of children with developmental language disorders were carried out after the children had reached school age, in part because of the difficulty involved in studying toddlers. Parents frequently do not recognize language disorders in preschoolers since the limits of delayed but normal acquisition of language, and those of delay which presages deviancy, are not necessarily clear-cut (11).

The etiology of developmental language disorders varies among children and is unknown in most cases. In some children, dysphasia probably reflects perinatal damage to the brain, especially when the history reveals significant neonatal anoxia or hypotension or when there is other evidence for brain dysfunction such as dysarthria, late walking, or a convulsive disorder. In other children, language disorders, presumably reflecting inefficient brain development, may have a genetic etiology since other family members are reported to have spoken late or indistinctly for a long time, or to have been dyslexic. Inefficient cerebral development may, in some children, manifest itself by lack of the usual pattern of a wider posterior hemisphere on the left than on the right (277).

A number of attempts have been made to define *the* pathogenesis of developmental language disorders. Some of these are reviewed in recent publications on developmental dysphasia (181,376,377,648). From the viewpoint of a clinician who is impressed with the diversity among children classified as being developmentally language disordered (6,292), and who has an even superficial experience with adult aphasia, it seems highly improbable that there is either a single etiology or a single pathogenesis for developmental language disorders.

Problems of Definition and Classification

There is no accepted definition of what constitutes a developmental language disorder (dysphasia) (376,489). Some definitions are essentially diagnoses by exclusion: According to many workers, a child has a language disorder if his verbal expression and/or his comprehension of language are judged deficient, provided this cannot be accounted for on the basis of hearing loss, motor deficit, mental retardation, gross brain damage, emotional disorder, or inadequate exposure to language. The vagueness of many of the terms in this clinical definition is only too obvious. Other definitions state that there is a language disorder when a child's verbal skills are 2 years below norms or at a level 50% below expectation. Such definitions are imprecise since by such criteria severity would vary depending on chronological age. Still another definition is that a child has a language deficit if his verbal IQ score is 20 or more points lower than his performance IQ score. This definition has the advantage of recognizing that a child may have a lowered IQ and have a language disorder as well, but it has other weaknesses:

a) It is not applicable to very young children since psychologic tests at that age do not provide legitimate IQ measures, that is, they correlate rather poorly with later IQ measures.

b) It is restrictive, since the language items on intelligence tests were not designed to study language itself but the efficiency of problem solving based on language use.

c) It says little or nothing about what aspects of linguistic performance might be deficient.

Having no satisfactory definition of developmental language disorders, it is not surprising that there is also no agreed upon classification for them. The most widely accepted classification derives from differentiating (a) disorders that affect expression alone or, more often, predominantly (192,402), from (b) those that affect reception primarily and expression as a corollary of defective reception.

This classification resembles the classification of adult aphasia. It satisfies the neurologist who views language as a system in which input operations must necessarily precede processing and in which speech output is the last link in a long chain (494). Deafness, auditory processing disorders, and verbal auditory agnosia (340,492,647) can be considered input disorders reflecting dysfunction in progressively more central relays in the auditory pathway, while phonologic programming disorders and dysarthria are their counterparts on the speech output side. Classification of "central" linguistic processing disorders is more difficult. There are children whose phonology and syntax are adequate but whose understanding of the meaning of linguistic messages is deficient despite apparently good nonverbal intelligence; children who can speak and have an adequate labeling vocabulary, but who neither ask questions nor understand them; and children with echolalia who parrot perfectly what they do not understand.

Attempts have been made to classify developmental language disorders according to linguistic rather than neurologic criteria. Within the context of disorders that affect production selectively, those that affect reception with production deficits as a consequence, and those that affect repetition, Aram and Nation (17) attempted to divide dysphasias into those that implicate *phonology* (the rules governing sounds used as linguistic symbols), *morphology and syntax* (the rules whereby words are modified and arranged into meaningful sentences), and *semantics* (the rules for attaching a meaning to individual words in the repository of word meanings or lexicon, and for extracting the idea or message in a sentence or longer utterance). Aram and Nation (17) used formal language tests and submitted the test results to factor analysis. They were able to isolate 6 syndromes among the 47 preschool children with developmental language disability they tested. These are summarized in Table 8A. At follow-up 5 years later, similar deficits persisted in some children, some had changed, and some had disappeared. Twenty of thirty children retested had persistant language or learning disability or both, while ten were functioning without problems and would be considered normal (642).

TABLE 8A. *Linguistic syndromes in children with developmental language disability: formal tests*[a, b]

Syndrome	Remarks
1. Generalized low performance	Comprehension and expression poor
2. Repetition strength	Comprehension impaired, parrot
3. Comprehension deficit	Expression and repetition fairly good
4. Phonologic comprehension-formulation-repetition deficit	Syntax clearly better than phonology
5. Nonspecific formulation-repetition deficit	Comprehension better than expression
6. Formulation-repetition deficit	Comprehension good

[a]On the basis of formal tests of comprehension, expression, and repetition.
[b]Adapted from data in Aram and Nation, ref. 17.

TABLE 8B. *Linguistic syndromes in children with developmental language disability: language use*[a,b]

Syndrome	Remarks
1. Verbal auditory agnosia (word deafness)	Mute and uncomprehending, can process visual language, behavior variable.
2. Semantic-pragmatic syndrome	Fluent, echolalic, anomic, impaired comprehension of discourse, often hyperverbal and tangential, behavior variable.
3. Mixed phonologic-syntactic syndrome	Nonfluent, comprehension better than expression, oromotor function variable.
4. Phonologic programming deficit syndrome (verbal apraxia)	Severe expressive disorder with adequate comprehension, oromotor function variable.
5a. Fluent autistic syndrome	Prosody, phonology, and comprehension variable; pragmatics severly impaired; echolalic.
5b. Nonfluent severe autistic syndrome	Virtually mute or severe phonologic deficit, severe comprehension deficit, nonlinguistic deficits usually severe.

[a]On the basis of communicative language use in parent-child interaction.
[b]Adapted from data in Rapin and Allen, refs. 489, 490.

If the assessment of verbal production is complex, the assessment of comprehension is more difficult still. It is easy to overestimate comprehension since language is highly redundant and since there are many visual cues in an interaction that help comprehension. Mothers regularly report that their child "understands everything," when what the child understands is single words and the communicative context. To judge comprehension, the investigator must rely on what the child does as well as what he says. Inferring that a child does not comprehend because he fails to respond or produces a "wrong" response may be fallacious since lack of response has other possible causes such as unwillingness to cooperate, distraction, not to mention an ambiguous verbal command. When the child does respond adequately and one can infer comprehension, it becomes necessary to vary the complexity of what is said in order to assess the adequacy of comprehension. This is done systematically in such tests of comprehension as the Carrow (94) and Reynell Scales (502). The Token Test (66) provides nonredundant verbal commands that do not require a verbal output. A special version has been designed for children (166) but it is not applicable below age five since it presupposes a knowledge of concepts like big and small, square and circle, colors, and prepositions. It also requires a memory span for strings of up to five words. It is sensitive to subtle comprehension deficits in children with learning disability as well as in speaking children with earlier deviant language acquisition.

Formal tests do not enable one to assess the richness of a child's verbal repertoire. Recording a child's spontaneous speech on videotape as he plays with his parents allows not only a formal linguistic analysis of the child's production using such measures as mean length of utterances (MLU), the number of different words in his vocabulary, the complexity of his syntax, and the semantic focus of his utterances, it also provides the opportunity to evaluate the *pragmatic* aspects or use of language in its verbal and nonverbal context (11). One can study the child's spontaneous productions: Are they requests, commands, or comments? How do they relate to the child's current activity? Does the child initiate communication? Does he answer questions? What is his ability to name and to repeat? Analysis can take into account nonverbal as well as verbal responses, for example, head nods, pointing, or the carrying out of commands.

Rapin and Allen (11,489,490) are currently conducting a longitudinal study of this type in preschool children with language disorders. They have tentatively isolated and characterized five syndromes (Table 9), some of which appear to correspond fairly well to those described by Aram and Nation (17) (Tables 8A, 8B). These five clinical syndromes should be considered tentative. They still lack the strength that will be provided by (a) systematic linguistic analyses of children's utterances, (b) neuropsychologic investigations that may illuminate pathogenetic mechanisms responsible for the children's symptoms and that may provide stronger diagnostic criteria for nosologic classification, and (c) electrophysiologic studies (23,173) that may enable one to differentiate patterns of cortical activity in normal and in incompetent speakers. This list of syndromes may not be exhaustive, for example, it does not include disorders of speech such as stuttering, an extremely

TABLE 9. Speech comprehension and production across dysphasic syndromes[b]

Syndrome	Phonology		Syntax		Semantics		Pragmatics	Fluency
	Comprehension	Production	Comprehension	Production	Comprehension	Production		
1. Verbal auditory agnosia	↓[a]	↓	↓	↓	↓	↓	N	↓
2. Semantic-pragmatic	±[a]	N	↓	N	↓	±	↓	↔[a]
3. Mixed phonologic-syntactic	±	↓	±	↓	±	N	N	↓
4. Phonologic programming deficit	N[a]	↓	N	±	N	N	N	±
5a. Fluent autistic	N	N	↓	N	↓	↓	↓	↔
5b. Dysfluent autistic	↓	↓	↓	↓	↓	↓	↓	↔

[a]N = normal; ↓ = abnormal or decreased; ± = variable; ↑ = increased.
[b]Adapted from data in Rapin and Allen, refs. 489,490.

common syndrome whose pathogenesis remains controversial. Because of variability of symptoms within syndromes, it may be necessary to break down some of the relatively common syndromes into subsyndromes.

Syndromes Among Dysphasic Children

Verbal Auditory Agnosia

The core symptom of verbal auditory agnosia (word deafness) is thought to be inability to decode phonology (203,414). Since phonologic decoding is the necessary first step for language comprehension (359), this deficit produces a devastating language disorder. The children understand little or nothing of what is said to them. As a result they are mute or their few utterances show gross phonologic distortions and misarticulations. Their syntax is rudimentary or nonexistent, that is, they speak in single words. A characteristic feature of some children with this syndrome is that they are eager to communicate, they may develop a gesture language, they can read facial expression, and they may be able to engage in such tasks as drawing (492). They play appropriately with toys, indicating that they understand their symbolic value. Many of these children develop severe behavior problems, either tantrums or withdrawal. This is especially likely to happen if the severity of their comprehension deficit is underestimated. They are rarely frankly autistic, however. These children characteristically have a spuriously low IQ if tested verbally or with instruments like the Stanford-Binet (576) that are linguistically loaded, while their scores on nonverbal tests like the Raven Matrices (497), Leiter (349), or the Performance Scale of the Wechsler batteries (612,613) may be average or near average. They profit greatly if they are educated as though they were deaf through the use of Total Communication (manual signs used simultaneously with speech). Some may learn to read and to do arithmetic computations at a time when their oral speech is still very poor. Nevertheless, their scholastic skills are usually defective as long as their linguistic skills remain grossly impaired. The outlook for these children is variable and depends on the nature and extent of their underlying pathology and on the appropriateness of the method used to educate them.

This syndrome has been identified most frequently in preschool children who, like many autistic children, lose their previously acquired verbal skills. Language deterioration often, but by no means always, occurs in the context of a convulsive disorder (341,492). The seizures may be typical complex partial absences or they may be generalized or focal motor seizures. The EEG usually shows bilateral atypical spike-and-wave activity. One child who presumably suffered from this syndrome was found at postmortem examination to have bilateral porencephalies affecting auditory and auditory association cortex of both temporal lobes (340). Another child who underwent a cortical biopsy had a chronic encephalitis (372). The outlook in 9 of these children followed into adult life (382) was surprisingly favorable, with subsidence of the seizures, improvement of the EEG, and the acquisition of serviceable speech in all; one patient had a mild persistent language disability and 4 had a moderate disability. This relatively favorable outcome is by no means universal. Correlation between seizure control or an improved EEG and improved language skills is lacking in many children. Some children never have seizures, some have normal EEGs, and in some cases the syndrome is developmental rather than acquired.

The pathogenesis of the children's comprehension deficit, as was just stated, seems to be an inability to decode phonology. Tallal and Piercy (572) discovered a specific processing disorder in a group of 12 children with developmental dysphasia for the brief rapidly changing acoustic signals that differentiate one consonant sound from another. Whether a more severe deficit of this type accounts for the syndrome of verbal auditory agnosia is uncertain but it has been suggested (203).

Semantic-Pragmatic Syndrome

Children with this syndrome have no difficulty decoding phonology or producing well formed sentences. Their deficit affects comprehension and use of language. They have trouble understanding discourse (491). Typically, they have a striking difficulty processing such sophisticated linguistic devices as embedded clauses, conditionals, and wh- questionforms. One can show that the deficit is linguistic rather than cognitive by reasking the child the question he could not answer in such a way that it requires a yes-no response and demonstrating in this way that he does know the answer. The children usually have an intact or superior auditory memory and are fluent. They may repeat whole sentences verbatim or recite TV commercials. While they often have no difficulty retrieving verbal labels for objects or pictures, they nonetheless have an anomia in spontaneous speech. As a result, some of their words miss the mark despite the fact that they belong to the appropriate semantic field. This gives their speech a loose, tangential, or somewhat inappropriate quality. Their train of thought appears illogical and difficult to follow. In some, this characteristic amounts to a thought disorder of frankly psychotic proportion.

The children may exhibit a variety of abnormal behaviors, they may be hyperkinetic and distractible, and display some autistic features, especially in early childhood. They are often unaware of the impact of their behavior on others, perhaps because of difficulty reading facial expression and tone of voice. It is not clear to what degree their behavior disorder is primary and a direct reflection of the brain dysfunction that has also affected their linguistic skills, and to what degree it is secondary to their inadequate comprehension of language and to the social consequences deriving therefrom.

The children's comprehension deficit is likely to be overlooked or underestimated because their spontaneous speech is so fluent and because they understand single words and simple phrases and are sociable. They use language conversationally but often more for the purpose of maintaining social contact than to convey information. Their speech has been compared to cocktail party chatter; it resembles quite closely the speech of adult patients with Wernicke's aphasia who also speak a lot even though they have little to say, use clichés rather than information-rich words, and have deficient comprehension at the level of semantic processing.

Like children with verbal auditory agnosia, children who suffer from the semantic-pragmatic syndrome tend to have much lower verbal than performance IQs. Some of these children learn to read despite their deficient verbal skills but their ability to understand what they read may be limited. It is important to test silent reading comprehension, which may be superior to their ability to answer oral questions, before labeling such children hyperlexic.

Infantile hydrocephalus is the best recognized etiology for the semantic-pragmatic syndrome. Hydrocephalic children have been called hyperverbal or chatter boxes. Swisher and Pinsker (569) found no strong relationship between the children's IQ and the number of words they produced; they stressed that the children's ability to produce syntactically adequate sentences may mask their inadequate comprehension. As a result, hydrocephalic children's cognitive deficit is likely to escape notice during casual office assessment. Surprisingly, the correlation between ventricular size and severity of cognitive and linguistic deficit is not as close as one might expect, although hydrocephalus occasionally results in frankly autistic behavior and mutism as well as profound retardation.

Ventricular enlargement usually predominates in the posterior part of the hemispheres in infantile hydrocephalus and damages the white matter more than the cortex. Severe hydrocephalus typically causes visual-spatial deficits as well as the semantic-pragmatic syndrome (553). Is it possible that these symptoms interfere with the connections of the angular-supramarginal region of both hemispheres with either subcortical targets, like the pulvinar, or with intrahemispheric corticocortical connections? Hydrocephalic children in whom both verbal and performance IQs are depressed can legitimately be considered globally retarded, yet the flavor of their speech is unmistakable and remarkably similar to that of much brighter children with the semantic-pragmatic syndrome whose visual-spatial skills may not only be intact but superior and who, perhaps, have lateralized rather than bilateral hemisphere deficits of unknown etiology.

There are no sharp boundaries between higher functioning echolalic autistic children, a condition DSM III (171) calls infantile autism residual state, children DSM III labels as suffering from childhood onset pervasive developmental disorder because their symptomatology was not present or not recognized until after 30 months, the arbitrary cut-off for making a diagnosis of infantile autism, and children who have the linguistic syndrome we have chosen to call the semantic-pragmatic syndrome. It may be reasonable to suggest that all these children share a common language deficit and that what distinguishes them is the presence and severity of their affective and behavioral aberrations.

Infantile Autism

Infantile autism, whose behavioral and affective aspects were discussed in Chapter 9, can be considered the most severe among the disorders of communication. Its prognosis is tied in part to the severity of the language disorder: Autistic children who remain mute after age 5 have an even bleaker prognosis than autistic children who learn to speak, although prognosis for independent functioning in adult life is always guarded, and linked with overall cognitive competence as well as with communicative competence (153,522). As stated in Chapter 9, the etiology and pathogenesis of autism are poorly understood and likely diverse.

Autistic children invariably are impaired in their use of oral language for communication, but it is equally striking that they do not enter into communicative interaction and do not appear to read body language, facial expression, or tone of voice. Since these latter skills are thought to engage nondominant hemispheric function, there is reason to believe that both hemispheres may be affected in autistic children, albeit to different degrees. Some children with autistic behavior have been found to have left temporal lobe atrophy, involving the limbic structures in its mesial aspect (260). Others are said to have atypical hemispheric asymmetry (277). A few have gross structural pathology on CT scans although the majority do not (142). A significant proportion will develop seizures as adults (153) and, in this writer's experience, enough of them have focal EEG abnormalities in childhood to call for an EEG as part of the initial diagnostic investigation. All mute autistic children require definitive assessment of hearing at intake in order to rule out a peripheral hearing loss. This usually mandates the recording of brain stem and cortical auditory-evoked responses. Abnormally long latencies of brain stem auditory-evoked responses have been found in some hearing autistic children (544,567). This observation is important for two reasons: It is one more piece of evidence indicating that autistic children suffer from brain dysfunction, and it suggests that an auditory processing disorder contributes to some mute autistic children's severe comprehension deficit for speech. When mute autistic children learn to speak, some have grossly deviant articulation and prosody. Their speech is monotonous, chopped, and robot-like. It may be that these children have an auditory processing disorder that resembles that of children with verbal auditory agnosia.

Other autistic children who acquire speech are fluent and echolalic. They have a good verbal memory and adequate, although not necessarily normal, phonologic skills, but are deficient at the level of syntactic and semantic decoding. Since they usually parrot exactly what they hear, they reverse pronouns and refer to themselves either in the third person, by name, or as "you." Their communication deficit resembles that of children with the semantic-pragmatic syndrome, with the notable exception that they are not as eager to communicate, have eye avoidance, and cannot interpret the nonverbal aspects of the communicative interaction. Their behavior is generally much more bizarre but has somewhat the same flavor as that of some of the children with the semantic-pragmatic syndrome.

Whether or not mute or almost mute autistic children and verbose echolalic autistic children should be separated into two subgroups, as proposed by Rapin and Allen (489), awaits further research. Mutism itself is probably not valid grounds for separating children with auditory processing disorders from those who do not have them since some mute autistic children become fluent while others remain severely dysfluent.

Echolalia should not be discouraged in autistic children, at least in the early stages, as it may provide the child with the opportunity to improve his comprehension and production of speech (26). A small proportion of autistic children are exceedingly proficient at decoding written language and become hyperlexic or preoccupied with numbers (141,289,407). Echolalic children and hyperlexic children are able to decipher the phonologic code but not the semantics of the message. Their impaired semantic processing is reflected by a lower verbal IQ than performance IQ, although such children almost always perform at a superior level on at least some subtests (splinter skills).

Hypotheses about the pathogenesis of autistic children's language deficits are easy to formulate but none has received definitive support from morphologic or electrophysiologic evidence (141,150): Pathology in the central auditory pathway subcortically or in the temporal lobes would explain acoustic phonologic processing and speech production disorders; posterior temporoparietal pathology in the dominant hemisphere, comprehension deficits involving semantics; nondominant temporal pathology, deficient processing of prosody and facial expression; and limbic pathology, impaired drive to communicate and blunted experience of pleasure and displeasure. Interruption in the connections between these various areas would be likely to produce similar symptoms. High functioning autistic children have islands of competence presumably denoting efficient operation of some cortical systems. For example, some autistic children are interested in music and can carry a tune. Extraordinary proficiency of some autistic children for putting together puzzles, taking apart mechanical toys, or decoding written texts may reflect the consequence of attention and learning being inordinately focused on nonverbal visual-spatial tasks to the exclusion of, or because of the lack of demand for, learning requiring verbal skills. Greater proficiency for visual than auditory processing of language has been capitalized upon and sign language has been introduced to supplement and clarify oral speech (96,377,526). Because Total Communication has enabled some autistic children to acquire a serviceable communication system and has been associated with behavioral improvement, this approach is worth trying with all mute or virtually mute autistic children. It is also being tried with severely retarded mute though nonautistic children.

Isolated islands of unusual proficiency or "splinter skills" do not necessarily presage a favorable prognosis for autistic children and should not be interpreted as evidence that the child's potential overall competence is high. Rutter (522) stresses, nevertheless, that IQ tests in autistic children, far from being unfair, provide valuable prognostic information: The more testable the child, the more tasks he is capable of doing well, the better the outlook, as is true for mentally deficient children in general; or, to put it differently, the better the child functions, the less severe and diffuse the brain dysfunction, the better the prognosis. This statement does not minimize the importance of the child's environment and of the schooling he receives. Autistic children do better if they can be taught to enter into communicative interaction, to obey commands, and to organize their activities. Presently, environmental manipulation and intensive work with the child and his parents are the best we can offer. It may make the difference between the occasional autistic child who is able to function independently and the majority who will end up institutionalized or dependent for life. While pharmacotherapy with such drugs as thioridazine has a place in the management of autistic children (91), its main value seems to be to make the child more available to educational intervention.

Mixed Phonologic-Syntactic Syndrome

This syndrome is the most common of the developmental dysphasias. Comprehension is always better than expression and may occasionally be normal, although more typically comprehension is adequate for routine situations but impaired for complex discourse. The children are nonfluent, they have a small vocabulary, their syntax is rudimentary or aberrant, and their phonology marred by omissions, distortions, and substitutions. Speech is used communicatively, in some children supplemented by pointing, head nods, and other gestures. Some children with this syndrome have signs of pseudobulbar palsy or oromotor apraxia. These are not severe enough to explain the children's inadequate speech production but reflect dysfunction in adjacent cortical areas. Like children with the previously described syndromes, children with phonologic-syntactic syndrome tend to have deficient verbal IQs. Those who have associated motor signs may score low on tests requiring graphomotor skills and may have somewhat depressed performance IQs as well. The children's behavior is variable. They may be frustrated by their inability to make their wants known and have temper tantrums. Since comprehension is fairly adequate, they tend to have less severe and less pervasive behavior problems than children with verbal auditory agnosia, with the semantic-pragmatic syndrome, or with autism.

No definite pathologic correlation has been made for children with this syndrome, but one can speculate that their dysfunction involves anterior brain regions having to do with language production. Prognosis in children with this syndrome is variable and depends on its severity. Children who are not too severely affected will often learn to speak adequately by school age or before, except for some persistent articulation deficits, curtailed syntactic skills, and word finding problems. They often reemerge in school with dyslexic linguistic problems (6,391,488).

Phonologic Programming Deficit Syndrome

Severe forms of this syndrome are rare. It is characterized by extremely deficient expression, amounting to mutism in some children, associated with normal or near normal comprehension of speech. What differentiates this syndrome from the preceding one is the striking discrepancy between expression, which is much worse in the phonologic programming deficit syndrome, and comprehension which is good. The children's cognitive competence is variable.

There are two variants of this syndrome. In one, the children are very nonfluent or even mute. They speak in single poorly articulated words or short phrases at best; in the other, the children are much more fluent and attempt to speak in sentences, but what they say is so distorted because of mispronunciations, phonemic substitutions, and sequencing errors as to render them virtually unintelligible except to the members of their immediate family or when the context serves to clarify what they are trying to say. Characteristically, children with this syndrome can produce speech sounds in isolation but not when they are embedded within a word. Many of these children invent an elaborate manual language even though they may have mild motor or apraxic deficits of their limbs. They profit greatly from the use of Total Communication which lessens their frustration and improves their behavior since it gives them a vehicle to make known their wants.

Referring to the severely dysfluent children, Ferry and collaborators (191) speak of a verbal apraxia (as opposed to a buccolingual apraxia), that is, of an inability to transform verbal images into the motor commands required for speech. The children may or may not have oromotor problems but these are not nearly severe enough to account for extreme dysfluency that verges on anarthria: While the children cannot speak they can often eat, lick, and wag their tongue quite well, and if they drool at all, it is much less severely than many cerebral palsied children with severe pseudobulbar palsy who struggle to produce some poorly intelligible strangled utterances. This is in striking contrast to the children under discussion who do not talk at all and hardly attempt to do so. Children with the speech programming deficit syndrome resemble patients with aphemia (520), an acquired syndrome that renders patients mute but does not interfere with their ability to write, unlike patients with Broca's aphasia who write much as they speak. The programming deficit in aphemia, and perhaps in the speech programming deficit syndrome as well, appears to be specific for speech and to occur at a later state of linguistic output programming than in Broca's aphasia and in the phonologic-syntactic syndrome. Typically, these children acquire some scholastic skills although rarely at a level commensurate with their normal peers. Whether deficient school performance reflects a true reading disability, cognitive incompetence, or an underestimate of the children's abilities because of their severely deficient expression remains to be determined.

While the neurologic basis of the phonologic programming deficit syndrome is rarely known, it is plausible to suspect that it may reflect a more limited anterior lesion than the one postulated to give rise to the phonologic-syntactic syndrome. One patient with this syndrome has two discrete porencephalies, presumed to have been acquired at age 9 months when he had an acute illness with encephalopathic manifestations, that involve both the territory of the frontal branches of the middle cerebral artery. Since the porencephalies affect both the cortex and the subjacent white matter, they readily account for the oromotor problems that complicate but do not explain the patient's severe expressive deficit. No doubt the etiology of this syndrome varies, but it is worth noting that McLaughlin and Kriegsman (402) describe severe speech articulation deficits in boys with the fragile-X chromosomal syndrome. The site of pathology in these boys is unknown.

Mild variants of this syndrome are difficult to differentiate from, or perhaps identical to, lags in the maturation of speech articulation in otherwise normal children. Whether it turns out to be useful to try to separate children with this syndrome from those with the phonologic-syntactic syndrome whose comprehension is good remains to be seen.

READING DISABILITY (DYSLEXIA)

The problems of definition, classification, etiology, and pathogenesis that beset developmental language disorders pertain equally to the disorders of written language. The literature on dyslexia is very large (e.g., 43,47,98,309,326,361, 452,509,515) and contains many contradictory statements. Some writers imply that there is but one syndrome of developmental dyslexia (133,415). This review, which attempts to relate deficiencies in complex behaviors to brain dysfunction or inefficiency, defends the position that there are several varieties of dyslexia.

Like speech, reading calls for a large number of skills, first and foremost, an adequate knowledge of oral language: The striking failure of congenitally deaf children to acquire serviceable reading skills (126,146) is a case in point. In order to read, a child must learn to segment speech into phonemic units, to associate grapheme with phoneme, and to synthesize syllables by blending individual phonemes. He must be able to retrieve words (as opposed to nonsense sounds) from his lexicon (repository of word meanings) and transcend the individual word to capture the sense of the message. Short-term sequential memory is called upon as multiple, parallel, and sequential, visual, auditory, and linguistic operations are performed on the text to be read. Second, reading requires adequate visual-spatial perceptual function (452). Although deficits in this area interfere with letter recognition and the acquisition of a look-say vocabulary, it is uncommon for these deficits to provide an adequate and sufficient explanation for dyslexia. Third, the child must be capable of attending to the task and be motivated to make the required intellectual effort. Finally, to show that he can read, he needs to have an output channel at his disposal, be it his voice and articulators for speech or his hand to point, write, or sign.

As one might anticipate, there are many levels of operations where things may go wrong and interfere with the child's ability to learn to read. Dyslexia may reflect brain damage or brain maldevelopment (205). In the latter case, it is either because of a prenatal insult or as the result of a genetic trait, or both. In some families, dyslexia is reported to show genetic linkage with chromosome 15 (546a). Dyslexia often occurs in families and may be inherited as a dominant trait (254). Dyslexia, like dysphasia, has a strong predilection for males. It is not clear whether this sex distribution reflects anatomic differences in hemispheric organization, brain maturation, or cognitive style (638,640), or differences in susceptibility to brain insult or in efficiency of recovery. Surprisingly, perhaps, there seems to be little if any relation in many dyslexics between the presumed etiology of the reading disability and the particular syndrome of dyslexia (391). What determines a child's difficulty appears to be what system is inoperative, not what produces the dysfunction. Defining each child's deficits and strengths is of paramount importance from the standpoint of prescribing a program of educational remediation geared to overcome or circumvent his particular difficulties (390,594).

Syndromes Among Dyslexics

A number of attempts have been made to identify specific syndromes among children who do not learn to read (65,195,320). Mattis (389,391) and Denckla (156,157) isolated at least four syndromes among dyslexic children based on an analysis of results of a neuropsychologic test battery, after they had excluded as irrelevant to reading those deficit scores that dyslexics shared with brain-damaged readers.

Language Disorder Syndrome

All of the children with this syndrome have an anomia or difficulty retrieving verbal labels, associated with at least one other sign of language impairment such as a disorder of comprehension, difficulty with sentence repetition, or deficient speech sound discrimination. Severely affected children have trouble acquiring the grapheme-phoneme correspondence so that they are forestalled from using a phonetic approach to reading; some children have difficulty blending phonemes into words. Because of their anomia, less severely affected children who can use the phonetic approach to reading may not recognize that their sound-blend has resulted in a neologism (nonword). Dysphasic dyslexic children tend to have lower verbal than performance IQs (391), some may have difficulty with motor coordination of the right hand or with speech articulation, and some with sequencing. Their reading and spelling tend to be very deficient and they may also have difficulty with mathematics.

Visual-Spatial Perceptual Syndrome

This syndrome is much less prevalent than the first and is associated with deficient visual-spatial perception and memory, without a language or sound-blending deficit. [Claims that poor coordination of the eye muscles or inadequate convergence is responsible for reading disability are unconvincing (59,361).] These are the children who confuse *p* with *q*, *d* with *b*, and *m* with *w*—a symptom called strephosymbolia by Orton (452). They too may have difficulty learning to associate the picture of a letter with its sound. They often fail to recognize even the most common word, like /the/, or /cat/, or /boy/. Their performance IQ tends to be lower than their verbal IQ (391). They are helped by learning to analyze words phonemically and to associate phonetic sounds with letters.

Articulation and Graphomotor Discoordination Syndrome

Children with this syndrome have an oromotor apraxia and difficulty with sound blending. They have trouble with fine motor coordination and, as a consequence, with writing. They usually acquire a look-say vocabulary but are hampered in phonemic decoding by their sound blending deficit. Their language skills and visual spatial skills are good but they have trouble with constructional tasks because of difficulty coordinating the two hands.

Sequencing Deficit Syndrome

This syndrome seems to result from an inability to deal with ordered sequences (156,389). The children have trouble repeating digits, words, and sentences, and with concepts like before-after, more-less. Their sequencing deficit impairs sound blending and progress toward a look-say vocabulary. For example, they may not differentiate /*saw*/ from /*was*/ or /*lighted*/ from /*delight*/. Children with sequencing deficits also tend to have difficulty with arithmetic.

*   *   *

It is tempting to speculate that children with the first syndrome may have dysfunction affecting (inter alia) the posterior language areas of the dominant (usually left) hemisphere; those with the second, right posterior dysfunction; those with the third, dysfunction affecting the foot of the left postcentral gyrus in an area responsible for the syndrome of phonetic disintegration of language and kinesthetic motor apraxia in adults (378); and those with the fourth, dysfunction in the region of the angular gyrus, or subcortical pathology affecting the left arcuate fasciculus or other areas responsible for conduction aphasia in adults (218). While there are essentially no data to support these speculations, Galaburda and Klemper (205) found that the planum temporale was unusually small on the left and that there were other areas of mild cortical dysplasia in the left hemisphere of a man with familial dyslexia who died accidentally. Another recent report (174) suggests that focal dysfunction in language areas of the brain plays a role in dyslexia: With special computer techniques, differences were detectable in the EEG and evoked responses of 9 dyslexic boys, compared to 10 controls, while they were engaged in visual and linguistic tasks. Differences were not limited to the language areas of the left hemisphere, however, but were more widespread; in particular, they involved the mesial-frontal region bilaterally. If dyslexia reflects inefficient language skills much more often than inefficient visual-perceptual skills, it will come as no surprise that reading disability is a frequent, not to say usual, sequella of developmental language disability (6,18,488,642).

Some children have signs pointing to more than one syndrome, and some may have other evidence of brain dysfunction, such as motor clumsiness, that is irrelevant, except by association, to the pathogenesis of their reading disability (391). By and large, the more widespread the brain dysfunction, the more severe the reading disability: Children with signs of two or more syndromes are likely to have subnormal IQs (389). Prognosis for functional reading is best in children with pure syndromes and a high IQ. How some of these children learn to read despite deficits that render most children dyslexic needs to be investigated since it might provide clues for remediation.

Others besides Mattis (389,391) and Denckla (156) have attempted to define neuropsychologic syndromes among reading disabled children. Although Benton (43,47) cautions that a coherent theory that explains reading disability satisfactorily has not been achieved, and that the multiplicity of abnormalities found to be associated with dyslexia in various studies is confusing, a consensus seems to be emerging that at least two main types of dyslexia exist, one reflecting linguistic inefficiency presumably associated with dominant hemispheric dysfunction, and one visual-perceptual inefficiency associated with nondominant hemispheric dysfunction (24,195,205). The Mattis and Denckla studies, along with a consideration of the types of acquired alexia encountered in adults (266), suggest that careful research is likely to show that there is more than one type of dyslexia associated with dominant hemispheric dysfunction (488).

DISORDERS OF WRITING, SPELLING, AND MATHEMATICS

When teachers complain that children have trouble writing *(dysgraphia)* the physician needs to know whether they are speaking of a problem with orthography, or one with motor control (discoordination, tremor, motor apraxia), or with visual-spatial perception (5). The importance of writing for learning to read and to spell has been stressed by Bradley (71). She notes that poor readers tend to be clumsy, which is certainly true of children with the graphomotor discoordination syndrome of Mattis (391), and may be true of some children with the dysphasic dyslexic syndrome. Bradley utilizes a remediation approach that consists of having the children write words of their choosing, spelling them out loud as they do so, then saying the word. She has them do this several times each day for six consecutive days. She finds that the children retain the ability to read and spell these words much longer than when only reading or spelling is used. One can speculate whether retention is facilitated because writing calls into play motor-kinetic learning that, as was seen in Chapter 5, seems to depend on different pathways than visual and auditory learning.

Inadequate reading will inevitably result in poor spelling *(dysorthographia)*. The type of spelling error made by dyslexics provides clues to the type of their reading disability. Boder (65) noted that the spelling of children who have difficulty with phonemic analysis and sound blending may be far off the mark (dysphonetic) while children whose deficit is visual or mnemonic tend to make educated guesses about how a word might be spelled that render their spelling more or less intelligible, though idiosyncratic (dyseidetic). Children with sequencing problems invert letters and syllables within words and telescope words, a problem that, in mild form, is common among normal persons.

There are children who learn to read but whose inordinately poor spelling indicates that they were potential dyslexics who were fortunate enough to have become readers. It is important to detect such children because reading often remains laborious for them. They may not come to attention until junior high or high school, when reading proficiency is assumed and their lack of fluency jeopardizes their ability to get at the ideas in texts they are supposed to read for information. This may lead to frustration, unexplained failure in subjects such as social studies or science, and secondary behavior disorders or dropping out of school.

Dyscalculia has received less emphasis than dyslexia. Our culture expects boys to be better at mathematics than girls (640), although the degree to which this reflects biologic, maturational, or cultural influences is still subject to debate. Even recent evidence suggesting that boys' superiority for mathematics is largely biologic (38) has not been accepted by all investigators. Certainly, many boys do well, or at least they are much better at mathematics than they are at reading.

If the teacher reports that the child has trouble with mathematics, the physician will want to determine whether the difficulty involves mathematical concepts (which may reflect a language problem), or the process of enumeration (217)—perhaps related to the Gerstmann syndrome (45), or sequencing, or the visualization of spatial relations. The latter problem may cause difficulty, not only with geometry and measurement, but also with calculation since one needs to know which operation to start on the right, which on the left, and how to line up numbers in order to proceed. The point is that mathematical ineptitude, like dyslexia, may reflect either verbal or spatial or memory or cognitive problems. As was the case for constructional apraxia (46) and dyslexia, different children may fail the same task for different reasons. Mathematical failure needs to be studied in detail, as has been done for dyslexia, in order to determine what it is that the child cannot do and when the deficit is sufficiently severe to suggest that it results from neurologic dysfunction. Mathematical performance can be assessed by using standard achievement tests or specialized tests such as the Key Math Test (124).

This list by no means exhausts the "learning deficits" one can encounter in school children as a result of cerebral pathology or inefficiency. It simply reflects those scholastic skills that children in our culture are expected to acquire. No one seems to worry if a child is inept in art and graphic skills although, paradoxically, the ability to draw and reproduce block patterns is included in every intelligence test battery. It is not required that every child be able to carry a tune or recognize melodies, play a musical instrument, or learn to dance. We saw earlier that in most people the right hemisphere is most efficient for processing nonspeech sounds (184,329), the melody of speech and tone of voice (32,513), facial expression (358,404), and emotion (35,593), as well as visual-spatial stimuli. Not surprisingly, it is also involved in many aspects of musical processing (54,134). One can surmise that children with total lack of proficiency for music or art may be suffering from lateralized inefficiency of the nondominant hemisphere. Conversely, the interest in music (and puzzles) of some mute autistic or dysphasic children who can carry a tune most likely reflects better right- than left-sided cerebral function.

FINAL COMMENT

School problems are extremely common (56,67,97,114,261,315,421). They will often be brought to the attention of the child's physician in the context of the new Right to Education Law (PL 94–142) (454) that mandates that every handicapped child be evaluated thoroughly in order that he may receive any special education he may require in the "least restrictive environment." The best way for the physician to get an idea of what might be wrong with such a child is not through his physical or even his neurological examination but by asking the child to read, write, and to do some arithmetic. How the child goes about these tasks often provides sufficient data to indicate that the child needs remedial education and will make it obvious whether or not further investigation is warranted. While we rarely know the etiology of dyslexia and other types of scholastic failure, it is rarely relevant for remediation to determine whether the learning deficit is the result of a genetic deficit, a maturational lag, or an acquired insult to the brain (314,315). Nonetheless, the rigidities of the educational system and of the requirements for funding are typically based, not on a statement of the child's deficit, but on a categorical diagnosis such as "brain damage," as opposed to "learning disability," that in many states requires a statement from a physician. We need not reiterate here that these labels more often than not have doubtful validity. Determining whether a child is right-handed, left-handed, ambidextrous, or has mixed dominance for eye, hand, and foot, is largely irrelevant unless it corroborates other signs indicating lateralized cerebral pathology. What the child needs is competent and individually designed remedial education (594). Children who do not read must not be robbed of the content of education: Let them do their work orally as long as reading is so difficult for them that it precludes their using it as an efficient way for gathering information. Let not this one scholastic failure poison every class of every day and prevent the child from learning about his culture and about science, and deprive him of exposure to stimulating material to expand his mind. Book learning is important, even crucial in our culture, but this is a recent development. The illiterate societies of the recent past indicate that a full and independent life is possible so long as a person has occupational and social competence. In any case, it is the very rare person indeed who will not be motivated to learn to read at least a few of the words of his native language that permeate our culture.

11

Cognitive Incompetence

DEFINITIONS

Cognitive competence may be defined as the capacity to process large amounts of information efficiently, and to program behaviors that will have favorable adaptive consequences, not only for the present, but for life. A somewhat more narrow definition might emphasize the ability to solve new problems thanks to the discovery of underlying principles (468). Dealing with complex situations flexibly and creatively presupposes the capacity and motivation to transcend immediate circumstances and previous learning in order to think out contingencies and possible solutions, that is, to anticipate the future before acting. If intelligent behavior implies an inherently efficiently functioning brain, it also implies a time dimension during which the person has interacted with his environment and has had a chance to develop increasingly effective response strategies. Cognitive competence, therefore, evolves as a result of the dynamic interplay between the genetic programs of a person's developing brain and the particular environmental circumstances that modify them.

Mental deficiency by these definitions might be characterized as the consistent adoption of maladaptive behaviors. Occasional maladaptive behaviors, or maladaptive behaviors limited to a narrow set of contingencies, would not fulfill this definition of mental deficiency. If mental deficiency denotes overall cognitive incompetence, this diagnosis is difficult to sustain in the face of impoverished environmental opportunity, of deficient sensors (e.g., blindness, deafness) (487) or effectors (e.g., spasticity, anarthria), or of focal brain pathology that impairs restricted aspects of cerebral processing. Strictly speaking, the term *simple mental retardation* refers to the failure to achieve one's cognitive potential because of a deficient environment, while mental deficiency, used synonymously with moderate to severe mental retardation, denotes lack of cognitive potential. In practice, the terms mental retardation and mental deficiency are used interchangeably (113,286). Severe mental deficiency implies generalized or multifocal brain dysfunction or pathology because of a static encephalopathy present from early life (344,589), whereas *dementia* denotes dissolution of intellectual competence as the result of a diffuse and progressive cerebral disease. If the disease is manifest *in utero* or in early infancy it may be impossible to differentiate profound mental deficiency, implying a static condition, from the dementia of a progressive illness that occurs so early that it precludes any meaningful development (485) (Fig. 23).

The term mental deficiency has often come to be defined in a narrow and highly artificial way as poor performance on intelligence tests in the face of what is deemed to be adequate environmental opportunity and lack of sensorimotor or gross "emotional" handicap. Such a definition implies that intelligence tests probe a sufficiently broad sample of behaviors to be fair mirrors of the brain's overall efficiency. Provided there are no mitigating circumstances, it also implies that the summary score or IQ is a valid measure of this efficiency or "intelligence." This assumption is not necessarily warranted since the IQ measures performance at a particular moment in time and since the predictive validity of the IQ is less than its concurrent validity, that is, its correlation with other measures of current competence (240,406,575). To put it differently, a child's IQ is a more reliable measure of his rate of development and present level of function than of his potential (286).

Conventional definitions of learning disability, dyslexia, developmental language disability, and minimal cerebral dysfunction also require that the deficit not be explainable on the basis of environmental deprivation (including inadequate teaching), sensory abnormality, gross brain damage, emotional factors, or mental retardation. These negative definitions stress poor achievement in the face of what appears to be "adequate" ability. What is meant by "adequate" ability is competence measured by a test instrument that will not be adversely affected by the child's particular handicap or deficiency. For example, blind children are tested verbally, deaf children are given ostensibly nonverbal tests (487), dyslexics are assessed with instruments that do not require reading or spelling, manipulative tests are avoided for cerebral palsied children, and socially deprived children are assessed with "culture free" instruments. While these accommodations appear reasonable and represent acceptable pragmatic compromises for testing in the face of deficits that do not reflect cerebral dysfunction, they violate one of the basic assumptions of intelligence tests batteries, the sampling of a broad and representative range of behaviors. These accommodations are based on the inference that all aspects of behavior are correlated because the single characteristic, intelligence, influences them all. This view contrasts with the thesis that intelligence is the result of a number of less strongly correlated special abilities. Curtailed intelligence tests are not "fair" when one is evaluating a child with deficits in complex behaviors since the disregarded areas of deficit may be a better gauge of the child's proficiency for real life than his restricted areas of competence. Even when a whole battery is administered, the summary score or IQ cannot be taken too seriously in children with circumscribed brain dysfunction since it does not describe the variance of subtest scores: Depending

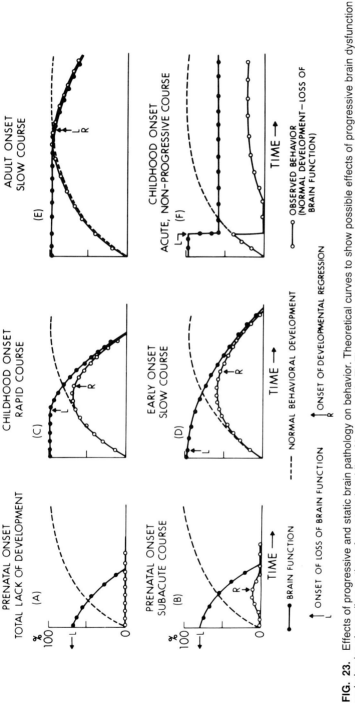

FIG. 23. Effects of progressive and static brain pathology on behavior. Theoretical curves to show possible effects of progressive brain dysfunction on behavior, depending on time of onset and rapidity of its course (A–F). The curve depicting observed behavior is the result of the difference between the curves indicating expected development and brain function. **(A)** Prenatal onset, with damage at birth so advanced that no development is observed, suggesting a severe static encephalopathy. **(B)** Prenatal onset, with damage at birth somewhat less severe. Development is minimal and markedly delayed but does appear to be taking place initially. **(C)** and **(D)** Onset at birth, with a less acute course. **(E)** Onset in adulthood. Note that in **B, C,** and **D,** the loss of milestones (R) may not appear until months or years after the onset of the illness, which will therefore not appear progressive unless it is realized that deceleration of development or developmental standstill implies deteriorating function. When a progressive disease starts after adolescence **(E),** loss of function should be less delayed and the disease recognized as progressive virtually from its start. A severe static lesion acquired postnatally **(G)** may produce total regression acutely, but development may be expected to resume until the time of puberty. (Reproduced with permission from Rapin, ref. 486.)

on the skills sampled by each battery, IQs derived from different tests may vary by 20 or more points in a given child with brain dysfunction (629).

GENETIC AND ENVIRONMENTAL CONTRIBUTIONS TO INTELLIGENCE

Cognitive competence increases during maturation as the stimuli and experiences provided by the environment mold the developing brain. Environmental accidents such as infections or trauma may have direct and drastically deleterious effects on brain development. The child with an IQ below 50 can be assumed to have some type of serious brain pathology (344,589), although a normal or bright-normal IQ by no means rules out structural brain damage or serious brain dysfunction. Even normal brains exposed to favorable environments vary in efficiency. The relative contribution of heredity and sociocultural environment to this variance is extremely difficult to ascertain because of heredity and environment covary (623). Recent research on identical twins indicates that genetics plays an important part in determining intelligence (506,634), even though studies of adopted children and epidemiologic surveys of large populations of children highlight the crucial influence of the parents' socioeconomic status and educational level for their children's intellectual competence (193,529). A raging controversy has arisen because of the lower performance, on the average, of black children than white children on standard intelligence tests (368). This is interpreted by some as evidence for genetic differences. Others attribute it to lack of education and social opportunity, or to the greater probability that a black child has sustained a biologic insult such as lead poisoning (440), intrauterine exposure to alcohol (566), or prematurity (634), or to the accident of his belonging to a subculture that is distinct from that of the designers of intelligence tests, thus rendering the test unfair. Data from the Perinatal Collaborative Study (78) indicate that there is no relationship between IQ and social class in children who sustained encephalopathic insults. Across a total sample of 26,000 children, a negligible portion of the IQ variance at age 4 was accounted for by insults directly associated with pregnancy and the perinatal period. While development was not correlated with socioeconomic and educational factors in infancy, these variables, especially as they affected the mother, predicted a substantial portion of the variance of the IQ at age 4. In contrast, in a longitudinal study of middle and upper class adults, McCall (396) found that for men, the father's but not the mother's educational achievement and occupational status predicted personal achievement and status as efficiently as the IQ after age 8; women were affected by both parents' standing; and IQ between the ages of three and seven years was not a good predictor for either sex. Further evidence from the Collaborative Study (443) indicates that MBD is less strongly related to perinatal insults than anticipated and that constitutional factors appear to play an important role in its occurrence.

The anatomic and physiologic correlates of intelligence are unknown. In animals, enriched environments during development increase cortical thickness (39) and foster dendritic growth (129), both of which denote more complex interneuronal connectivity and, presumably, more efficient cortical function. Impaired dendritic growth is not pathognomonic of a detrimental environment (595) since grossly distorted dendrites are observed in the brains of some infants with severe congenital mental deficiency or genetic-metabolic dementia (482). Relatively invariant stages in the maturation of the fetal brain and in the unfolding of infants' motor and adaptive skills bear witness to the genetic programs controlling the anatomic development of the brain (634). Resilience of brain function in the face of all but the most extreme malnutrition (560) and lack of stimulation (605), and in the face of some severe pathologic insults reflects fail-safe built-in systems that we call plasticity (192,558). Lack of blatant functional consequences following acquired cerebral injury in early life does not necessarily bespeak recovery, however (263,294).

INTELLIGENCE TESTS

Assessing the competence of a person to function in his environment requires the sampling of a large number of skills. Many specialized instruments have been designed to this end. Intelligence tests are more or less well standardized and validated instruments that purport to measure the efficiency of complex behaviors by sampling responses in a variety of contrived situations.

Tests designed to measure other skills besides intelligence have been developed: Personality tests are intended to assess a person's affect and behavioral style and the dynamics of his interpersonal relations. Developmental scales have been devised to gauge children's maturity by noting how they deal with manipulative and social situations of everyday life (34,199,328). Achievement tests measure specialized skills, in particular scholastic ones (124,243,298,644). Aptitude tests attempt to predict proficiency at particular jobs or avocations (240).

Intelligence Test Batteries

Originally designed to predict children's success in school, intelligence test batteries are now viewed as a means for assessing the cognitive competence of persons of all ages. In existence for three-quarters of a century and used in millions of individuals from early childhood throughout adult life, they are better standardized than most other psychologic instruments, and have been the subject of vast amounts of research in terms of what it is they are measuring (validity), their reliability, predictive value, and diagnostic efficacy (136).

If intelligence is the capacity to process information efficiently and to program behaviors that will have favorable adaptive consequences, and if one's goal is to assess a person's intelligence, one must sample a broad and representative range of behaviors. This requirement was obvious to the developers of intelligence tests who devised many different subtests. Each subtest was contrived to tap different intellectual capacities, some requiring verbal skills for solution, others not. The mean score of the aggregate of these subtests or IQ was designed to discriminate among normal persons with different capabilities.

Only those capacities tapped by the various subtests contribute to the IQ score. For instance, standard tests do not call upon musical ability, artistic talent, flexibility in interpersonal relations, initiative, creativity, and a myriad of other skills that may have as much or more to do with successful adaptation to life's opportunities than the skills they do assess. Be that as it may, as a result of the routine IQ testing of school children, many exceptionally bright children coming from underprivileged families have been identified and placed into academically challenging classes, while reasons other than bad behavior were found to explain the academic failure of others.

The use of psychologic tests for assessing brain function, as opposed to making comparisons between ostensibly normal individuals, is a relatively recent development (44). A detailed study, using a variety of tests, of soldiers with well-defined brain wounds and known premorbid IQ scores demonstrated conclusively that the effects of focal brain pathology on behavior may be quite discrete (378,533,578). A considerable effort was then devoted to studying the effects of lesions in defined brain locations on standard intelligence batteries, and to developing specialized tests sensitive to particular types of lesions (378,480,501,533,578). Present awareness of the specialization of the two cerebral hemispheres not only for verbal versus visual-spatial tasks, but also for serial versus holistic processing of information calls for a revision of our methods for assessing global intelligence (308).

EFFECTS OF AGE AT TESTING

Intelligence tests have become so widely used that in many people's minds high intelligence has become synonymous with a high IQ score. Because the IQ takes the age of the child into account (the IQ is the ratio of scaled score or mental age to chronologic age), the IQ is assumed to be essentially constant over a person's life span. This is clearly not the case in childhood since the IQ reflects not only a person's native ability but also his environmental opportunity. Furthermore, the IQ does not measure the same abilities at all ages because different aspects of cognitive competence mature at different ages, and because the rate and order of maturation are not invariant across children (395).

The concept of general intelligence is not applicable to infancy. During the first year of life, the earliest skills to mature are sensorimotor skills. The infant explores his world with his eyes, his ears, and his other senses, and learns to manipulate objects with his hands and to displace himself. He will acquire the notion of the permanence of objects and learn to pursue objects that disappear from sight, but at that stage he remains limited to the particular data provided by his senses. Infant scales, therefore, are limited almost exclusively to measuring sensorimotor skills. Expressive language emerges during the second year, as the child acquires a symbolic system and becomes capable of evoking internal images or memories that he learns to manipulate in "mind experiments." This, according to Piaget (467,468), marks the child's first steps toward the development of the complex cognitive operations that will enable him to start detaching himself from the here and now and that deserve to be called "intelligence."

After the age of 2, intelligence tests not only sample linguistic and manipulative skills, they begin to explore problem solving capacities. They rely to a much greater degree than earlier on the use of verbal instructions, even for nonverbal tests. More and more, test performance will be colored by the child's life experience (learning), as well as by his innate skills. Reasons for the weak correlation of scores on infant tests with scores on intelligence tests in later childhood are obvious: They measure very different aspects of behavior (357,629). Sensorimotor maturation, which depends on subcortical as well as cortical activity (19,79,151,387), has relatively little to do with maturation of the skills required for complex intellectual operations which engage late-maturing areas of association cortex. The older the child, the better test results will predict success in school and adult intellectual competence, but the more sensitive they become to the cultural and social environment of the child and to his linguistic skills (396).

Because tests do not measure the same skills at each age level, comparing the scores yielded by corresponding subtests in the same child across ages, or in different children, may in fact be comparing different aptitudes since the children may have used different strategies for solving the same problem (631). For example, verbal skills facilitate performance on such an ostensibly nonverbal task as Picture Arrangement, a subtest of the Wechsler Intelligence Scale for Children or WISC (612) requiring that a series of cards be arranged in sequence so that they tell a story.

Infants and toddlers must be tested on their own terms. Their willingness to "play the game" is the major limiting factor for data collection. The cooperation and attention of preschoolers may be equally difficult to enlist, especially if they are tested in an unfamiliar environment by an unfamiliar person. Psychologists trained to work with children are acutely aware of this limitation and take great pains to put the child at ease, use appropriate behavioral techniques to reward him for cooperation, and break-up testing into multiple short sessions. The designers of tests for preschoolers were quite lenient in specifying acceptable responses and methods of administration (34). In older children, and especially in adults, motivation to perform is taken more or less for granted, and behavior is assumed to be under the verbal control of the examiner. These assumptions may not be warranted when testing children from alien cultures or subcultures, and children with brain dysfunction in whom distractibility and impulsivity may interfere seriously with the predictive validity of test scores, even though the score may in fact be describing current performance quite accurately. Motivation cannot be taken for granted, of course, when evaluating persons with severe behavioral or psychiatric conditions or those with nonorganic deficits.

SCREENING TESTS

Intelligence tests were standardized on the basis of administering the whole battery. Administering the entire battery to a young handicapped child may take several hours and is therefore expensive. This makes test batteries unsuitable for screening purposes. Much effort has been expended toward developing special purpose efficient screening instruments; some of them, like scholastic achievement tests, are suitable for group administration in order to pick out children with exceptional ability and children in need of specialized services. One needs to reiterate here that screening tests are just that, a first pass designed to identify children who need more definitive testing. They are not reliable measures of cognitive competence.

Cost-effectiveness is an important consideration when using any test for diagnosis. Cost-effectiveness depends on the validity, reliability, specificity, and sensitivity of the test. Every test will yield some false-positives, i.e., will misclassify some normals as abnormals, and some false-negatives, i.e., will miss some abnormals (196). The more specific the test, the greater its diagnostic efficiency and the reliability of its results on retest. But even sensitive tests have a threshold effect. Setting the threshold or sensitivity of the test will depend on the circumstances of its use. If the condition to be detected is very rare in the population screened, a very sensitive test will miss few affected individuals but will yield a large number of false-positives who will need to be retested for confirmation. This may be acceptable if the condition is very serious and one is unwilling to miss even one affected individual, for instance a child with phenylketonuria or congenital hypothyroidism (434). If the condition to be screened for is common, one may decide that it will be more cost-effective to miss a few affected individuals in the interest of minimizing the number of false-positives. For example, educational administrators may defend this position when screening for children with learning disability, if they want to avoid flooding special classes with children whose learning disability is mild and who may be able to "make it" without specialized intervention.

Screening for Intelligence

Screening for intelligence rests on the premise, mentioned earlier, that man is endowed with a fundamental quality, "intelligence," that influences virtually every aspect of behavior. It is assumed, therefore, that even a limited sampling of behaviors provides a valid gauge of intelligence. Among favorite screening instruments, the Peabody Picture Vocabulary Test (175) requires that a child point to one of four pictures in response to a verbal label. This test is often used·in children with severe motor handicaps or speech deficits. While quite highly correlated with the results of such batteries as the Wechsler and Stanford-Binet scales, this test tends to overestimate intelligence in children from culturally enriched environments and to underestimate it in children from deprived or different cultural settings. It is unsuitable for children with hearing losses or language disorders. The Raven Progressive Matrices (498), developed to screen for officer candidates among enlisted men in England during World War II, is a test of nonverbal analogic reasoning. It was designed to be culture-free and not to depend on skills acquired in school. A colored version for children (497), while unsuitable for children with impaired visual-spatial skills, is widely used as a nonverbal screening test, for example, among the deaf (126,231). These and other screening tests of intelligence are often utilized to evaluate environmental effects such as malnutrition (605), birth order (653), and other circumstances whose effects are weak and that require efficient testing of a large number of persons in order to obtain statistically reliable data. One must keep in mind the limited validity of screening instruments and curtailed batteries for this purpose as well as for evaluating the competence of handicapped persons.

Screening for Brain Damage

A popular use of screening tests has been to detect "organicity" (604). The search for a single instrument to detect brain damage rests on an oversimplistic, unitary concept of brain damage. Most of the tests used for this purpose tap visual-spatial or visual-motor skills that, while they do assess the skill of the preferred hand, are particularly sensitive to nondominant hemispheric dysfunction. The search for organicity goes back to the time when children with these types of deficits were likely to be labeled "brain injured" (564,565), and those with language deficits mentally retarded. Lower performance IQ than verbal IQ was widely used as evidence for organicity, since performance items are less culturally dependent than verbal ones and therefore were thought to be particularly sensitive to dysfunction of an innate or neurologic type. This practice is questionable since lower verbal than performance IQ may reflect language disorder as well as cultural deprivation. A wide discrepancy between Performance and Verbal IQ does suggest the need for more probing neuropsychologic investigation, as does marked scatter between subtest scores.

Poor performance on Digit-Symbol or Coding, a timed subtest of the Wechsler scales calling for rapid substitution of an arbitrary figure for a digit, is a favorite screening test for brain damage since it requires sustained attention as well as adequate visual memory, visual-perceptual, and graphomotor skills (604). The most widely used screening test for brain damage in children is the Bender Gestalt (331), which demands that the child copy and then reproduce from memory a series of complex geometric figures. The test is rendered more sensitive if the child has to draw them on paper with a "noisy" background of wavy lines (2). Indices of organicity include rotations, perseveration, fragmentation, distortions, poor integration of parts, and substitution of lines for dots (331,604). The ability to draw a diamond, an item on the Stanford-Binet at the 7-year level, is often used in the pediatric clinic as a quick screening test for perceptual-motor deficits; another is the ability to reproduce block patterns. The Purdue Pegboard Test (209,625) is very sensitive to cerebral dysfunction producing general or lateralized motor deficits, deficient eye-hand or intermanual coordination (493).

Despite a very large literature indicating that children with brain damage do less well than those without on such screening tests, these tests are not sensitive to all forms of brain damage, and failure may have other explanations since complex performance is always multidetermined. Among children with learning disabilities, the validity of screening tests for differentiating those whose brain dysfunction or inefficiency is not demonstrable by neurologic testing and who are thus labeled "developmentally" disabled, from those with a documentable brain lesion is seriously questioned.

NEUROPSYCHOLOGIC TESTING OF CHILDREN WITH BRAIN DYSFUNCTION

Since focal brain lesions affect many aspects of behavior discretely, psychologic tests can be used as a more sensitive way of probing for brain dysfunction than the clinical techniques used by neurologists. In fact, neuropsychology grew out of attempts by physicians to study patients with brain lesions (44).

This use of psychologic tests is clearly different from their use to measure cognitive competence or intelligence. The children have already been identified as neurologically impaired by various symptoms and by screening procedures, for example, a medical evaluation, poor development of language, failure to learn to read, or motor clumsiness. The purposes of testing are (a) to provide a detailed inventory of what it is that the child can and cannot do, in order to arrive at a precise and tailor-made prescription for remediation, and (b) to attempt to diagnose the location and, perhaps, the nature of the underlying brain dysfunction responsible for his symptoms. One is no longer probing the relative efficiency of a normal brain but attempting to define areas of strength and dysfunction in a child who is known or assumed to have a pathologic nervous system. Two types of neuropsychologic tests will be discussed: clinical tests and formal tests.

Neuropsychologic Investigation of Deficient Performance

Clinical Neuropsychologic Tests

Clinical neuropsychologic tests are ad hoc procedures that resemble those used by neurologists for diagnosis. Their role is to define a deficit whose presence is suggested by other findings in the examination. For instance, the neuropsychologist who suspects frontoparietal dysfunction may want to know whether the patient can name objects, bisect a line, sort cards, draw the face of a clock, or recognize his right side from his left. In this type of test, the administration and scoring are rarely standardized, but the patient's performance is usually easily distinguished from that of normal subjects. Although some tests of this type yield numerical scores, many do not.

Most aphasia batteries (556), tests for nondominant hemispheric and frontal lobe dysfunction, for apraxia, neglect, and cross-modal coordination, and other special purpose tests are of the ad hoc type (49,215,271,369,378,604). New tests are continually being developed by investigators of higher cerebral functions. Specialized tests of verbal memory (86,611) and tests to probe the function of a single hemisphere such as the tachistoscopic presentation of stimuli to a single visual field or the delivery of competing acoustic stimuli to the two ears (dichotic stimulation) fall into this category (164,216,329). This type of test may yield data that are of crucial diagnostic importance for illuminating the location and severity of the pathology responsible for the patient's deficit.

Formal Neuropsychologic Tests

A second approach to neuropsychologic testing is to start with one of the well standardized intelligence batteries mentioned earlier (e.g., 279,398,612,613). Instead of ending with a summary score or full-scale IQ that reflects the weighted mean of scores on verbal and performance subtests, the neuropsychologist will scrutinize the scores on each of the subtests to highlight areas of deficit. He will then choose other subtests or specialized instruments in order to delineate as closely as possible what it is the child cannot do. These data can guide the choice of educational approaches (390). The neuropsychologist's ultimate goal is to delineate specific syndromes of behavioral dysfunction which will enable him or her to make hypotheses about underlying derangements in cerebral function.

In order to define cognitive skills required for performance, scores on test batteries have been submitted to factor and cluster analyses (282,285,583). Subtests that share substantial amounts of variance are assumed to call upon common skills which may be teased out by further examination of the demands made by these subtests. By expressing children's performance on subtests from different batteries with a common numerical scoring system, for instance standard scores or centiles, and by grouping correlated subtests, psychologists can use a common system of coordinates to plot each child's performance on a wide variety of instruments. The resulting profile is convenient for making visual comparisons across children and across tests. Wilson and coworkers (628,629) have pioneered the use of profile analysis to characterize the neuropsychologic deficits of preschool children with developmental language disorders and of school-age children with learning disabilities (Figs. 24 and 25). They have shown that children with ostensibly similar complaints, for instance, school failure, may have very different neuropsychologic profiles and, by implication, a different pathogenesis. Their findings are consonant with the findings of Mattis (389,391), Denckla (156), and Fisk and Rourke (195), discussed earlier, who delineated at least four discrete neuropsychologic syndromes among dyslexic children. Profile analysis highlights for the psychologist and educator a particular child's areas of deficit (e.g., visual memory, visual perceptual skills, sequencing, verbal fluency, naming). This information is required in complex cases in order to design an individualized educational program to meet the child's particular needs, as required by Public Law 94-142, the Education For All Handicapped Children Act (454). It can also be used to group children with similar difficulties for whom similar remedial approaches may be beneficial. This should increase the efficiency of remedial classes.

Tables 10 and 11 list the neuropsychologic batteries currently used by Wilson and coworkers (628,629 and personal communication) for preschool and school-age children with learning disabilities and other chronic neurologic syndromes. Note that for the older children, psychologic tests are supplemented by tests of scholastic

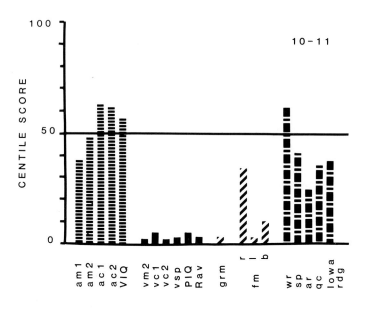

FACTORS :   AUDITORY   VISUAL   MOTOR   ACHVMT

FIG. 24. Neuropsychologic profile of an 11-year-old girl referred for testing because of increasing academic difficulty and behavior problems in school. She was born prematurely with a birth weight of 2,200 g and remained in an incubator for over 3 weeks. She required extra help in first grade but did learn to read. Behavior problems in third grade were attributed to "poor self-image, lack of confidence, and dependency." Psychotherapy was prescribed but did not improve matters. Family history positive for a father who had difficulty learning to read, a mother with visuomotor difficulties (both parents are college graduates), and a brother with a language deficit. Neurologic examination shows "soft signs." CT scan and EEG normal. Refer to Table 11 for the composition of the factors whose mean scores are depicted by the bars. On a centile scale, 50 represents average performance. The scale is not linear: scores one standard deviation from the mean fall at 16 and 84, two standard deviations from the mean at 2 and 98. The scale thus emphasizes differences in the middle range of performance and minimizes differences at the end of the scale. Nevertheless this display provides a convenient way to illustrate patterns of strengths and weaknesses across tasks. Note the marked discrepancy in this child's scores for tasks dependent on auditory processing and those dependent on visual processing, and between verbal and performance IQ scores. Note also deficient performance of the left hand compared to the right on the Purdue Pegboard Test (fm), a finding that strengthens the impression of right hemispheric dysfunction. Abbreviations: ac = auditory cognitive; achvmt = achievement tests; am = auditory memory; ar = written arithmetic; fm = fine motor (r = right hand, l = left hand, b = both hands together); grm = graphomotor; lowa rdg = lowa reading test; PIQ = Wechsler performance IQ; qc = quantitative concepts (oral arithmetic); Rav = Raven matrices; sp = spelling; vc = visual cognitive; VIQ = Wechsler verbal IQ; vm = visual memory; vsp = visual spatial; wr = word recognition. (Courtesy of B. C. Wilson.)

achievement. Not every test or subtest is used in every child but items appropriate to each child's deficit are selected.

Use of Neuropsychologic Testing to Define Brain Dysfunction

Less progress has been achieved toward this second goal of neuropsychologic testing in the pediatric age group than toward its use for delineating performance

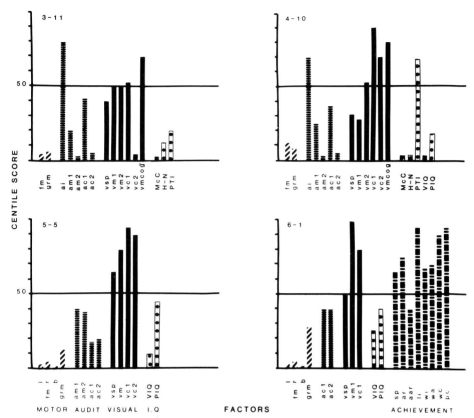

FIG. 25. Neuropsychologic profiles over time in a preschool boy with developmental language disability who has significant receptive problems. Past history, family history, and motor milestones unremarkable. Neurologic examination and EEG normal. Refer to Tables 10 and 11 for the composition of the factors whose means are depicted by the bars. Note generally lower scores for tests dependent on acoustic processing than those dependent on visual processing and the variability of IQ scores depending on the test chosen. The shape of the profile remains relatively stable over time with some variations. Abbreviations: aar = acoustic arithmetic; ac = auditory cognitive; ai = acoustic integration; am = acoustic memory; fm = fine motor (l = left hand, r = right hand, b = both hands together); grm = graphomotor; H-N = Hiskey-Nebraska; li = letter identification; McC = McCarthy; pc = passage comprehension; PIQ = Wechsler performance IQ; PTI = Pictorial Test of Intelligence; sp = spelling; vc = visual cognitive; VIQ = Wechsler verbal IQ; vm = visual memory; vm cog = visual motor cognitive; vsp = visual spatial; wa = word attack; wc = word comprehension; wi = word identification. (Courtesy of B. C. Wilson.)

deficits. As mentioned earlier, there is every reason to believe that the fundamental organization of children's brains is similar to that of adults. Consequently, similar lesions should have similar consequences, with the possible qualification that plasticity of cerebral organization is greater in childhood, and that recovery of function on the basis of the use of alternate strategies and of anatomic reorganization in undamaged portions of the brain is more efficient than in adults (192,558). Indeed, profiles of dysfunction observed in children with known brain lesions parallel those

TABLE 10. *Tentative neuropsychologic battery for profile analysis in preschoolers[a,c]*

Name of Factor	Subtest	Test	Source
Fine Motor	Right hand, left hand, both hands	Purdue Pegboard	Wilson, et al. (625)
Graphomotor	Geometric Design	WPPSI[b]	Wechsler (613)
	Draw a Design	McCarthy Scale	McCarthy (398)
Acoustic Integration	Auditory Closure	ITPA[b]	Kirk, et al. (322)
	Sound Blending	ITPA	Kirk, et al. (322)
Auditory Memory	Verbal Memory 1	McCarthy Scale	McCarthy (398)
	Verbal Memory 2	McCarthy Scale	McCarhty (398)
	Verbal Fluency	McCarthy Scale	McCarthy (398)
	Number Questions	McCarthy Scale	McCarhty (398)
Auditory Cognitive	Auditory Association	ITPA	Kirk, et al. (322)
	Opposite Analogies	McCarthy Scale	McCarthy (398)
Auditory-Visual Cognitive	Size and Number	McCarthy Scale	McCarthy (398)
	Counting and Sorting	McCarthy Scale	McCarthy (398)
	Grammatic Closure	ITPA	Kirk, et al. (322)
	Picture Vocabulary	Pictorial Test of Intelligence	French (202)
	Information Comprehension	Pictorial Test of Intelligence	French (202)
Visual-Motor Cognitive	Manual Expression	ITPA	Kirk, et al. (322)
Visual Spatial	Puzzle Solving	McCarthy Scale	McCarthy (398)
	Block Building	McCarthy Scale	McCarthy (398)
	Block Patterns	Hiskey-Nebraska Test	Hiskey (279)
	Drawing Completion	Hiskey-Nebraska Test	Hiskey (279)
Visual Memory 1	Memory for Color	Hiskey-Nebraska Test	Hiskey (279)
	Visual Memory	ITPA	Kirk, et al. (322)
	Immediate Recall	Pictorial Test of Intelligence	French (202)
Visual Memory 2	Visual Attention Span	Hiskey-Nebraska Test	Hiskey (279)
Visual Cognitive 1	Form Discrimination	Pictorial Test of Intelligence	French (202)
	Picture Identification	Hiskey-Nebraska Test	Hiskey (279)
Visual Cognitive 2	Picture Association	Hiskey-Nebraska Test	Hiskey (279)
	Visual Association	ITPA	Kirk, et al. (322)

[a]Indentification of neuropsychologic factors and the choice of subtests composing them were arrived at on the basis of repeated factor and cluster analysis of test results in normal and developmentally delayed children. Subtests that did not provide substantial variance or whose contribution was redundant were excluded after preliminary analyses. Definitive choice of subtests is pending the testing of a larger number of children.

[b]Abbreviations: ITPA = Illinois Test of Psycholinguistic Abilities; WPPSI = Wechsler Preschool and Primary Scale of Intelligence.

[c]Adapted from data provided by B. C. Wilson and J. J. Wilson *(personal communication)*, and from data in Wilson, Wilson, and Davidovicz, ref. 629.

of adults; profiles of dysfunction in children with developmental neurologic syndromes, like specific learning disabilities (MBD), whose anatomic basis is unknown also resemble them (629). Is it not likely that the child with MBD whose profile is similar to the profiles of children with overt pathology may be suffering from dysfunction in corresponding systems?

One should not assume that there is complete agreement among neuropsychologists as to the localization of lesions responsible for particular syndromes of dysfunction (308). Nevertheless, anterior lesions are likely to interfere with the execution of motor programs, and posterior lesions with perceptual tasks. In most persons, left hemispheric lesions impair linguistic and sequencing skills and right posterior lesions the performance of visual-spatial tasks. Right temporal lesions interfere with visual learning and the recognition of melodies and faces, left temporal

TABLE 11. *Tentative neuropsychologic battery for profile analysis in school-age children[a,c]*

Name of Factor	Subtest	Test	Source
Fine Motor	Right hand, left hand, both hands	Purdue Pegboard	Gardner (209)
Graphomotor	Bender Gestalt Test		Koppitz (331)
	Bender Gestalt Test with BIP[b]	Canter BIP[b]	Adams (2)
Auditory Discrimination	- in quiet	GFW[b]	Goldman, et al.
	- with noisy background	GFW	(236)
Acoustic Integration	Sound Blending	ITPA[b]	Kirk, et al. (322)
	Auditory Closure	ITPA	
Auditory Cognitive 1	Vocabulary	WISC[b]	Wechsler (612)
	Information	WISC	
	Auditory Reception	ITPA	
Auditory Cognitive 2	Similarities	WISC	
	Comprehension	WISC	
	Auditory Association	ITPA	
Auditory Memory 1	Digit Span	WISC	
	Digit Span	NCCEA[b]	Spreen and Benton (556)
	Digit Span	ITPA	
Auditory Memory 2	Sentence Repetition	NCCEA	
	Paired Associates	Wechsler Memory Scale	Wechsler (611)
Auditory Memory 3	Token Test, part 4	Token Test	di Simoni (166)
Word Retrieval	Word Fluency	NCCEA	
	Word Fluency	McCarthy Scale	McCarthy (398)
Verbal IQ	Verbal Subtests	WISC	
Visual Spatial	Block Design	WISC	
	Object Assembly	WISC	
	Right-Left Orientation Test	Benton-Spreen Test	Benton and Spreen (49)
	Embedded Figures Test	Benton-Spreen Test	
	Block Patterns	Hiskey-Nebraska Test	Hiskey (279)
	Spatial Reasoning	Hiskey-Nebraska Test	
Visual Cognitive 1	Picture Completion	WISC	
	Picture Identification	Hiskey-Nebraska Test	
	Drawing Completion	Hiskey-Nebraska Test	
	Visual Reception	ITPA	
	Form Discrimination	Pictorial Test of Intelligence	French (202)
Visual Cognitive 2	Picture Arrangement	WISC	
	Picture Association	Hiskey-Nebraska	Hiskey (279)
	Picture Analogies	Hiskey-Nebraska	
	Visual Association	ITPA	
Visual Memory 1	Memory for Color	Hiskey-Nebraska	
	Visual Sequential Memory	ITPA	

TABLE 11. *(cont'd)*

Name of Factor	Subtest	Test	Source
Visual Memory 2	Visual Attention Span	Hiskey-Nebraska Test	
	Immediate Recall	Pictorial Test of Intelligence	
Auditory-Visual Cognitive	Grammatic Closure	ITPA	
	Picture Completion	WPPSI[b]	Wechsler (613)
	Picture Vocabulary	Pictorial Test of Intelligence	
	Information and Comprehension	Pictorial Test of Intelligence	
	Similarities	Pictorial Test of Intelligence	
Performance IQ	Performance Subtests	WISC	
Raven Score	Raven Coloured Progressive Matrices	Raven Coloured Progressive Matrices	Raven (497)
Achievement Measures	Word Recognition	WRAT[b]	Jastak and Jastak (298)
	Oral Reading	Gray Oral Reading Test	Gray (243)
	Spelling	WRAT	
	Quantitative Concepts (verbal arithmetic)	WISC	
	Written Arithmetic	WRAT	
	Letter Identification	WRMT[b]	Woodcock (644)
	Word Attack	WRMT	
	Word Identification	WRMT	
	Passage Comprehension	WRMT	

[a]Identification of neuropsychologic factors and the choice of subtests composing them were arrived at on the basis of repeated factor or whose contribution was redundant were excluded after preliminary analyses. Definitive choice of subtests is pending the testing of a larger number of children.

[b]Abbreviations: BIP = Background Interference Procedure; GFW = Goldman Fristoe Woodcock Test of Auditory Discrimination; ITPA = Illinois Test of Psycholinguistic Abilities; NCCEA = Neurosensory Center Comprehensive Examination for Aphasia; WISC = Wechsler Intelligence Scale for Children; WPPSI = Wechsler Preschool and Primary Test of Intelligence; WRAT = Wide Range Achievement Test; WRMT = Woodcock Reading Mastery Test.

[c]Adapted from data provided by B. C. Wilson and J. J. Wilson (personal communication).

lesions with verbal and sequential learning. Most complex tasks probably call for the transcallosally integrated activity of both hemispheres. For example, reciting a string of digits backwards requires verbal sequential skills and the ability to visualize symbols. Placing pegs in holes with both hands simultaneously (Purdue Pegboard) (209,493,625) calls for the coordination of motor programs originating in the frontal cortex of each of the hemispheres, but is also very sensitive to deficits in subcortical systems such as the basal ganglia, cerebellum, and spinal cord.

Up to the recent past, neuropsychologists were mostly concerned with delineating syndromes of dysfunction that reflected pathology in the cerebral cortex. These syndromes had as prominent features aphasias, agnosias, and apraxias. More recently, neuropsychologists working with adults have identified syndromes of neuropsychologic deficit pointing to pathology in subcortical systems (9). Typically these include alterations in mood and personality, impaired memory, defective ability to manipulate acquired knowledge, confusion, and slowness in processing information. These symptoms are seen in patients with diseases of the basal ganglia such as parkinsonism or Huntington's chorea, and in patients with midline tumors affecting the thalamus or limbic structures. Some of these symptoms resemble those of patients with prefrontal lesions who may be inappropriately euphoric, impulsive and boastful, or apathetic and lacking in initiative (271,378,480,604). This resemblance attests to the close connection between limbic structures and the orbital frontal lobe, and to their role in choosing among complex behavioral strategies (459). Neuropsychologic syndromes of subcortical dysfunction have not been well studied in children although it is widely assumed that the hyperkinetic syndrome may reflect dysfunction in subcortical catecholaminergic systems (316,536).

12

Methods of Investigation

Tools at the clinician's disposal to detect and characterize brain dysfunction and, in every case, to consider the possibility of a progressive illness or one in need of specific treatment, include the history, physical examination, ancillary investigations of the structure, physiology and chemistry of the brain, psychologic tests, and consultations. Converging information from independent sources greatly improves the reliability of a diagnosis, but physicians need to know which source is most likely to provide useful data in a given child.

ANAMNESTIC DATA

Hospital Records

Most historic data provide only circumstantial evidence concerning the cause of a child's dysfunction, because the information is usually retrospective and its reliability and relevance are difficult to assess unless hospital records are obtained. The reliability of hospital records themselves may be less than satisfactory since items that later prove to have been of crucial importance may not have been recorded. Nevertheless, good medical practice demands that birth records (both the mother's and the child's), records from clinics or physicians who followed the child, and particularly records of hospital admissions for illnesses which may have had encephalopathic implications be obtained. Even reliable records do not always clarify the relevance of a particular item in the history to the child's current problem: By no means are all small prematures or all children who required exchange transfusions for hyperbilirubinemia brain damaged. Nonetheless documentation of a difficult birth, eclampsia in the mother, or a severe febrile illness in infancy provides at least suggestive etiologic information when the child later develops seizures or a learning problem in school. There is ample evidence to indicate that the probability of brain dysfunction is greatly enhanced by many pathologic events of the pregnancy, delivery, and neonatal period (78,327,442). Even though statistics do not apply to the individual, historical evidence for an etiology can be accepted as presumptive. In some cases, a definite etiology will be found. Negative information, of course, does not rule out an encephalopathic episode which may have gone unrecognized or unrecorded, or the severity of which may have been underestimated at the time.

Developmental Milestones

Developmental milestones such as age at smiling, sitting, walking, first words, speaking in sentences, and toilet training are revealing if accurate. Mothers who kept infant books should be encouraged to bring them, inasmuch as parental memory regarding particular milestones is likely to be unreliable, with the possible exception of age at walking (483). Grossly deviant milestones should be reported since they may be the only corroborative evidence for neurologic dysfunction going back to early life. Questions concerning social behavior and play may be equally enlightening (342). Data about sleep patterns, level of activity and organization, unusual habits such as head banging, tantrums, or destructiveness, and unusual swings in mood and affect are often highly informative. The Denver Developmental Screening Test (199) is one of several useful devices to help physicians obtain a broad developmental history. Promising leads should be followed with more detailed questions.

Family History

The family history is just as important as the history of the child. For deficits with the high probability of a genetic etiology such as febrile seizures, hearing loss, reading disability, language disorders, or unexplained mental retardation, it is essential to draw up a family tree and to inquire about consanguinity. The physician can draw an adequate family tree of at least the immediate family as part of his routine history taking. When the child has an unusual facies or minor anomalies, or when the family history is very complex, he may need to request the help of a geneticist in order to clarify the diagnosis and to furnish data on recurrence risks.

PHYSICAL AND NEUROLOGIC EXAMINATION

Physical Examination

The physical examination may provide the major clue to the diagnosis of a genetic metabolic disease or intrauterine infection responsible for the child's neurological deficit (485,486). An unusual looking facies, organomegaly, and abnormalities in bones, joints, or skin may suggest a storage disease. Hair with an unusual texture or color, cataracts, cloudy corneas, optic atrophy, or retinal pathology mandate detailed investigation since these signs are not typical of children with routine static encephalopathies. Depigmented macules, adenoma sebaceum, and chagrin spots are pathognomonic of tuberous sclerosis, multiple café au lait spots of neurofibromatosis, while hemangiomas suggest other neurocutaneous syndromes.

Neurologic Examination

The findings on neurologic examination encompass changes in head circumference, motility, motor coordination, visual acuity, eye movements, the retina, speech and language, and mental status (247,464,587). Again, the physician is seeking evidence that either will point to a particular syndrome or specific diagnosis known to be associated with brain pathology or dysfunction, or to the existence of a focal brain lesion. In discussing motor deficits, we mentioned the useful distinction made by Denckla (156,157), among others, between minor neurologic signs that would be abnormal at any age ("pastel classic" neurologic deficits that indicate focal brain dysfunction), and deviance that would be normal at an earlier age, the latter being likely, though not entirely reliable, evidence for a maturational lag rather than focal brain pathology (314). Finally, the medical evaluation of every child must include a screening evaluation of the *mental status*—alertness; orientation; interpersonal behavior; language; judgment; memory for digits, words, and sentences; vocabulary; information; and drawing—and of scholastic skills like reading, writing, and arithmetic.

At this point in the investigation, the physician should have a relatively clear idea of the child's level of functioning, of the probability of detecting a specific deficit in brain function, and of the need for further tests and/or consultations with other specialists such as a neurologist, geneticist, neuropsychologist, audiologist, speech and language pathologist, or psychiatrist. A medical evaluation that is adequately comprehensive will greatly decrease the need for multiple and expensive consultations or for an often time-consuming multidisciplinary evaluation which, ideally, should be reserved for complex cases. In the majority of children with learning disabilities, careful medical evaluation by an experienced physician, coupled with the testing provided by the school, may be sufficient to arrive at a diagnosis and to make recommendations regarding class placement. Special education is the backbone of management, with medication and counseling as adjuncts.

LABORATORY TESTS

The purpose of laboratory tests is (a) to clarify the diagnosis, hopefully by specifying the etiology of the child's illness, (b) to exclude a condition in need of a specific therapy, or (c) to illuminate the pathogenesis of the child's symptoms. The choice of tests to be performed will depend on the historical data and findings on examination. As always, the physician must keep in mind the possibility that the child's symptoms signal the start of a progressive illness. Among progressive illnesses that may present insidiously with learning disability, the physician needs to consider genetic-metabolic conditions (486), hydrocephalus, a slow virus infection such as SSPE or subacute rubella encephalitis, and, remotely, a neoplasm. How vigorously the physician will pursue such diagnoses will depend on the strength of his suspicion after he has taken a history and examined the child.

Screening Tests for Metabolic Errors

Screening tests for metabolic errors have a low yield in children with seizures, mild mental deficiency, learning disability, and behavior disorders. Nevertheless, because of the implications of metabolic illness for genetic counseling and the low cost and ready availability of screening tests for inborn errors of amino acid and carbohydrate metabolism, these should be obtained in children with unexplained developmental delay, especially if it is severe (Table 12). Enzyme tests for lysosomal deficiencies on white blood cells or skin fibroblasts grown in tissue culture are expensive and time consuming; they should be reserved for children in whom there is a high index of suspicion on genetic or clinical grounds. The obvious importance of detecting metabolic errors is that a few are treatable; for example, some of the acute amino acidurias and organic acidurias of infancy, lead poisoning in preschool children (440), and, in school age children and adolescents, Wilson's disease, which may present as clumsiness, slurred speech, bizarre behavior, or a school problem. Wilson's disease is eminently treatable so that having a high index of suspicion for it is appropriate.

Chromosome Studies

Chromosome studies are clearly indicated in children with atypical facial features or multiple congenital anomalies. Their yield has increased dramatically with modern banding techniques (401), but remains low in unstigmatized children. Most genetic conditions inherited as single mendelian traits are not detected by chromosome analysis but may be suspected on clinical grounds (400,545). One exception is a recently described X-linked mental deficiency syndrome with speech deficit called the fragile-X syndrome (402,590).

Titers for Intrauterine Infections

Titers for intrauterine infections such as toxoplasmosis, cytomegalovirus, herpes simplex, syphilis, and rubella provide corroborative evidence when the clinical picture suggests the diagnosis. Rubella titers are useless in children who received the rubella vaccine, and the usefulness of all of these titers decreases with age since many asymptomatic individuals can be shown to have had an acquired inapparent infection.

Radiologic Examination

Radiologic examinations include plain X-rays of the skull and computerized transaxial tomography scanning (CT scan). *Skull X-rays* are cheaper than CT scans and do not require the sedation needed to obtain adequate CT scans. They allow the detection of skull asymmetries, for instance, thickening and smallness of the skull overlying an atrophic hemisphere, of the deformities caused by premature closure of sutures (craniosynostosis), or the intracranial calcifications of tuberous sclerosis (239) and intrauterine infections such as toxoplasmosis and cytomegalo-

TABLE 12. *Tests for genetic-metabolic diseases*

Test	Purpose
Automated blood chemistries (SMA 6, 12), blood gases, serum ammonia, etc.	Screening for a variety of metabolic diseases and dysfunctions.
Urine tests	Metabolic screening for elevated excretion of amino acids, carbohydrates, mucopolysaccharides, porphyrins, etc.
Quantitative assays in blood or urine by gas-liquid chromatography, mass-spectroscopy	Measurement of amounts of amino acids, carbohydrates, organic acids, and other metabolites.
Spinal fluid examination (protein, cells, immunoglobulins, etc.)	Screening for certain illnesses (eg., leukodystrophies, demyelinating illnesses).
Measurement of heavy metal content in blood, urine, liver, or hair	Copper: Wilson's disease, copper malabsorption syndrome. Lead poisoning, other intoxications.
Electromyography, nerve conduction velocity	Screening for peripheral neuropathy (some leucodystrophies), and involvement of muscle or anterior horn cells.
Evoked responses, electroretinography	Screening for some diseases that affect electrophysiology (e.g., some storage diseases).
CT scans	Detection of areas of increased or decreased density, of brain atrophy, etc.
Microscopic examination of white blood cells, skin, bone marrow	Screening for certain storage diseases.
Chromosome analysis in white cells	Detect a trisomy (extra chromosome), translocation (piece of one chromosome attached to another), or deletion (missing chromosome or piece of chromosome). Most useful in children with unexplained mental deficiency and multiple anomalies.
Enzymatic assays in white cells, cultured skin fibroblasts, liver, muscle, other tissue, or amniotic cells	Definitive diagnosis of genetic diseases whose biochemical basis is understood. Used in prenatal diagnosis.
Brain biopsy	Very rarely indicated, only after all other tests have failed to yield a diagnosis.

virus. They may be informative when the skull is too large, too small, or deformed. With the advent of CT scanning, however, the indications for skull X-rays have become very limited since they rarely yield enough information to arrive at a specific diagnosis.

CT scanning (1,297) is a powerful technique because it provides images of the brain without the need for the injection of air into the spinal fluid pathways or the intraarterial injection of dye (intravenous injection of contrast material is used when it is important to visualize the cerebral vascular tree). CT scanning has replaced pneumoencephalography and ventriculography, which were invasive procedures that carried a definite risk and required hospitalization. Cerebral angiography is still needed in some cases of vascular disease and to confirm some surgical lesions detected by CT, but today it is almost never required for children in whom static brain lesions are suspected. Radionucleide brain scanning, which even earlier had very limited usefulness in children suspected of static brain damage, is no longer indicated except under very unusual circumstances.

CT scanning is the procedure of choice to help decide whether a child with an unusual pattern of head growth is suffering from hydrocephalus or megalencephaly (Fig. 26). CT scanning discloses focal or generalized brain atrophy, structural developmental anomalies of the brain, tumors, and other brain lesions like abscesses, arteriovenous malformations, extradural and subdural collections, hemorrhages, infarctions, acute posttraumatic cerebral contusions and brain swelling, acute plaques

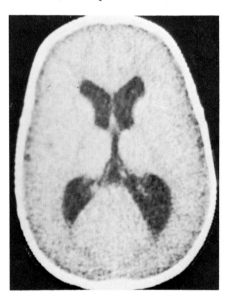 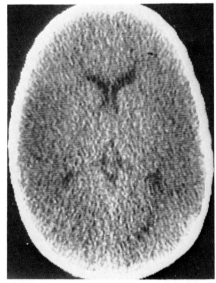

FIG. 26. CT scans in two infants with big heads. Black areas represent spaces filled with cerebrospinal fluid, gray areas brain, white areas bone; differences in texture of the CTs indicate that different scanners were used. The scan on the left shows dilated frontal and occipital horns of the lateral ventricles indicating hydrocephalus, while the one on the right shows small ventricles, denoting megalencephaly. (Courtesy of A. Danziger.)

of demyelination, the reduced density of the white matter characteristic of some leukodystrophies, intracranial calcifications, cysts, and other lesions visible to the naked eye (Fig. 27). It does not, of course, enable the detection of microscopic lesions.

One should not obtain a CT scan on every child with focal seizures or in whom the neurologic examination or neuropsychologic tests suggest a focal brain lesion. Nonetheless, it is occasionally helpful to document a static lesion and to exclude a progressive one. Its indiscriminate use in every retarded, learning disabled, cerebral palsied, or epileptic child is deplored because of the high cost and low yield of abnormalities requiring therapy or providing a definitive diagnosis.

The amount of radiation to the head to obtain a CT scan is small and there are no risks when contrast material is not used (contrast material is rarely required in children with static lesions), and when sedation is unnecessary. Therefore, CT scans are safe enough to be used for research purposes, for example, to try to validate focal deficits suggested by the EEG or pattern of neuropsychologic scores. In most, but not all, right-handed persons without neuropsychologic deficit, the posterior portion of the left hemisphere is wider than the right (206) (see Fig. 1D). This asymmetry is lacking in some persons with developmental language disorders, including autism, or with reading disability (206,277), although the significance of departure from the usual pattern is difficult to interpret in the individual case.

Positron Emission Tomography, Cerebral Blood Flow, and Nuclear Magnetic Resonance

PET (336,465) consists of computerized imaging of the relative brain uptake of positron emitting isotopes incorporated into metabolites, antimetabolites, or drugs. Upon injection of these compounds, one can visualize areas with increased or decreased metabolic activity in a pathway involving the compound, for example, glycolysis. This approach to studying focal changes in cerebral metabolism coupled with the performance of specific behavioral tasks has great potential but is still in the realm of research and will probably find limited application in children who do not have a serious neurologic condition. The same statement can be made for the measurement of cerebral blood flow by the inhalation of radioactive inert gases like xenon (343,346). As stated earlier, this technique has provided stunning confirmation of inferences about localization of brain function that were based on neuropsychologic test patterns in patients with known cerebral lesions. Nuclear magnetic resonance is a technique based on the use of nonradioactive compounds whose metabolic fate can be mapped by imaging (386). It is only at the stage of development but it may largely replace X-ray and radioisotope methods of brain imaging in the future.

Electroencephalogram

The most widely used and informative test of neurophysiologic function is the EEG. It is important to stress that the EEG is not a test for brain damage but rather

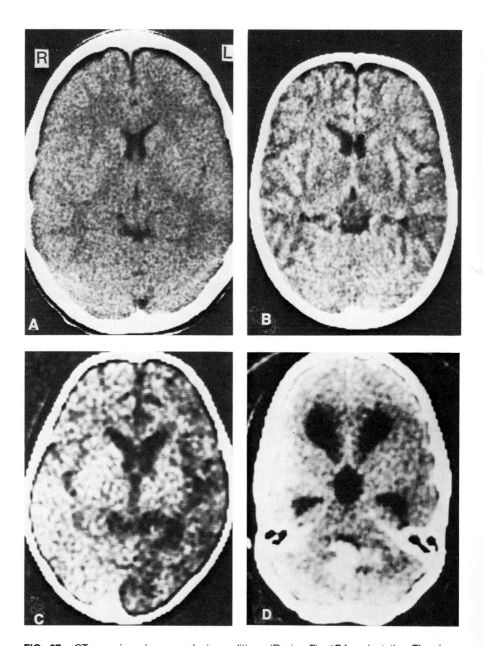

FIG. 27. CT scans in various neurologic conditions. (Review Fig. 1E for orientation. The plane of each CT cut is close to but not exactly that of the anatomic brain slice and varies somewhat across patients. Differences in texture of the CTs indicate that different scanners were used.) **(A)** Normal CT in a 10-year-old boy. Note the generally higher density of gray than white matter. **(B)** CT in a one-year-old retarded boy showing pathologically decreased density of the white matter. Biopsy showed spongy degeneration of the brain (Canavan disease). **(C)** CT in a child with a right sided infantile hemiparesis. Note diffusely decreased density of much of the left hemisphere (right side of the picture) with slight enlargement of the lateral ventricle. **(D)** CT in a young child with a dense midline cerebellar tumor mass (irregular white areas in the back of the head) compressing the fourth ventricle (and aqueduct) and producing acute hydrocephalus with dilatation of the third as well as the lateral ventricles.

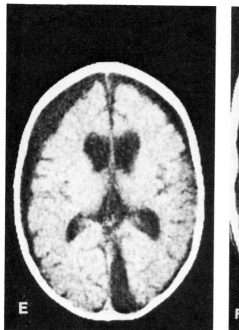 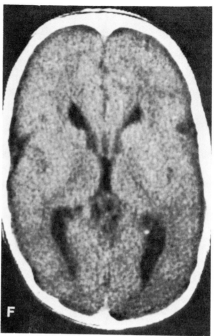

FIG. 27. *(continued)* **(E)** CT in an infant who was resuscitated following a cardiac arrest three months earlier. Ventricular enlargement and marked widening of the subarachnoid spaces denote brain shrinkage or hydrocephalus *ex vacuo*. The dark area to the left of the midline in the back of the head reflects left occipital destruction due to compression of the posterior cerebral artery by the herniated uncus of the hippocampus; this suggests that the original insult produced brain swelling and raised intracranial pressure. **(F)** CT scan in an 8-year-old profoundly retarded boy with a grossly enlarged head since infancy and in whom no diagnosis has been made. There is mild hydrocephalus *ex vacuo* and megalencephaly with probable dysgenesis.(Courtesy of A. Danziger.)

for electrophysiologic dysfunction. Its information value in children with learning disability who do not have seizures is low. Non-neurologists need to be aware that there are pitfalls in the interpretation of children's EEG records. The interpretation of children's EEGs is more difficult than that of adult records because EEG patterns change dramatically with age. There is a tendency for some neurologists who are not highly trained in reading children's EEG records to overinterpret them (234). For example, EEG reports often state that the EEG is somewhat too slow for the child's age: This does not provide reliable evidence for either immaturity or brain damage since mild slowing is present in a sizable proportion of normal children. Normal children's EEGs contain a variety of patterns, such as asymmetries, temporal slow waves, and even some sharp waves that are not seen in adult records and have little if any clinical significance. Some small children require sedation to be testable. EEG patterns are altered by drowsiness and sleep: Paroxymal slowing in drowsiness and vertex sharp waves in sleep should not be mistaken for seizure discharges.

Because of inadequate sampling, short records are unreliable at all ages but especially so in children. Finally, the technical quality of records obtained in doctors' offices is unpredictable and occasionally substandard according to established criteria of evaluation.

In children suspected of brain dysfunction, the EEG is most useful for detecting unsuspected seizure discharges. As discussed in Chapter 4, convulsive disorders, even those not associated with an acute metabolic derangement, do not necessarily denote brain pathology, however. This is notably the case of febrile seizures (441), of classic petit mal (103,412), and of some focal seizures, especially those affecting the face in sleep that are associated with Rolandic or midtemporal spikes (353). Unexpected temporal lobe foci in children with intermittent behavior abnormalities (470), and more particularly bilateral paroxysmal discharges in some children with receptive language disorders (492), autistic features, or unexplained mental deficiency suggest that an EEG be obtained in children with these symptoms. A severe EEG abnormality of this type calls for a trial of anticonvulsants even if clinical seizures have not been recognized. Almost continuous spike-and-wave activity is occasionally seen in children with ataxia (40,75), and in others whose dullness reflects clouding of consciousness (absence stupor) rather than severe retardation or autistic behavior (14,75). Appropriate anticonvulsant medication may improve such children's behavior dramatically.

Specialized electrophysiologic techniques may be helpful in particular cases. EEG monitoring during a whole night of sleep has occasionally enabled the diagnosis of a specific sleep-associated disorder with daytime dullness such as sleep apnea, sleep walking, or nocturnal seizures (249). Telemetering the EEG enables the child to move around and is useful in cases where one is seeking to correlate an unexplained behavior with a possible seizure disorder (55,296).

Averaged Evoked Responses

Averaged evoked responses to sound, light, and somatosensory stimulation have their place in the evaluation of handicapped children with delayed language, visual impairment, in certain diffuse encephalopathies such as hypsarrhythmia, in children with autistic behavior, and in those whose hearing cannot be tested reliably because of their age or inability to cooperate with standardized behavioral techniques. Brain stem evoked responses have become the method of choice for audiometry in early childhood (438). Sophisticated electrophysiologic measures reflecting perception and decision-making may eventually provide powerful tools for understanding the neurophysiologic basis of complex behaviors (90,161,278). Statistical computer analyses of EEG and evoked response records [neurometrics, brain electrical activity mapping (BEAM)] (23,173,174) are new approaches whose clinical usefulness in the individual child is not well validated at this time. Therefore, these procedures must still be considered research techniques. Their future appears bright, especially when combined with special neuropsychologic techniques such as dichotic auditory stimulation (52,291,329), tachistoscopic stimulation of half of the visual field, and reaction time, to name a few (164,216,418,652).

PSYCHOLOGIC AND NEUROPSYCHOLOGIC TESTING

To reiterate what was said in Chapter 11, general intelligence is a construct of limited validity in the face of focal brain dysfunction. The purpose of psychologic testing is therefore not to measure the IQ, which is a meaningless summary score in the face of substantial subtest variability since it reflects neither the areas of competence nor those of incompetence; its foremost purpose is to delineate functional areas of strength and deficit in order to prescribe appropriate remedial education. By so doing, it may also be possible to group children with similar deficits into syndromes that provide insight into underlying pathogenetic mechanisms. Validation of hypotheses about the presumed location and severity of brain dysfunction responsible for particular clusters of symptoms may thereby be facilitated.

In the United States today, virtually every child's achievement is assessed periodically in school, usually through the use of standardized group pen-and-pencil tests. Ideally, children who fail should be referred for individual testing, as should children whose behavior causes concern. School psychologists are more sophisticated in their use of test results and are less likely than in the past to be satisfied with the IQ as a sufficient measure for deciding on class placement and remediation. Other professionals too are less prompt to assume that the IQ is immutable and are more aware of its limitations for predictive purposes.

Middle-class children with delayed language acquisition, clumsiness, and school failure rarely go unnoticed, in fact, they are often overdiagnosed and overtested. The child whose need is more likely to be unmet is the quiet child from a deprived family whose problems, if they are noticed, are ascribed to his social environment, especially if his family is non-English speaking. Low achievers with behavior disorders may also go unreferred unless it is realized that their behavior problems may not be the cause of their inadequate scholastic performance; rather both behavioral and learning problems may reflect underlying brain dysfunction, or the behavior problems may be a reaction to the social consequences of poor achievement caused by a learning disability. Still another group of children who may not be referred for testing but who would profit greatly from it are intelligent learning disabled youngsters whose deficit goes unrecognized because the child has managed, somehow, to compensate for it, often at the cost of considerable effort, frustration, and low self-esteem. Exceedingly poor spelling, slow reading, math failure, or unexplained behavior problems in a patently bright child should be considered clear indications for referral to the psychologist.

Physicians, as well as school professionals, refer children for testing. They need to know enough about psychologic tests so as to be able to evaluate test results and the appropriateness of the instruments chosen for a particular child, and so as to have some idea of the probable validity of the psychologist's interpretation of the results (373). Physicians who received training in child development and in assessing handicapped children and those with learning disabilities will want to ask the psychologist for subtest scores as well as summary scores in order to scan the child's performance themselves. They will know that a test like the Stanford-Binet (576) or Peabody Picture Vocabulary Test (175) is inappropriate for a child with a language deficit. They will look for discrepancies between verbal and performance IQ scores and for subtest scatter on the Wechsler scales. They will be aware that the Leiter Test (349), a nonverbal test recommended for use in deaf, language-disordered, and culturally deprived children, requires the manipulation of small blocks and may penalize clumsy children and those with apraxia or visual-spatial deficits. In other words, such well informed physicians are capable of looking at the results of psychologic testing with a neuropsychologic eye. The idea is not to make psychologists out of physicians but to make them informed consumers of the data provided by psychologists, and enable them to integrate these data with their own medical and historical data. This will allow them to discuss test results intelligently with the psychologist so that they can offer a useful interpretation to the parents who are bound to consult their physician about the tests and about the appropriateness of recommendations for school placement or of referrals for further consultation or therapy.

CONSULTATIONS

The need for certain consultations is obvious: *Orthopedic* consultation for the child with contractures, scoliosis, or limb deformity; consultation with a *physiatrist* when braces, wheel chairs, or exercises are required; consultation with an *otologist* when a hearing loss is suspected; or with an *ophthalmologist* when the child has a strabismus or does not appear to see well, or when retinal pathology was suspected on ophthalmoscopy. Discussion is limited here to indications for consultation with child neurologists, developmental pediatricians, clinical geneticists, and child psychiatrists, and for referral to a multidisciplinary facility for comprehensive evaluation.

Child Neurologist

The child neurologist will be most helpful in cases in which there are doubts concerning the static or progressive nature of the child's neurologic condition. Typically, the neurologist attempts to make a specific diagnosis rather than be satisfied with an inventory of the child's deficits. He will usually have definite ideas concerning the need for an EEG, CT scan, or tests for metabolic diseases. He can help decide whether or not the child is having an unusual seizure disorder that might account for part or all of his aberrant behaviors. Because of their neuropsychologic training, many child neurologists will provide a useful consultation when test results raise the question of focal brain dysfunction despite the absence of "hard" neurologic findings, a history of seizures, or an acquired encephalopathy. Some child neurologists are very knowledgeable about language disorders and what to do for children with autistic behavior. Many child neurologists will be well informed about specialized school placements and remedial tutorial resources in their community. All child neurologists will be familiar with the use of anticonvulsants, cerebral stimulants, and tranquilizers. Child neurologists, like developmental pediatricians, may be members of multidisciplinary teams that evaluate and manage handicapped children and may serve in a consulting role to school systems. Physicians who function in such teams are likely to take a broad view of the consequences, for the child and his whole family, of mental deficiency, motor and sensory handicaps, and behavior problems, and to make suggestions that encompass social and educational as well as strictly medical manipulations.

Developmental Pediatrician

The competencies of the child neurologist and the pediatrician with special training in child development and in the care of handicapped children (developmental pediatrician) have large areas of overlap. Both are likely to carry out similar examinations and to make similar recommendations for the evaluation and management of children with cerebral palsy, learning disorders, mental retardation, and other nonprogressive neurologic conditions. Differences are not so much in clinical approach as in point of view: The developmental pediatrician's main concern is to mitigate the impact of the child's handicap, while the child neurologist will, in addition, attempt to diagnose the illness or type of brain dysfunction responsible for the handicap. Many child neurologists are oriented primarily toward the care of acute neurologic emergencies and the diagnosis of rare diseases, and may be less eager than developmental pediatricians to manage static conditions. The developmental pediatrician's training stresses routine interaction with nonmedical professionals. He is likely to know more than some child neurologists about modes of physical and occupational therapy, speech and language therapy, infant stimulation programs, and other educational resources in the community. He will be well informed about psychologic testing but may not be as familiar as the neurologist with the goals of neuropsychologic testing. In truth, when it comes to the care of statically handicapped children the choice of consultation with a child neurologist or a developmental pediatrician is largely one of availability.

Clinical Geneticist

Clinical geneticists are particularly helpful when the child has an unusual appearance or several minor abnormal physical features ("stigmata"). In such cases geneticists are often able to identify a particular syndrome (400,545). They will draw up detailed family trees and, in suitable cases, obtain dermatoglyphics, chromosome studies, and appropriate tests to screen for metabolic conditions in the child, in other family members, or in unborn siblings by amniocentesis. They will counsel families regarding recurrence risks. Most physicians should be able to provide genetic counseling themselves when the definite diagnosis of a disease caused by a single mendelian trait has been made. When the genetics are unclear, for example, in sporadic malformations such as spinal tube defects that are probably multidetermined, geneticists are likely to be much more knowledgeable than the average physician about recurrence risks. Geneticists also tend to have given a lot of thought to the ethical implications of amniocentesis and genetic counseling; this may be of great help to the families of handicapped children.

Child Psychiatrist

In the days when the Freudian influence dominated American psychiatry, child psychiatrists were reluctant to get involved with children suffering from organic brain dysfunction, mental retardation, or other serious handicaps because such children were felt to be poor candidates for psychotherapy. The emergence of liaison-psychiatry in pediatric departments and the availability of more effective psychotropic drugs have changed this attitude. It is now common for psychiatrists to belong to multidisciplinary teams that evaluate handicapped children. They help parents gain insight into their reactions to having a handicapped child; this is often beneficial to all family members. In the case of intelligent children with low self-esteem because of a learning disability or other handicap, the psychiatrist may work with the child himself or refer him to a social worker or psychologist for play therapy or counseling. Child psychiatrists provide invaluable consultations when other physicians have difficulty deciding whether a child's behavior is but a facet of his neurologic defect, the reflection of a psychosis, or a behavioral reaction to his awareness of his handicap. They often make very useful suggestions regarding the handling of children with difficult behavior. Psychiatrists manage their share of children with learning disabilities and ADD since patterns of referral to them, to psychologists, to child neurologists, to developmental pediatricians, and to multidisciplinary clinics overlap.

The Multidisciplinary Clinic

The greatest advantage of the multidisciplinary clinic is that it provides almost all needed consultations in one place. If the clinic works efficiently, evaluation of a child may be expedited, provided there is flexibility built into the system and provided an experienced member of the team screens the child at intake to determine which of the services he will need. Appointments need to be given promptly and kept by the family. Ensuring that this happens requires close monitoring and well-organized clerical systems. The collecting of information from outside sources and the collating of new information provided by the team must be done expeditiously so that the team can discuss the case, relay its recommendations to the family, and make the appropriate referrals for educational placement, special therapies, or medication without undue delay. The key to a successful multidisciplinary clinic is the effectiveness of its data management and communication systems.

Multidisciplinary clinics, in addition to the services of physicians, psychologists, speech and language pathologists, and physical and occupational therapists, can supply the invaluable input of social workers, educational consultants, and specialists in infant development—professionals who are rarely available in other medical settings. Since the clinics provide the opportunity for the viewpoint of various specialists to be shared and integrated, the care received by children who go through them is often of high quality.

They do have drawbacks, however, chiefly their cost, the delay they almost inevitably introduce before a referral for management can be made, and the possibility that the child will become lost in the shuffle. These drawbacks become very serious when less than adequate management practices are used and when children are accepted unselectively, depriving those children who need the services of the clinic the most. The importance of adequate screening, flexibility, close monitoring to minimize burdensome and expensive redundancies, and effective communication with parents is clear. Ideally, each child should get just what he needs and no more. The problem is that it is often difficult to predict what the child will need until he has been evaluated.

A final problem with multidisciplinary clinics is that their role may be ambiguous. While their primary mission is to evaluate handicapped children, manage some aspects of their care, and refer them to appropriate agencies in the community for other aspects of care, they often have the additional mission of educating students, physicians, and other professionals. Unless carefully supervised, this second mission often increases the inefficiency of the clinic and the cost of an evaluation to the patient or the community, and threatens the efficiency with which test results and recommendations are communicated to the child's family and other interested parties.

13

Management

The goals of management are harmonious development, optimal use of available sensorimotor, emotional, and intellectual assets, and socially acceptable behavior. Available tools include pharmacologic agents, surgery, manipulation of the environment, counseling and psychotherapy, and remedial education, not to mention physical, speech and language, and other specialized therapies not considered here. These measures are aimed at diminishing hyperactivity and distractibility, alleviating emotional disturbances and preventing the development of additional ones, and compensating for perceptual and learning disabilities.

The role of the physician is not limited to making a diagnosis, prescribing drugs, and referring the child to an appropriate school or remedial program. He must follow the child and his family long-term so that he is aware of new problems that emerge as the child matures and can alter management appropriately.

DRUG, SURGICAL, AND DIETARY THERAPY

The most important applications of drug therapy in children with brain dysfunction are (a) seizures, (b) abnormal involuntary movements, and (c) hyperkinetic behavior, distractibility, and other behavior problems. We do not yet know enough about the neurochemistry of memory to prescribe drugs to improve learning or the retrieval of memories. As far as we know, any beneficial effect of drugs on cognitive abilities and scholastic achievement is indirect and long-term studies indicate that they are modest at best (29,557).

Anticonvulsant Drugs

Details regarding the use of anticonvulsants in seizure management are beyond the scope of this book and are readily available elsewhere (e.g., 99,365,445,461). A brief overview of the most commonly used anticonvulsants is provided in Table 13. A few general rules concerning their use follows:

a) If at all possible, use a single drug and monitor blood levels to ensure compliance and to avoid toxicity and discarding a drug as ineffective before therapeutic blood levels have been achieved.

TABLE 13. *Anticonvulsants in common use*

Drug	Usual dose (mg/kg/day)	Therapeutic level (μg/ml serum)	Main toxic side effects
Phenobarbital[a]	3–5	15–40	Drowsiness, hyperkinetic behavior
Phenytoin[a]	4–7	10–20	Rash, gum hypertophy, ataxia
Carbamazepine[a]	20–30	5–12	Gastric, bone marrow, liver
Primidone[a]	10–25	8–12[f]	Drowsiness, ataxia, behavior disorder, anemia
Ethosuximide[b]	20–30	40–100	Gastric, bone marrow
Valproic acid[b,c]	30–60	50–100	Gastric, liver, bone marrow
Clonazepam[b,d]	0.01–0.2	.013–.072	Drowsiness
Trimethadione[b]	10–25	—	Kidney, bone marrow
Diazepam[b,d,e]	0.3	—	Drowsiness

[a]Drugs for major motor, focal motor, and complex partial seizures.
[b]Drugs effective against minor seizures, especially petit mal absences.
[c]May make phenytoin levels go down and phenobarbital levels go up.
[d]Useful in infantile spasms and in some forms of myoclonus.
[e]Used intravenously as first drug in status epilepticus.
[f]Primidone also breaks down to phenobarbital.

b) Drugs like phenobarbital, phenytoin, primidone and carbamazepine that help major motor, focal motor, and complex partial (psychomotor) seizures may make petit mal absence seizures worse and vice versa. Drugs likely to help absence seizures include ethosuximide and other succinimides, valproic acid, and clonazepam. Trimethadione (Tridione®) is also helpful for absences, but is rarely used today because of bone marrow and kidney toxicity. In children with both generalized and petit mal seizures, it is usually necessary to use one drug from each category, although valproic acid may be sufficient to control both seizure types in some children.

c) Keep the number of anticonvulsants used in a patient down to no more than two if at all possible. Manipulate the dosage of one drug at a time, using blood levels as a guide, and do not change dosage too frequently so as to have an adequate time sample to observe therapeutic effects. Be aware of drug interactions (461) since adding a second drug may affect the blood levels of the first.

d) Be familiar with the pharmacokinetics of drugs in order to give adequate doses, especially in acute situations where a prompt effect is desired.

e) Do not quarrel with success, especially in a child whose seizures have been difficult to control. Whatever drug or combination of drugs in whatever dosage achieves the desired affect without toxicity or unacceptable side effects is the regimen to continue for that particular child.

f) Except under special circumstances, chronic seizure medication should not be stopped suddenly, lest sudden withdrawal of anticonvulsants precipitate a flurry of major seizures or status epilepticus.

g) Measures other than anticonvulsants that may be helpful in intractable convulsive disorders of infancy and early childhood include ACTH, steroids, and the ketogenic diet (365).

h) When seizures are intractable, reconsider their etiology, think of an undiagnosed metabolic illness or possibly a neoplasm.

i) Convulsive disorders are chronic conditions that require treatment for several years after seizure control has been achieved. A conservative rule is four years on medication seizure-free before attempting gradual withdrawal of anticonvulsants (182). Children who are seizure free but whose EEG remains highly abnormal and children whose seizures were very difficult to control are less likely to remain seizure-free off medication than children with less severe convulsive disorders.

In children with seizures, there is little evidence that anticonvulsants alter behavior or learning, provided blood levels are kept in the therapeutic range and the prescription of multiple drugs can be avoided. Large doses of anticonvulsants have sedative effects and thus interfere with learning. There is some experimental evidence in immature rats that high doses of phenobarbital reduced brain growth; low doses did not, but appeared to increase motor activity (163). Phenobarbital clearly worsens the behavior of some hyperkinetic children (347). When drugs with less sedative effects, like carbamazepine (Tegretol®), are substituted for phenobarbital, scholastic achievement has been reported to improve in some children (527). Unfortunately, carbamazepine has drawbacks, including cost and risk of toxicity. Since experience with relatively new anticonvulsants like carbamazepine and valproic acid (Depakene®) is much less extensive than with phenobarbital and phenytoin (Dilantin®), definite statements about their advantages must await further evaluation.

Rarely, prolonged ingestion of large doses of anticonvulsants, in particular phenytoin, results in a clinical picture resembling a dementia, occasionally complicated by dystonic movements and increased frequency of seizures (370). Reduction in dose or substitution of another drug may reverse the child's symptoms and improve cognitive performance.

The use of anticonvulsants in children who do not have clinical seizures but whose EEG contains paroxysmal features in the hope of improving cognitive efficiency is controversial. Anticonvulsants were stated earlier to be indicated in children whose grossly abnormal EEG includes very frequent or continuous spike-and-wave or slow spike-and-wave complexes, since their dullness or ataxia may reflect subclinical seizure activity (14,75). Anticonvulsants may be tried in autistic children or those with verbal auditory angosia who do not have clinical seizures but whose EEG contains paroxysmal features since bitemporal or limbic epileptic activity may contribute to their communication deficit (341,492). While a few patients may improve with drugs, in most the correlation between EEG and clinical state is weak. It would seem, unfortunately, that in most of these children both the paroxysmal discharges and the clinical symptoms are the common consequences of the cerebral dysfunction rather than the symptoms reflecting the recruitment of potentially normally functioning cortex by the epileptic activity.

Treatment of Motor Disorders

Physical and Occupational Therapy

Physical and occupational therapies aimed at strengthening and stretching muscles, improving posture and hand use, and preventing contractures are clearly helpful in children with significant motor disorders (64,170). Their use in clumsy children is more controversial. These therapies fall under the purview of physiatrists who prescribe them, as well as necessary braces and appliances.

Drug Therapy

Tourette or multiple tic syndrome (535), believed to result from an imbalance in neurotransmitters (perhaps increased dopamine activity in the basal ganglia) is associated with a learning disability in some children (375). Therapy is warranted if the tics are severe enough to render the child conspicuous and result in social ostracism, especially if vocal tics and coprolalia (swearing) are prominent. The most effective drug is haloperidol, a postsynaptic dopamine blocking agent. Haloperidol should be started in small doses (0.5 mg/day) and increased progressively until the tics are reduced to an acceptable level. The usual dose required is of the order of 3 to 5 mg/day, but some children may require and tolerate much larger doses. The dose should be titrated frequently, the goal being to administer the smallest dose that will produce the desired effect. If large doses are required, it may be necessary to add anticholinergic drugs like trihexyphenidyl (Artane®) or benztropine (Cogentin®) to prevent side effects which include dystonia, sometimes associated with buccolingual dyskinesia and oculogyric crises, or a parkinsonian-like syndrome. Acute reactions can be ameliorated rapidly with intravenous diphenhydramine (Benadryl®). Because haloperidol has very prolonged effects, diphenhydramine may have to be given orally for several days to prevent recurrences. Other drugs such as clonidine and pimozide are being tried on an experimental basis in Tourette syndrome, but there is a paucity of experience with their use.

There is no drug with a reliable effect to ameliorate *athetosis*, although carbamazepine at anticonvulsant doses (blood level 5 to 12 μ/ml) may be worth a trial. Its effect may be related to its stimulation of GABA receptors. *Dystonic syndromes* also respond poorly to drugs. The phenothiazines chlorpromazine and fluphenazine (Prolixin®), which are dopamine blockers, reduce the dystonia of some children, as does carbamazepine. Large doses of trihexyphenidyl and benztropine should also be tried. Some children's dystonia is made much worse by L-DOPA, while occasionally a child will improve with this drug. *Chorea* may also respond somewhat to the phenothiazines and perhaps to some cholinergic and gabergic agents (541). We have as yet no effective drug to reduce the *intention tremor* and ataxia of neocerebellar dysfunction. In some patients *postanoxic intention myoclonus* responds to the administration of 5-hydroxytryptophan and carbidopa (579). *Benign essential* tremor does respond to the β-adrenergic blocker propranolol, usually in large doses (up to 160 mg/day); it is not clear whether its peripheral or central action is beneficial in essential tremor. Although there are drugs on the market whose indication is the reduction of *spasticity*, for example, dantrolene (Dantrium®) and baclofen (Lioresal®), their effectiveness in children with spastic cerebral palsy is limited.

This brief and somewhat pessimistic review of drugs that can be used to mitigate motor consequences of cerebral dysfunction reflects primitive understanding of the neuropharmacology of motor control. As more information becomes available, one can hope that better and more specific pharmacotherapy may be developed.

Surgical Therapy

Because of the failure of drugs and physical therapy to ameliorate most motor symptoms, other therapeutic approaches have been tried. One of them is *chronic electrical stimulation* with electrodes implanted over the cerebellum or dorsal columns of the spinal cord (507) in the hopes of relieving spasticity, abnormal involuntary movements such as dystonia and athetosis, and, in the case of cerebellar stimulation, of controlling intractable seizures (128). Surgical lesions produced by freezing, electrical currents, or other means in the thalamus or cerebellum, usually with stereotaxic methods under local anesthesia, have had limited success in some patients with cerebellar tremor, dystonia musculorum deformans, and, in the days before the advent of L-DOPA therapy, parkinsonism (127).

Each of these surgical approaches triggered an initial wave of enthusiasm. Following reports of acute and long-term complications and of less optimistic long-term effects than had been anticipated, the clinical use of these procedures has waned. At this time they cannot be recommended as accepted treatments because their indications and real therapeutic value have not been fully evaluated. None of them is a panacea. Functionally meaningful improvement has undoubtedly been achieved in some patients (127), but success is unpredictable for the majority, and complications occur and can be serious. Chronic electrical stimulation and stereotaxic surgery are still considered experimental, invasive, and highly controversial approaches to therapy (41).

Management of Behavior Disorders

In contrast to the relative dearth of studies concerned with the pharmacotherapy of motor symptoms, the literature concerned with the treatment of children with behavior disorders, especially hyperactive and distractible children, is very extensive (e.g., 12,29,183,227,316,557,618). Interpretation of results is beset with many problems: There are no agreed upon criteria to define hyperkinetic behavior. One result is that teachers, parents, and physicians frequently disagree on whether a child should be considered pathologically hyperactive or distractible (420). Another problem is that investigators use vastly different criteria when selecting children for study. Hyperkinetic children are often treated as though they constitute a homogeneous sample, even though hyperkinetic-impulsive, hyperkinetic-anxious, hyperkinetic-aggressive, and hyperkinetic-psychotic children may respond differently to pharmacologic agents and behavioral therapies (194,316,618). Children with learning disabilities and motor clumsiness (so-called MBD) are also treated as though they were suffering from a single condition. Furthermore, in many studies (e.g., ref. 536), the terms MBD and hyperkinesis (attention deficit disorder or ADD with or without hyperkinesis, in current parlance) are considered synonymous, despite the evidence that MBD and ADD most likely reflect different types of brain dysfunction that coexist in some but by no means all children. Owing in part to this confusion, indirect effects on cognitive or learning tasks are often used to measure the effectiveness of treatments directed at enhancing attention or vigilance.

Drug Therapy

Investigators have interpreted a favorable response to stimulant drugs as evidence that hyperkinesis is the result of brain damage or dysfunction. This circular type of reasoning has been discredited by studies showing that a proportion of normal children (495) and adults (574) respond to stimulants in much the same way as hyperactive children, with improved performance on reaction time and cognitive tasks, calmness, or even sedation.

When considering the results of attempts to alter behavior, the following question should be asked: What were the criteria by which clinical subjects were selected? What was their age? Were matched control subjects used? Was the performance on the same children compared under treatment and no treatment conditions, using a double-blind protocol? How long was the therapeutic trial? What indicators were used to measure treatment effects? Was the effect of treatment specific or nonspecific?

One needs to consider treatment effects on alertness and vigilance, on attention (distractibility, ability to focus attention, length of attention span), on motor activity (frequency and characteristics of movements of the whole body or seat, of the limbs, and face), on impulsivity, motivation to perform, and mood. Some studies have pointed out that stimulant drugs do not decrease the activity levels of hyperkinetic children in all situations, but do so most dramatically in structured situations (29). Better performance with stimulant drugs has been variously attributed to increased alertness, lessened distractibility, control of impulsivity, improved social relations, mood elevation, and heightened motivation. In any case, all that drugs can do is to improve the availability of the child to the educational process; they are not a treatment for learning disability as some would almost have us believe.

The possibility of nonspecific treatment-associated effects must always be considered, especially when double-blind procedures are not used. Any intervention may improve performance over nonintervention conditions *(placebo effect)*. Moreover, a nonspecific effect is more likely with drugs (or treatments) that produce a subjective effect than with those that do not, even if the effect has no direct relevance to the task (557). This is explained by the subjective perception of an effect of the treatment, leading to the expectation of improvement which, in itself, is therapeutic. Expectation of improvement by the parent, teacher, or observer may result in improved performance because of a change in attitude toward the child *(Hawthorne effect)*. Beneficial treatment effects may be directly related to the therapy without being specific, for example, increased alertness will improve the performance of any task. Finally, measurable improvement in the laboratory does not always imply improvement in real life, yet there may be real improvements that are difficult to measure objectively.

The reliability of reports of behavioral changes by teachers, parents, and other professionals can be improved if they are asked to respond to standard questionnaires (581). In double-blind protocols, teachers and parents are requested to fill out questionnaires on several drug and placebo days. Results are tabulated before the code is broken. (Detailed behavioral questionnaires are used frequently as a means for cataloging children's symptoms in the diagnostic phase of the investigation or for assigning children to particular treatments). Some acute drug studies are limited to a comparison of half-a-day on and half-a-day off the drug (316). More typical double-blind protocols last one or more weeks under each treatment condition. Very few studies have used well standardized tests to measure drug effects over a period of months or years. Double-blind placebo studies can also be used during the course of therapy to adjust dosage or to determine whether therapy has retained its effectiveness.

Among the drugs used in hyperkinetic children, two classes have received the most attention: (a) the cerebral stimulants, notably dextroamphetamine and methylphenidate, and (b) the tranquilizers or psychotropic drugs, the most widely used of which are chlorpromazine and thioridazine. Other drugs such as the antihistamine diphenhydramine, and anxiolytic drugs like the benzodiazepines diazepam and chlordiazepoxide (Librium®), and hydroxyzine (Atarax®) are prescribed to some hyperkinetic children, but usually with limited success. Sedative drugs, notably the barbiturates, far from having beneficial effects may increase the child's hyperactivity, irritability, and sleep disorder (347).

Cerebral stimulants

The beneficial effect of amphetamine in hyperkinetic children was discovered accidentally by Bradley in 1937 (70). This effect remained unexplained for years despite many clinical studies that indicated that dextroamphetamine, methylphenidate and, more recently, pemoline (Cylert®) may decrease motor restlessness, increase attention span, and improve behavior in school to the point where learning is facilitated and teachers and parents find the child much easier to live with. Current psychopharmacologic research suggests that stimulants may exert their effects by altering neurotransmitter metabolism (552). Amphetamines have multiple effects on the brain: They act as agonists of norepinephrine and dopamine, both of which are predominantly inhibitory neurotransmitters. They increase the release of catecholamines from presynaptic terminals and inhibit their reuptake and degradation by monoamine oxidase, thereby increasing their availability. Shaywitz and co-workers (536) have suggested that hyperkinesis results from dopamine depletion, but others point out that it may be the balance of neurotransmitters that is altered.

A recent report of lowered levels of hydroxyindoles in the blood and platelets of some hyperkinetic children and of a beneficial effect of pyridoxine administration to this subgroup of children (122), will, if substantiated, support the view that ADD is not a unitary condition. It is likely that several different neurotransmitter alterations, resulting from a variety of brain insults or genetic traits, may result in hyperkinetic behavior as a final common symptom. Other symptoms that accompany the hyperkinesis and biochemical markers in the urine or blood may eventually enable us to sort out the pathogenesis of this symptom in each patient, permitting individualized pharmacologic therapy.

Dose and administration. Indications for the use of stimulants are not entirely clear; therefore a trial of therapy, if possible using a double-blind placebo procedure, is frequently indicated. Methylphenidate enjoys greater popularity than dextroamphetamine although their action is similar. Dextro-amphetamine in coated spherules (Spansules®) and pemoline can be tried when sustained action is especially desirable. The action of amphetamine and methylphenidate is quite brief, usually lasting about 4 hrs, with onset of action within 30 min. The usual procedure is to start with small doses, 2.5 to 5 mg for dextroamphetamine, and 5 to 10 mg for methylphenidate, administered in divided doses in the morning and at midday. The drugs are rarely prescribed in the evening so as not to interfere with sleep, although a few children will have less trouble falling asleep with the drug than without. The child's response is monitored, preferably with a questionnaire spelling out particular behavioral changes to observe. The drug is increased every few days (or at the end of the defined trial period) until the desired effect, or side effects, occur. The usual maintenance dose is 2.5 to 30 mg for dextroamphetamine, 5 to 60 mg for methylphenidate, and 56.25 to 75 mg for pemoline the effects of which may be delayed for up to 21 days. These doses may be exceeded in some children. Occasionally a child who does not respond to one of these drugs will respond to another, but children who become even more hyperactive or who are weepy and oversensitive on small doses should be considered poor candidates for stimulants.

Some clinicians make it a practice to administer stimulants only on school days and to omit them on vacation days and weekends. This makes sense for children whose parents do not view them as pathologically hyperkinetic while their teachers do, but does not make sense for children who respond dramatically to drugs. Intermittent administration allows the child to experience the drug-free state and provides time during vacations for catch-up growth since stimulants, amphetamine especially, may stunt growth (523). Concern about drug abuse in adolescence or adulthood seems not to be warranted since it appears to be no more frequent in children who have received stimulants than in normal persons (618). Drug-free periods are often used to try to determine whether the child still needs the medication. It is important to keep in mind that, since drug effects and hyperkinesis vary with the child's environment, trials off medication for this purpose are better scheduled during school periods than holidays.

How long to treat hyperkinetic children is an open question. Hyperkinesis decreases in adolescence in some children but persists in others, although with altered manifestations. In fact, Weiss and Hechtman (618), as well as others, report that adolescence is a very difficult period for many of these children but that many settle down as adults and exhibit less chaotic and antisocial behavior. According to Wender (619) and Bellak (37), ADD may persist into adult life. Some of these adults respond favorably to stimulants, others may benefit from antidepressant drugs like imipramine (Tofranil®) or amitriptyline (Elavil®) (643). Antidepressants have been prescribed to an occasional hyperkinetic child with limited success. Caffeine has been tried, but its effectiveness is also limited (211).

Contraindications and side effects. In small doses, amphetamine produces euphoria and a hyperalert state and decreases REM sleep and appetite. In larger doses, it produces signs of peripheral sympathetic stimulation with tachycardia, hypertension, and jitteriness. In large doses, it may precipitate a psychosis with motor stereotypes, hallucinations, and paranoid ideation. In fact, amphetamine psychosis has been considered a possible model for paranoid schizophrenia (549).

Side effects of stimulants in hyperkinetic children may include sleep disturbance although, as just noted, the opposite may occur, as well as appetite suppression with weight loss and failure to grow (523). Some susceptible children may develop chorea (614) or tics, and the stimulants may unmask or precipitate Tourette syndrome (232). Consequently children with both Tourette syndrome (which is thought to reflect excess dopamine or dopamine sensitivity in the striatum) and MBD should not be treated with stimulants. In general, hyperkinetic children with aggressive and antisocial behavior do not respond well to these drugs (316). Frank psychotic symptoms and autism are also considered relative contraindications (91). Stimulants should be avoided in toddlers and preschoolers, and in any case, they have not been found to be very effective in that age group (618).

When methylphenidate is administered to children who are also receiving anticonvulsants, in particular phenytoin, it is important to monitor anticonvulsant blood levels since metabolic interactions can occur and phenytoin intoxication has been reported at least once (212). Oversedation, weepiness, heightened aggression, irrational irritability, and hallucinations, as well as tics, mandate discontinuation of the drug and a trial of other agents like the phenothiazines.

Tranquilizers and anxiolytic agents

Three tranquilizing agents are prescribed most frequently to children with brain dysfunction, chlorpromazine, thioridazine and haloperidol. These antipsychotic agents are thought to exert their effects by blocking catecholamine or, more specifically, dopamine receptors. Aside from differences in doses and side effects, definitive studies that demonstrate the superiority of one or another of these drugs in children with brain dysfunction are not available (362). Small doses, especially of thioridazine, are often prescribed to children who respond poorly to stimulants, but the effectiveness of these small doses tends to be overrated. It is uncertain whether beneficial effects of tranquilizers in children with brain dysfunction are due to their sedative or antipsychotic effects, or to other specific pharmacologic actions. Their use should be considered in hyperactive-aggressive children and especially in hyperactive-psychotic children. Large doses are often prescribed to severely retarded children with autistic behavior who mutilate themselves, but the rate of success is limited and behavior modification approaches may be less dangerous and at least as effective. The danger of producing parkinsonian or dystonic side effects and, with prolonged use, tardive dyskinesia must be kept in mind. Other complications of treatment include cholestatic jaundice, photosensitivity, blood dyscrasias, and, rarely, acute yellow atrophy of the liver.

It was pointed out earlier that anxiety may contribute to the development of hyperkinetic behavior and attentional defects. The benzodiazepines diazepam and chlordiazepoxide have been advocated for children with phobias and various neurotic behavior disorders (226). Their efficacy for long-term management of children with brain dysfunction is questionable, although they may provide a useful adjunct during the early stages of counseling.

Dietary Manipulations

The efficacy of dietary management of severe genetic conditions affecting the brain such as phenylketonuria, maple syrup urine disease, and galactosemia, to name a few, is impressive. So is the efficacy of pharmacologic doses of vitamins B_1, B_6, and B_{12} in other rare genetic diseases of infancy. The ketogenic diet (365), sometimes induced with the use of medium chain triglyceride (MCT) oil (290), is occasionally spectacularly successful in preschoolers with minor motor seizures. Perhaps as a result of these favorable results, there are many reports in the lay press and in the educational literature suggesting that nutritional deficiences or imbalances aggravate hyperkinetic behavior. Both hypoglycemia and excessive intake of refined sugar have been implicated! The Feingold diet (189) stressing avoidance of "junk" foods and synthetic food colors has achieved particular notoriety, as has the administration of vitamins in very high doses ("megavitamins") and of trace metals like magnesium (130). None of these claims has been corroborated by reports in the medical literature that rest on scientifically acceptable evidence. A recent report does suggest, however, that food dyes, in large doses, may impair learning in hyperkinetic, but not in normal children (568). Another report indicates that an artificial dye, erythrosin B, inhibits the uptake of dopamine by nerve synaptosomes (isolated nerve terminals) of the rat caudate nucleus *in vitro* (337). This effect seems to be nonspecific and its relevance to children's behavior remains uncertain (381).

The best one can say is that the recommended dietary manipulations are harmless, albeit expensive. Although most physicians will not feel they can recommend them, they will have little reason to discourage parents who started them on their own and who claim they have observed beneficial effects since they know that it may be impossible to differentiate specific from nonspecific therapeutic effects.

Surgery

A few brain damaged children with epilepsy and uncontrollably aggressive behavior, temper outbursts, or self mutilation unresponsive to large doses of tranquilizers or behavioral management approaches have been treated with bilateral amygdalotomies (437). Lesions are placed in the medial amygdala by stereotaxic methods and satisfactory results, without associated intellectual, cognitive, or autonomic side effects, are described. A small number of hemiparetic children in whom these behaviors occurred as a result of unilateral pathology have been treated by hemidecortication (hemispherectomy), that is, the removal of the entire neocortex of the affected hemisphere (13,31,633). Improved behavior has been attributed to the removal of the epileptogenic cortex that was formally driving secondary epileptic activity (mirror foci) in the contralateral hemisphere. Some patients, in whom epileptic activity and behavior abnormality were ascribed to unilateral temporal lobe pathology, have been treated successfully with temporal lobectomy (186).

The number of children for whom such drastic surgical methods should be contemplated is small. Since favorable results have been reported with these surgical approaches in well-selected cases, physicians caring for children in whom all other therapeutic attempts have failed and who face institutionalization on behavioral grounds need to be aware of these additional therapeutic modalities. The ethics of their use have been the subject of extensive discussion (592), and they should never be recommended without due consideration to nonmutilating alternatives.

COUNSELING

The primary physician is but one of many professionals and educators who will interact with the neurologically handicapped child and his family. He may be the one with the most sustained contact, spanning the years from infancy to late adolescence. His help will be needed again and again for new problems that arise as the child matures and the circumstances of his life change. The importance of this continued relationship cannot be stressed enough. The physicians's role is not only to take care of current illnesses, follow-up on medication, and reexamine the child to make sure there is no change in physical status, and no new signs that would force reconsideration of the diagnosis, his role is always to counsel. The physician's intimate knowledge of the child and his family will facilitate sensitive discussion of such topics as conflicts with peers and siblings, feelings of inadequacy, problems in school, the need for financial aid, and vocational options. The physician can bring up subjects such as the need for placement in a chronic care facility if he perceives that it would clearly be to the advantage of the whole family and appropriate for the child. In severely affected children, it may be advisable for the physician to discuss the possibility or probability of the death of the child and the need for an autopsy in order to determine, finally, what condition or disease was responsible and, perhaps, to advance scientific knowledge concerning it. A definite diagnosis will provide a firm basis for genetic counseling and, quite often, afford parents the solace of knowing that their severely handicapped child's life had the unique significance, by contributing to medical knowledge, of helping other families with problems similar to theirs (485). However painful, such topics are better discussed in advance, at a time when they are theoretical possibilities for the future rather than a crushing fact; advanced planning and consideration of reality will ultimately ease some of the family's distress.

Counseling by the physician encompasses three main areas: (1) providing factual information, (2) providing advice regarding outlook and management, and (3) providing therapeutic counseling and psychotherapy.

Factual Information

First and foremost, parents want a diagnosis, an estimate of prognosis, and advice about management. It is not sufficient to give out a diagnostic label; that label has to be defined and explained, otherwise parents will be confused since they will no doubt encounter diverse professionals over the years, some of whom may use terms different from the physician's to describe what is in fact the same condition. Clarification is particularly important when the best the physician can offer is a term such as cerebral palsy, mental retardation, ADD, brain damage, learning disability, convulsive disorder, or autism; each of these terms is a symptomatic label rather than a diagnosis. He must explain that these vague terms cover our ignorance of underlying pathogenesis, and stress that they do not say anything about the severity of the condition. Cerebral palsy, for example, is a term that is likely to be misunderstood; it is often viewed as a dangerous disease rather than a label for any static brain condition incurred in early life that produces a motor deficit. Parents need to know, when an IQ label is attached to a preschooler who has been tested in order to be admitted to a special program, that this label may be an unreliable predictor of future performance (78,357,396), and that it may be almost meaningless in a child with a circumscribed neurologic deficit (629). Parents should be told that mental retardation does not mean that the child will make no progress. At the same time, it should be explained that catch-up to complete normalcy will not occur or is extremely unlikely unless the deficit is very mild. Knowing that autism is the result of an abnormality of brain function and not an emotional problem for which they may have, unwittingly, been responsible will take a load off of the parents' minds. The need for counseling of parents whose children have seizures is particularly acute because of the frightening nature of seizures, their unpredictable occurrence, and their severe and unwarranted social consequences (338).

If the physician can make a definite diagnosis, it is extremely important that he provide the parents with the unvarnished truth and that he discuss the implications of the diagnosis. His explanation must include a discussion of pathogenesis, otherwise parents may carry a burden of unnecessary guilt for years. Very few parents understand that one can have a genetic illness with a totally negative family history and that, in fact, this circumstance is the rule when the trait is recessive. It is crucial to point out that autosomal recessive traits come from both sides of the family, that both parents are carriers, and that there was no way to detect the trait before the birth of the affected child. Recurrence risks for subsequent pregnancies and virtual lack of risk for other family members must be stressed. For dominant traits with possibly serious implications, like tuberous sclerosis or neurofibromatosis, examination of both parents, all siblings, and other willing family members is clearly in order, together with a discussion of the genetic implications, variability of phenotypic expression, and very high recurrence risks.

If the physician believes that his patient's condition is clearly acquired he should say so and explain the evidence on which he bases his judgment. He should be cautious in cases in which perinatal damage seems likely, inasmuch as a bad outcome does not necessarily reflect obstetrical negligence. He must be quite sure of his grounds since, if the parents decide to bring suit, he may be called upon to defend his opinion in court. When no explanation for the child's condition can be found, the physician should state this clearly and point out to parents that medical knowledge is woefully inadequate, and that it is common either to have no explanation or, sometimes, to have several possible ones and not to know which one was responsible.

The physician will of course discuss the medical implications of the condition, what medication may be advisable, what further tests may be needed now or in the future, and their purpose. He will also detail the steps to be taken and what consultations may be needed to provide additional information and why. In appropriate cases he should advise parents of the requirement for follow-up and plan the next appointment relatively soon as parents will undoubtedly have heard only a fraction of what he had to say.

Advice on Outlook and Management

After he has discussed diagnosis, the physician will speak of management and of the future, that is, of outcome. This is the part of the interview that will determine whether or not the parents will keep their next appointment and allow the physician to follow their child. The message to put across is that the reality and permanence of the brain dysfunction do not mean that nothing can be done. Therapeutic nihilism has no place when a diagnosis of brain dysfunction is first made, especially if the child is very young. Experienced physicians know that a case is hopeless only when the diagnosis of a progressive and invariably fatal condition has been made enzymatically or pathologically as well as clinically, or when damage is so profound as to preclude all possibility of development. Experience brings with it modesty: We have all seen children who did much better than predicted, and others who did much worse. The key is to be somewhat noncommital as to prognosis, to indicate that things look bad (or hopeful as the case may be) and to state that probable outcome will be clearer after follow-up indicates how the child responds to therapeutic intervention. Making definite statements as to probable age at walking or speaking is particularly dangerous since age at attainment of these milestones is unpredictable, even in normal children.

Even when the physician knows the situation to be hopeless, he must resist the temptation to abandon the patient. There are resources for such children and help for their families through specialized clinics and community agencies such as the Association for the Help of the Retarded Children, and United Cerebral Palsy centers. These agencies, and others, run day programs for even the most severely retarded brain damaged children. They attempt to develop such skills as chewing, independent feeding, toileting, dressing, and walking. In addition, parents are provided with guidance and counseling regarding day-to-day management problems at home. Many of these agencies have physiatric consultants who prescribe special wheelchairs, walkers, and other helpful aids. Other agencies such as the Muscular Dystrophy Association help defray the cost of clinic visits and of special appliances for selected patients, and provide recreational programs and social groups. The physician can suggest visiting nurse services if that seems advisable. He can make sure that the child is placed on disability so that his family may receive Social Security funds and Medicaid. In appropriate cases, he should ensure the child has been officially declared legally blind so that his parents may claim an extra exemption on their federal income tax return and so that the child may receive the services of an itinerant teacher for the blind and have free access to recorded Talking Books.

Toddlers and preschool children with a developmental disability, or at risk for one, must be referred to an appropriate educational program (454). There are now infant stimulation programs and preschool programs as well as special classes in schools. As mentioned in earlier sections, the long-term efficacy of such programs is difficult to measure scientifically (143), yet the benefits derived by parents of preschoolers who are in these programs are obvious, and the children profit by becoming more independent and self-assertive. Behavior modification is often used to foster toilet training and self-help for feeding and dressing, and to discourage self-mutilation, eye avoidance, or tantrums (210,333,339). The children are exposed to other children and learn critical social skills, for example, taking turns, looking at the teacher's face and listening when she speaks, and understanding that there are times when adults mean business and they had better do as they are told.

For the school-age child, the importance of placement in an appropriate school program has been stressed. The physician can often help achieve this by serving as a buffer and interpreter between the child's family and the school or the Committee on the Handicapped. A phone call to the teacher, guidance counselor, or school psychologist may clear up a problem and defuse a conflict. Physicians are often asked by schools to prescribe drugs which the physician may feel are inappropriate for a particular child with behavior problems. Telling the school why, after listening to their side of the story, may be extremely helpful.

When the child becomes an adolescent, counseling needs to be directed more and more to him or her, rather than to his parents, or mainly to his parents. He will need factual information about his condition, its implications for his life, his children, and his future. This is the time to bring up the problem of birth control for the cognitively handicapped, to give genetic counseling to the affected adolescent who is capable of profiting from the information, and to be concerned with vocational counseling and the prospects for independent or semi-independent living.

The informing part of counseling necessarily covers a broad territory and touches on many subjects besides strictly medical ones. Experienced physicians may be able to pack all this information into one interview, but how much of what the physician has said the family understands is problematic. One way out of this bind is to schedule a repeat visit of both parents without the child. Sufficient time should be allocated so that the physician can go over, once again, what he covered before, urging the parents to ask whatever questions have occurred to them. Such open-ended conferences are effective for the family and extremely informative for the physician who will get a much better picture of what is going on in the family than on a first visit. After the conference, some physicians may choose to send the parents a note summarizing the high points of the discussion and listing the diagnosis, whatever steps are to be taken, and how and where to get help. Considering that the child has a problem that will probably have lifelong consequences, it is appropriate to give it this much attention early on. Hopefully, this effort will ensure that the child has early access to whatever remediation services he needs and will ward off unnecessary problems. It may also discourage parents from running from one consultant to the next and from one untried therapy to another. It may lay the foundation of a trusting relationship because the physician has been both honest and sensitive and has expressed willingness to continue to care for the child and to help the family cope with the day-to-day problems they are experiencing, however bad they may be.

Advice About Behavior

In many young children, the kinds of problems that trouble parents the most are self-mutilating behaviors (head banging, biting), aggressive behaviors, tantrums, and sleep problems. In school-age children, hyperkinetic behavior, with or without other manifestations of the attention deficit disorder, come to the forefront. Parents frequently bring up other problems such as quarreling, excessive shyness, school phobias, heedlessness, and acting out. In adolescents, the focus shifts to inappropriate sexual conduct, including masturbation and promiscuity, antisocial behavior, dropping out of school, refusing to take medication, and rebellion against parents.

The physician can often advise the parents, reassuring them and pointing out some of the child's obvious needs such as praise and consistent management, and the value of rules and routines. He may have a suggestion regarding a change in the home situation or tell the parents how to find an after-school program or how to arrange a change of classes. However, with very difficult children, much more is needed than can be provided by the primary physician.

Psychologists and educators have become proficient in applying to handicapped children many of the laboratory techniques found to be effective for altering behavior. The best known is *behavior modification* (210,333,339). This consists of systematically rewarding desired behaviors while ignoring those one wishes to extinguish. To be effective, behavior modification has to be implemented by professionals who have special training in its use. Simply telling the parents about this approach will accomplish very little. By applying these methods while the child attends a remedial program that encourages parents' participation, psychologists or specialists in early childhood education can demonstrate their efficacy to parents and teach them how to use these methods in the home and apply them to other troublesome behaviors.

Behavior modification is but one approach for improving conduct. Parents can be taught how to communicate more effectively, how to listen more carefully to what the child is trying to convey, and how to avoid being manipulated by the child. the child can learn that certain behaviors are unacceptable and that methods he used to rely on to get his way no longer work. This type of goal is clearly an educational one, one that requires time and repeated contact and is thus best provided in the context of an educational program. What the physician needs to be aware of is not the details of what can be done, but the availability of such programs so that he will think to refer problem patients.

The utility of *psychotherapy* was touched upon earlier. There is no doubt that play therapy or other psychotherapies may be very helpful, as part of the management plan, with children in whom an unfavorable environment, interpersonal conflicts, or poor self-image complicate the symptoms of brain dysfunction. Individual psychotherapy for parents, parent groups, family therapy, and play therapy or counseling for siblings are adjuncts that may help tide over an entire family stressed by the presence of a neurologically handicapped member. These modalities are more time consuming and more expensive than drugs, but one must keep in mind that behavior has to be learned and that learning takes time, while all that drugs can offer is to make the child more available for whatever intervention may be deemed effective.

REMEDIAL EDUCATION AND TRAINING

The cornerstone in the management of children with brain dysfunction is remedial education (education taken in its broadest sense). The theoretical basis for this approach is that the function and fine structure of the brain are shaped by environmental experience (39,129,595). Through prolonged and repeated practice, proficiency in playing a musical instrument, skiing, or discriminating among flavors of teas can be dramatically enhanced in individuals with particular aptitudes; deaf children become remarkably visually attentive and blind children evolve highly proficient tactile, acoustic, and olfactory senses (487). The brains of individuals with such special talents must be different, at some submicroscopic level of organization, from the brains of individuals who do not have such skills. Children with hemiparesis may learn to tie their shoes with one hand; their right hemisphere may subserve speech and writing even though their left hemisphere would normally have programmed such tasks (31). While recovery of function after brain damage depends in part on restitution of the anatomic and physiologic state of the brain as the acute effects of the lesion subside, later improvement reflects reorganization in spared areas and the acquisition of new ways to achieve a particular behavioral goal. To what degree this reorganization includes redirecting of severed axons, reinnervation of denuded synaptic sites, changes in receptor sensitivity, or other anatomic and physiologic alterations is not well known in man (192,558).

The goal of special education and training is functional competence. This may be achieved by two main approaches: (1) improving a given skill through practice, and (2) teaching substitute skills for attaining particular goals.

Depending on the degree of handicap, improved mobility can be achieved through gait training, muscle strengthening exercises, and the use of biofeedback to teach relaxation of antagonist muscles, or through bracing and the use of crutches, or through the use of a wheelchair and a car with manual controls. The realization that practice can improve the deficient performance of some handicapped persons engendered the optimistic assumption that training is always beneficial. Intensive programs in which exercises to improve crawling, fine motor coordination, balance, or visual tracking and convergence were practiced extensively became popular. These programs were offered rather indiscriminately to children with severe mental retardation and motor deficits, as well as to some children with learning disabilities and minor motor deficits, in the hopes of improving their cognitive as well as their motor skills (147).

Assessing the efficacy of such training is difficult: It is never very clear whether improvement, if it occurs, is the direct consequence of training, reflects improvement because of maturation that would have occurred anyway, or represents a placebo effect caused by the expectation of success in both the child and his caretakers (100).

The extent and location of pathology are rarely known, especially in children with nonprogressive cerebral dysfunction. Even if known, they are rarely considered when prescribing therapy. Children with "soft signs" probably would do well without intervention, while children in whom effector pathways are massively affected will not do well, no matter how much training they receive; in them the goals of intervention should be to avoid secondary consequences of motor deficits such as scoliosis, contractures, painful joints, and disuse atrophy. Rather than spending hundreds of hours in exercises that will not give them functional motor skills, time might be spent more profitably teaching such children to use electric typewriters, communication boards, or motorized wheelchairs. Children whose cognitive skills and alertness are extremely limited are not good prospects for the learning of substitute skills or for training aimed at improving their limited skills.

Inability to forecast the extent of functional deficit several years hence interferes with assessing the efficacy of intervention. Nonetheless, there is little to lose, besides money, time, and effort, in prescribing special training for handicapped children and those perceived as being at substantial risk for developmental delay. As a result of PL 94-142, implemented in October, 1977, there are now "free" (i.e., supported by taxpayers) remedial programs available for handicapped children of all ages, from infancy to 21 years of age (454). "Child Find" programs strive for the early identification of children in need of special education. Primary care physicians, pediatricians, public health nurses, educators, other professionals, and parents can refer children who will be placed in what are hoped to be adequate and effective programs as soon as they have been evaluated and their eligibility has been determined (454). Yearly monitoring is mandated in order to determine the appropriateness of the program for the particular child, to define goals for the next academic year, and to determine whether there is a continuing need for services. Parents are given a strong voice in the choice of a program and the evaluation of its benefits. Formal procedures have been set up to protect the rights of children and to mediate, in cases of disagreement, between the child's guardians and the professionals who make the educational referrals.

As a result of PL 94-142, a formidable educational and testing industry has arisen and will no doubt grow even further. It behooves physicians and other professionals to be on the alert for children in current need or who are likely to experience future need for special programs. Nondetection of handicap, or referral to an inadequate or inappropriate program, occasionally becomes a grounds for lawsuit. The physician must be informed about the quality and appropriateness of the program which his patient attends. The rapid proliferation of programs since the law was enacted in 1975 has meant that the quality and efficacy of some are marginal and need evaluation.

Programs for children with such single well-defined handicaps as deafness, blindness, moderate retardation, spasticity, and dyslexia are quite widely distributed and readily available. Day programs mentioned earlier may help even the most severely retarded brain damaged children receive needed therapy and training. Some attempt to use Total Communication (sign language together with speech) with nondeaf nonverbal children, for example, autistic and severely retarded youngsters (92,526).The trend toward deinstitutionalization has spawned some humane and imaginative programs like halfway houses, supervised group living, camps, and respite facilities which permit families of severely handicapped persons living at home to have a vacation from caring for them (117). Remaining residential institutions, which will continue to be needed for the very severely handicapped and those without families, have been upgraded and offer more remedial programs than they did in the past.

Children for whom it is most difficult to find good programs are those with multiple handicaps, for example, deaf-retarded, deaf-autistic, or blind-spastic children, and those whose handicap is either uncommon or difficult to diagnose or whose management is still experimental. For example, children with severe language disorders are likely to be misdiagnosed as globally retarded or as suffering from a primary emotional disorder, while fluent children with a milder disorder may be overlooked for years. In any case, there are a few good programs for preschool children with language disorders (they are rarely served adequately with one or two half-hour sessions of "speech" therapy a week). No one knows yet what constitutes an adequate and efficacious school program for autistic children.

Good programs for infants and preschoolers, whatever the child's handicaps, are directed toward the parents or caretaker at least as much as toward the child. Part of their therapeutic value is to educate parents regarding milestones of development and behavior management techniques, in addition to teaching them special exercises they can do at home and providing them with devices like walkers, standing tables, or spoons with thick handles that will facilitate care of the child. Another benefit is that parents meet the parents of other handicapped children. They share problems and workable techniques, thus gaining a more realistic perspective into their own problems. Through counseling, parents often lose some of the irrational guilt feelings they inevitably suffer. They learn about available resources and can plan more realistically for their handicapped child's future. Because the child is out of the home for part of the day, or at least for a few hours a week, parents are able to devote more time to their normal children and to the fulfillment of their own needs. Parents of severely handicapped children often become less depressed when their child attends an appropriate program and they start to experience its many benefits. They no longer feel hopeless and helpless. They gain feelings of competence as therapists enlist their help as cotherapists of their child and, often, of other children in the program. A not insignificant number of mothers with children in good programs have gone back to work or to school, some to become professionals in the care of handicapped children.

For the school-age child, one of the issues is whether he should attend a special school or be "mainstreamed", that is, placed in a school with normal children and provided with the remedial help he requires either by attending a special class in that school for all or part of the day, or by receiving individual instruction in deficient areas. Literal interpretation of PL 94-142, which specifies that the child be educated in the least restrictive environment, favors mainstreaming. For children with severe handicaps such as congenital deafness or verbal auditory agnosia, one can argue that the least restrictive environment is one where everyone uses Total Communication. Mainstreaming school age deaf children who have serviceable oral language skills may be advantageous socially and for the development of speech, but may mean an impoverished educational experience, despite the availability of a resource room teacher of the deaf for one period a day, because the child may miss much of the informal exchange taking place in the normal classroom. Decisions about mainstreaming clearly must be individualized.

Intelligent children with a learning disability usually attend most classes with their normal peers and are provided with special tutoring for one or more subjects and, sometimes, with private tutoring after school to help them with their homework. If the learning disability is severe and if the child remains functionally illiterate after the elementary grades, he may profit by attending a special school geared to using methods other than reading to present the content of the curriculum. More commonly, such children remain in normal classes, but teachers of subjects like social studies, mathematics, and science will have to make special accommodations for their dyslexic pupils. For example, the child may need to be allowed to take examinations orally, to prepare recorded rather than written reports, and to have someone read aloud to him the material he is to learn or the problems he is to solve. Dyslexics are now entitled to use the Talking Books recorded for the blind and made available through the Library of Congress. Unless these accommodations are made, severely dyslexic children are likely to miss out on the content of education. Beyond elementary school, the ability to obtain information by reading is taken for granted. "Dyslexics" who can read but do it very slowly and inefficiently spend so much energy in the deciphering process that they are likely to miss the content of what they read. Unless this barrier to learning is removed, such children will often be "turned off" by school, they will stop listening, and may become behavior problems in junior high school, and school dropouts in high school.

Hyperkinetic children present special problems for their teachers. They often disrupt the classroom and interfere with other children's education as well as their own. Strauss (564,565) was one of the first to point out that the children's hyperkinesis tends to abate if extraneous stimuli are removed. He advocated placing each child in a partially enclosed cubicle with bare walls painted a neutral color. Materials were to be presented one at a time; for example, in reading, most of the text was to be masked with the exception of the line the child was actually reading. Hyperkinetic children do better when routines and procedures are explicit. Open classrooms, where children have the freedom to choose one of several activities taking place simultaneously in different "corners" of the room and to set their own pace, are generally inappropriate for hyperactive distractible children. Familiar and orderly classroom routines produce an environment that is predictable and comfortable because of its stability. Hyperkinetic children need to be given the frequent opportunity of controlled motor activity after they have completed a task; for example, they might distribute materials to their classmates, wash the blackboards, run errands, or simply stand up and stretch.

Volumes have been written to provide teachers with techniques that are helpful to learning-disabled and distractible children (e.g., 67,98,261,315,452,564,565,594). These are based on such principles as making abstract relationships concrete in order to promote insight into the process being taught; breaking down operations into smaller steps; minimizing perceptual confusions; providing three-dimensional and realistic examples that the child can manipulate rather than two-dimensional pictures and diagrams; and encouraging the child to verbalize what he is doing or what has to be done in order to minimize impulsivity, to make the operation explicit, and to strengthen perception, particularly in children with better verbal than visual-spatial skills (408,420,618). All of these approaches, and many others, ideally should be used with the full knowledge of each child's neuropsychologic profile so that teaching can be individualized (390).

The danger for the older learning-disabled pupil is to give too much emphasis to drill in the three R's. If proficiency has still not been achieved, attention should shift from these scholastic skills, for which the adolescent may or may not eventually acquire a modicum of competence, to the acquisition of practical skills important in adult life, for example, how to use a checkbook, pay a bill, ask for information, and behave during a job interview. Many vocational programs expose the handicapped adolescent to a variety of shops in the hope of finding a trade or skill that appeals to him and that he can master sufficiently well to earn a living, if not in the open market, at least in a sheltered workshop. Some of these vocational programs are very good, but others do not have the resources to provide a wide range of options or to keep up with the technologic changes of the marketplace. Finding a niche for handicapped workers is difficult. It requires the continuous seeking out of potential employers who have the requisite personnel resources to supervise a handicapped worker and the imagination to fit him comfortably and profitably into their operation. State departments of education or social services have offices concerned with vocational rehabilitation and the placement of handicapped workers. Their effectiveness varies widely.

OUTCOME

Information concerning what happens to children with neurologic dysfunction as adults is sparse. The idea that MBD and hyperkinesis abate in the teens and disappear by adulthood is not invariably true (618,619). Bellak (37) stresses that the hyperkinetic child of yesterday may be the sociopathic adult of today. He recommends that severely affected individuals continue to use stimulant drugs in adulthood. Since school is, for the majority of persons, the most severe test of their cognitive abilities, many brain-damaged and mildly retarded persons will be less conspicuous as adults than as children (102,586,635). Those who have acquired adequate social skills, learned a trade, and found a niche in the marketplace that does not penalize them too severely for their deficits, and those who do not have severe emotional problems, and do not engage in antisocial behavior are likely to disappear into the population. This will not happen for the most severely handicapped, of course, but how many of those identified in childhood as learning disabled "make it" as adults is not known at this time. It is clear, however, that severity of deficit and overall cognitive competence are but two variables in the equation, and that personality and such environmental circumstances as family cohesion and resourcefulness, the efficacy of remedial education, and the availability of employment opportunity may play just as crucial a role in determining outcome.

Glossary

ABSENCE SEIZURE—Brief loss of consciousness without loss of posture tone, often associated with fluttering of the eyes or minor automatisms. Absences may be the result of petit mal seizures (q.v.)* or complex partial seizures (q.v.).

ACETYLCHOLINE—An excitatory neurotransmitter that is widely distributed throughout the central nervous system, at the neuromuscular junction, and in the autonomic nervous system. For example, "upper" and "lower motor neurons" are cholinergic cells. There are two types of cholinergic synapses, nicotinic and muscarinic. Cholinergic drugs acting predominantly on nicotinic synapses have prominent sensorimotor effects; those acting on muscarinic synapses, autonomic effects.

ADD—Attention deficit disorder (q.v.).

ADRENALIN—Epinephrine (q.v.).

AFFERENT—Input to a neuron or neuronal system.

AGNOSIA—Failure to perceive or recognize a previously familiar stimulus. One can have an auditory angosia, tactile agnosia, visual agnosia, or agnosia for more complex stimuli such as faces.

AGRAPHIA—Loss of the ability to write as a result of focal damage to the dominant hemisphere. Agraphia is often associated with aphasia and with alexia.

AKINESIA (HYPOKINESIA)—Paucity of movement and associated movements, characteristically seen in patients with parkinsonism and those who are overdosed with phenothiazines or other dopamine blocking agents.

ALEXIA—Loss of the ability to read in a previously competent reader as a result of an acquired brain lesion, usually affecting the dominant hemisphere. Alexia may or may not be associated with agraphia. There are several syndromes of alexia, depending upon the location of the lesion.

AMBIDEXTROUS—Without established hand preference for skilled acts like writing.

---

*q.v. *(quod vide)*: Refer also to the term immediately preceding q.v., in this case, petit mal seizures.

AMNESIA—Inability to remember and to learn.

Retrograde amnesia is the inability to retrieve previously stored items. Occurs most often in the acute phase following a cerebral concussion.

Anterograde amnesia is the inability to learn new material. While it may result from either failure of items to pass from short-term memory to long-term memory or from inadequate consolidation, failure to retrieve is thought by some to be responsible for most cases of anterograde amnesia. It is characteristically caused by bilateral lesions of the hippocampus and mesial temporal structures, or by bilateral pathology affecting the mammillary bodies of the posterior hypothalamus and dorsal medial nucleus of the thalamus. The most common cause of this latter pathology is chronic alcoholic encephalopathy (Korsakoff syndrome or psychosis).

AMNIOCENTESIS—The removal of amniotic fluid for the prenatal diagnosis of a chromosomal anomaly or genetic-metabolic disorder of the fetus, of an open neural tube defect (spina bifida, anencephaly), or to determine the maturity of the fetus or his well being, in cases of RH incompatibility, for example. Amniocentesis can be performed from 14 to 16 weeks of gestation until term. The procedure involves little danger to the fetus, especially with ultrasound examination of the uterine contents. New developments are examination of the fetus through a fetoscope, and the ability to treat certain diseases of the fetus *in utero*.

AMPHETAMINE (DEXEDRINE®)—A stimulant drug. Prescribed for some children with ADD. It is thought to exert at least some of its effects by increasing catecholamine levels in the brain.

AMYGDALA—A large nuclear complex situated within the mesial temporal lobe. It is an important limbic relay. Some of its inputs come from the olfactory system, cingulate gyrus, and inferior temporal cortex. Its main outputs project to the hypothalamus and other limbic areas, and via the thalamus, to the prefrontal cortex.

ANARTHRIA—Inability to speak. It is most often caused by pseudobulbar palsy (q.v.), bulbar palsy, or another nonlinguistic motor deficit affecting the buccolingual musculature. It may also result from a global or very severe expressive aphasia or from aphemia (q.v.).

ANENCEPHALY—A malformation incompatible with survival in which a baby is born with an open skull and lacks most of the structures of the cerebral hemispheres.

ANGIOTENSIN II—A peptide that constricts blood vessels and has effects on the kidney. It is also found in the brain where it stimulates drinking behavior.

ANGULAR GYRUS—Gyrus located at the posterior end of the first temporal sulcus, adjacent to the occipital cortex. Involved in linguistic operations, *inter alia*.

ANOMIA (AMNESTIC APHASIA)—Difficulty retrieving words from the lexicon. It is usually tested for by asking the patient to name an object presented visually. Patients with anomia may use circumlocutions for words that escape them. They can usually pick out the correct word from a series. Retrieval of the target word may be enhanced by supplying the sound of the first letter of the word or a phrase of which the target word is an obligatory part.

ANOXIA—Lack of oxygen.

ANTEROGRADE AMNESIA—See AMNESIA.

ANTICONVULSANT DRUGS—Drugs prescribed to prevent the occurrence of epileptic seizures or to control them. Major anticonvulsants effective against generalized, partial complex, and focal motor seizures include phenytoin (Dilantin®), phenobarbital, carbamazepine (Tegretol®), and primidome (Mysoline®). Major anticonvulsants effective against absence seizures with bilateral EEG synchrony and against some myoclonic seizures include ethosuximide (Zarontin®), valproic acid (Depakene®), and clonazepam (Clonopin®).

ANTIPSYCHOTIC DRUGS—Drugs like the phenothiazines, lithium, reserpine, and the butyrophenones that are effective in the major psychoses and are thought to exert their effects by their interactions with cerebral neurotransmitters.

ANXIOLYTIC DRUGS—Drugs that help reduce anxiety. The diazepines, e.g., diazepam (Valium®) and chlordiazepoxide (Librium®), are thought to exert their effects by stimulating GABA receptors.

APHASIA—Impaired oral linguistic skills in a person with previously competent language as a result of an acquired brain insult. Aphasia is usually due to damage lateralized to the fronto-temporo-parietal language areas of the dominant hemisphere, usually the left. Some agreed upon aphasic syndromes include receptive (fluent) aphasia, expressive (nonfluent) aphasia, anomia (word finding difficulty), conduction aphasia (inability to repeat), and word deafness (verbal auditory agnosia). Inability to read (alexia), and to write (agraphia) may or may not be associated with these various aphasic syndromes.

APHEMIA—An acquired expressive language deficit which is extremely severe or total for speech (anarthria) but which spares writing. Some view it as an apraxia for the gestures required for speech articulation. It is caused by an inferior frontal lesion of the dominant hemisphere.

APRAXIA—Inability to retrieve motor commands for complex movements. In order to diagnose apraxia, one must have ruled out paralysis, sensory loss, or inability to understand the command to move. It is often tested by having the patient imitate a movement.

AQUEDUCT OF SYLVIUS—A narrow channel in the center of the mesencephalon (midbrain) for the passage of cerebrospinal fluid between the third and fourth ventricles of the brain.

ARCHITECTONICS—Detailed microscopic anatomy of the cortex.

ARCUATE FASCICULUS—A pathway joining the posterior (temporoparietal) to the anterior (frontal) language areas.

ASSOCIATION AREAS—Areas of the neocortex where discrete lesions do not produce discrete effects. These are areas assumed to participate in higher order processes such as perception, language, decision making, etc. Sensory association areas (secondary and tertiary sensory association areas) are regions to which neurons from the primary sensory areas project and which are thought to be involved in perception.

ASTEREOGNOSIS—Inability to recognize an object by palpation.

ATAXIA—Loss of balance and of fine motor control, usually because of dysfunction in cerebellar circuits, less often because of loss of proprioceptive inputs to the cerebellum and somatosensory cortex, or of vestibular dysfunction.

ATHETOSIS—A movement disorder involving the limbs and face predominantly in which slow writhing movements of the fingers and grimacing are superimposed on dystonic postures. The children often have truncal hypotonia and poor head control. Athetosis is often the consequence of neonatal hyperbilirubinemia (kernicterus) when it is characteristically associated with hearing loss, or of neonatal asphyxia involving the basal ganglia (status marmoratus).

ATTENTION DEFICIT DISORDER (ADD)—A syndrome characterized by distractibility, short attention span, and disorganization. Children with ADD tend to be impulsive and to have a labile affect. ADD may or may not be associated with hyperkinesis or motor restlessness (hyperactivity, q.v.) or with a learning disability (q.v.), but this is an associated symptom rather than being due to ADD. The syndrome may persist into adult life. Some children are helped by the administration of stimulants like methylphenidate or dextroamphetamine. The differential diagnosis of ADD includes anxiety, boredom, psychosis, and temperamental high energy level.

AUDITORY CORTEX—Situated in the horizontal or superior temporal region of the temporal lobe (planum temporale), tucked within the Sylvian fissure, which is the major fissure on the lateral aspect of the cerebral hemispheres.

AURA—A subjective sensory illusion or hallucination resulting from a focal seizure discharge in the corresponding part of the cortex. Because auras may be the prelude to a generalized seizure, they are often called warnings by the patient, although auras are seizures and provide useful information for localizing the site of origin of the seizure.

AUTISM (AUTISTIC SYNDROME)—A symptom complex first described by Kanner characterized by (a) inadequate communication through verbal and nonverbal channels, (b) affective, and (c) cognitive deficits. Frequent symptoms include gaze avoidance, aloneness, aberrant behaviors such as repetitive rituals, clutching on to objects, avoidance of change, flattened affect with lack of expression of pleasure and displeasure, improverished play, etc. Some autistic children are echolalic, using language non communicatively, at least at times, while others speak little or are mute. Autism is not a single condition or disease but a syndrome or symptom complex. While autism is no longer believed to be caused by aberrant life experience but rather by cerebral dysfunction of unknown type and location, there is no doubt that some autistic symptoms, for instance, gaze avoidance and destructive behaviors, can be ameliorated by environmental change. The behavior of some mute autistic children is said to improve if sign language is used to supplement speech. Long-term outlook in autism is guarded.

AUTONOMIC NERVOUS SYSTEM—Parts of the nervous system that control vegetative functions such as the caliber of blood vessels, gastrointestinal motility and secretion, heart rate, pupil size, sweating, and many others. The autonomic nervous system is classically divided into the sympathetic and parasympathetic systems, both with central and peripheral divisions.

AUTOSOMAL DOMINANT and RECESSIVE GENETIC TRAITS—Traits under the control of genes located on one of the 22 pairs of nonsex chromosomes. In autosomal dominant traits, mutation of a single gene on only one chromosome of a pair is expressed. If the mutation is an unfavorable one it results in disease. The person is said to be heterozygous for the trait when he carries two nonidentical genes for that trait. With autosomal recessive traits, mutation must affect both genes of a pair for the trait to be expressed. The patient is homozygous for the trait. His or her parents are obligatory heterozygotes, that is, each of them is a carrier for a trait that neither of them manifests, because expression of the abnormal recessive gene is prevented by the normal dominant gene. Autosomal traits affect both males and females, as opposed to X-linked traits that affect males selectively.

AXON—The long process of neurons that carries the nerve action potential away from the cell body toward the axon terminals when the neuron fires. Axons may branch fairly close to their origin, along their length, or close to their termination. Recurrent axon collaterals are axon branches that terminate on other neurons close to their neuron of origin. Axon terminals have specialized presynaptic membranes that release neurotransmitters and, presumably, neuromodulators across the synaptic cleft toward the post synaptic receptor membrane of the cell the axon innervates. Axons may or may not be myelinated. Conduction along axons is all or none, depending upon whether or not the neuron has become depolarized and has generated an axon potential.

BABINSKI REFLEX—Dorsiflexion of the big toe and fanning of the other toes in response to stimulation of the lateral aspect of the sole of the foot. This reflex denotes pyramidal tract pathology (q.v.) and is often associated with spasticity (q.v.)

BALLISMUS—Abnormal involuntary movements consisting of violent flinging of the limbs on one side of the body. Ballismus suggests pathology in the contralateral subthalamic nucleus or its pathways.

BALLISTIC MOVEMENTS—Movements that are thought to be preprogrammed, perhaps in cerebellar circuits, because they are executed too rapidly for proprioceptive feedback to control them.

BASAL GANGLIA—Large paired nuclear masses in the depth of each hemisphere comprising the neostriatum (caudate nucleus, putamen) paleostriatum (globus pallidus—with an external and internal segment), subthalamic nucleus (in the diencephalon), substantia nigra (in the mesencephalon), and their connections. The basal ganglia are the hub of an important motor control circuit (frontal premotor-striatal-pallidal-thalamic-frontal). Lesions produce contralateral motor symptoms. The basal ganglia are also thought to play a role in the control of complex behaviors, in part because of the extensive projections they receive from the nonspecific thalamic nuclei and from the cortex, notably the prefrontal cortex; this idea is speculative at this point.

BEHAVIOR MODIFICATION—A technique based on operant conditioning methods used in children to shape desired behaviors by rewarding them and to extinguish undesirable behaviors by ignoring them or, in some cases, by punishing them.

BIOGENIC AMINES—A class of compounds acting as neurotransmitters, notably the catecholamines—norepinephrine, epinephrine, and dopamine; and the indolamine, serotonin (5-hydroxytryptamine). They are thought to play an important role in the control of sleep, affect, many other complex behaviors, and perhaps in the pathogenesis of the psychoses.

BRAIN DAMAGE—The implication of this label is that the cause of brain dysfunction is, potentially at least, detectable with current technology, that it has resulted in an anatomic lesion. There is often a tacit assumption that "brain damaged" children have motor deficits, "hard" motor signs, and particular behavior and psychologic test patterns. Such assumptions do not withstand critical scrutiny.

BRAIN ELECTRICAL ACTIVITY MAPPING (BEAM)—Computer generated maps of changes in particular EEG frequency bands, or changes in evoked responses across scalp areas during given behavioral tasks such as reading, speaking, moving, making sensory discriminations, etc.

BRAIN STEM—The core of the hindbrain comprising the midbrain (continuous with the diencephalon), pons, and medulla (continuous with the spinal cord). It contains many tracts, the nuclei of the cranial nerves, and other nuclei such as the reticular formation, respiratory center, locus coeruleus, raphé nuclei, and other vital centers concerned with vigilance, sleep, motor tone, autonomic function, etc.

BROCA'S (EXPRESSIVE) APHASIA—An acquired aphasia produced by an anterior (frontal or frontoparietal) lesion of the dominant hemisphere. Comprehension is completely or largely spared. Expression is meaningful but effortful, sparse, and telegraphic. Syntax and phonology are impaired. Small words (functors), e.g., articles, prepositions, and auxillaries, are dropped. Language consists mainly of verbs and nouns. Patients tend to make the same errors in writing as in speech but reading comprehension is spared.

BUFFER—A term borrowed from computer science where it refers to a part of the memory or core that can be used again and again for ephemeral intermediate computational operations because the information it contained is dumped after an answer is arrived at, thus freeing it for other purposes. By analogy, buffer is used in neuroscience, for instance, for circuits involved in short-term memory operations.

BULBAR PALSY—Weakness of the muscles of the face, mouth, and pharynx owing to "lower motor neuron" involvement.

BUTYROPHENONES—A group of potent antipsychotic drugs or major tranquilizers the best known of which is haloperidol (Haldol®). They are thought to exert at least some of their effects by blocking dopamine receptors. Haloperidol is helpful in some patients with Tourette syndrome whose symptoms have therefore been tentatively attributed to excess dopamine in the basal ganglia.

CALCARINE CORTEX—Primary cortical projection area of the visual system, located in the mesial occipital lobe.

CARBAMAZEPINE (TEGRETOL®)—An anticonvulsant drug that is effective in major motor, focal and, especially, in complex partial or psychomotor seizures for which many consider it the drug of choice. It is generally ineffective against petit mal absences and myoclonus. In some children, it may have troublesome gastrointestinal side effects, and in toxic doses produces ataxia and drowsiness. Rarely, it produces liver or bone marrow toxicity.

CATALEPSY—A movement disorder characterized by the prolonged and apparently effortless maintenance of unusual postures, including those imposed by an examiner. It may be seen in some catatonic patients and can be produced in experimental animals by large doses of dopamine blocking agents.

CATECHOLAMINES—Dopamine, norepinephrine (noradrenalin) and epinephrine (adrenalin). They act as neurotransmitters.

CAUDATE NUCLEUS—Part of the basal ganglia (q.v.).

CEREBELLUM—A large structure located dorsally to the brain stem and forming the roof of the fourth ventricle. It comprises two hemispheres and a midline portion called the vermis. It is a major system concerned with motor control. It receives inputs from the spinal cord, inferior olivary nucleus, vestibular oculomotor, auditory, and visual systems as well as from the prefrontal cortex via the pontine nuclei. These inputs terminate in the cerebellar cortex. The cortex in turn projects to the deep cerebellar nuclei. The main output of the cerebellum is directed upward via the ventrolateral thalamus back to the sensorimotor and premotor cortex. Lesions of the cerebellar hemispheres produce ipsilateral motor deficit, those of the vermis interfere with stable posture of the head and trunk, and with gait. The cerebellar cortex contains two main types of cells, Purkinje cells, which are very large, and granular cells which are very numerous, as well as a variety of other interneurons.

CEREBRAL BLOOD FLOW STUDIES—Measurement, with the use of isotopes and computers, of the blood flow to the brain. Such methods enable one to record changes in blood flow, reflecting increased or decreased local brain metabolism, as a function of particular activities such as moving the hand, thinking, speaking, reading, etc.

CEREBRAL CORTEX—Outer layers of the brain containing the cell bodies of neurons that are arranged in defined horizontal layers and orderly vertical columns. The fine structure of the cortex varies greatly across cortical areas (architectonics). In general, the superficial layers receive inputs to the cortex, the deep layers contain output cells (in particular large pyramidal neurons). Various areas of the cortex are connected through local circuits and through longer fibers traveling in the white matter. Corresponding (homologous) areas of the two cerebral hemispheres are connected through commissural fibers. The cortex receives fiber tracts from many subcortical structures, notably the thalamus. It projects back to many subcortical structures, in particular the basal ganglia, to many nuclei in the brain stem, and directly to the spinal cord through the corticospinal (pyramidal) pathway.

CEREBRAL MANTLE—Cerebral cortex and subjacent white matter.

CEREBRAL PALSY (CP)—Motor deficit reflecting nonprogressive brain damage acquired in the perinatal period or in early life. The term says nothing about the type or location of the motor deficit or about its severity or cause.

CHIASM—OPTIC CHIASM (q.v.).

CHOLESCYSTOKININ—A gastrointestinal peptide also found in large amounts in the brain, notably the cortex. In the hypothalamus, it appears to play a role in the control of feeding behavior.

CHOLINERGIC—A compound that mimics the effects of acetylcholine (q.v.). Cholinergic cells or synapses release acetylcholine as a neurotransmitter. Cholinergic receptors bind acetylcholine.

CHOREA—Rapid irregular abnormal involuntary movements of the face and limbs that are nonrhythmical, of varying amplitude, and may at times appear bizarre or quasi-voluntary. Chorea is caused by pathology in the striatum (basal ganglia).

CHOREOATHETOSIS—A movement disorder usually seen in the context of cerebral palsy where choreic, dystonic, and athetotic movements are combined with a profound disorder of body posture and tone.

CHUNKING—Organizing data according to some rule that will enable them to be processed more efficiently. Categorizing items into superordinate classes is a common chunking strategy. Chunking is a term borrowed from computer science that is applied to the organization of material for storage in long-term memory.

CLONAZEPAM (CLONOPIN®)—An anticonvulsant drug useful against myoclonic jerks, including infantile spasms, and with some activity against absence seizures. It is generally ineffective against other seizure types. Because it may produce drowsiness, it is tolerated best if introduced in slowly increasing doses.

CLONIC MUSCLE CONTRACTION—Involuntary jerking movements separated by periods of relaxation. Clonic movements during a seizure indicate that inhibitory influences are starting to reassert themselves.

CLONUS—Self-perpetuating phasic contractions in muscles whose motor neurons have lost inhibitory control. Often precipitated by eliciting a stretch reflex. Clonus is a sign of increased excitability, and it often suggests pathology in "upper motor neurons." Clonus is but one sign of spasticity.

COLLICULI—Nuclei of the tectum of the midbrain. The superior colliculus is concerned with directing the eyes toward visual targets, the inferior colliculus with audition and sound localization.

COMA—A state during which a person has decreased or absent responses to sensory stimulation and is unconscious, often but not invariably with eyes closed. Coma is usually associated with marked decrease in movement and often with abnormal postures. The EEG is abnormal in coma. Patients do not remember what happened to them while they were comatose, and often for a variable period during the recovery phase (amnesia).

COMMISSURES—Bundles of fibers linking homologous brain regions of the two hemispheres. The two major commissures are the corpus callosum (q.v.) and the anterior commissure which contains fibers that link anterior portions of the temporal lobes and olfactory pathways. The anterior commissure is located in the diencephalon in the anterior wall of the third ventricle, below the most anterior end (rostrum) of the corpus callosum and above the optic chiasm.

COMMISSUROTOMY—Severing of the interhemispheric commissures, for experimental reasons in animals, or for the control of intractable epileptic seizures in patients. As a consequence, each of the hemispheres becomes functionally independent.

COMPLEX PARTIAL (TEMPORAL LOBE, PSYCHOMOTOR) SEIZURES— Seizures with complex symptomatology such as automatisms (e.g., picking at the clothes, humming, walking, chewing), and clouding of consciousness. Some patients experience strong emotions such as fear, sadness, or elation. Some patients can speak during such seizures and have sensory hallucinations, or illusions such as the feeling that they are reliving a previous experience in familiar surroundings (déjà vu), and many others. Some patients are amnesic for their seizure but others can describe their experiences. Most complex partial seizures originate in the temporal lobe. Those originating in the uncus of the hippocampus and associated with olfactory hallucinations and a dreamy state are called uncinate fits.

CONCUSSION—Brief loss of consciousness following an acute head injury. It is a reversible state and has been attributed to malfunction of the reticular activating system. Prolonged loss of consciousness after a head injury denotes more severe dysfunction than concussion, for example, cerebral contusion, brain swelling, or structural brain stem pathology.

CONDITIONING—A training technique in which a stimulus in one modality is regularly followed by one in another. The animal or person learns to associate or connect the second stimulus with the first and will produce a response normally associated with the second in response to the first.
Classic conditioning pairs a neutral stimulus with one that produces an autonomic response.
Operant conditioning uses a rewarding stimulus to foster response to an otherwise neutral stimulus.
Avoidance conditioning allows an animal to escape a noxious stimulus by responding to a warning stimulus.

CONDUCTION APHASIA—Inability to repeat. It is typically brought out by asking the patient to repeat the phrase "no ifs, ands, or buts." Also called subcortical aphasia because it has been ascribed to a lesion affecting the fibers that connect the posterior with the anterior language areas of the dominant hemisphere. Comprehension and expression are usually adequate although the patients often make paraphasic errors.

CONFABULATION—The recounting by suggestible amnesic patients of often improbable or self-contradictory events to fill in the void of their recent past which they cannot remember.

CONSTRUCTIONAL APRAXIA—A visuospatial-motor disorder that impairs the performance of such tasks as reproducing block patterns.

CONVULSIVE DISORDER—Epilepsy (q.v.). Paradoxically, one may speak of a convulsive disorder even in cases where patients have minor seizures such as absences and do not have convulsions. Convulsive movements result from involuntary rhythmical contractions of muscles driven by the paroxysmal discharges of the cortex.

COROLLARY DISCHARGES—Information about the firing of a neuron provided by axon collateral branches to targets outside of the main target of its axon. This information may be distributed as feedback to interneurons in the immediate vicinity of a pyramidal neuron of the motor cortex, for example, to neurons in the sensorimotor cortex due to receive feedback from the effectors of the motor command, or to subcortical loops concerned with motor control. Corollary discharges have often been compared to carbon copies of a letter distributed inhouse for informational use.

CORPUS CALLOSUM—A major bundle of transverse fibers linking homologous areas of the neocortex. It is situated between the two cerebral hemispheres above the diencephalon and third ventricle. It extends from the posterior frontal region anteriorly (genu) to the parieto-occipital region posteriorly (splenium).

CORTICOBULBAR TRACT—Part of the pyramidal tract (q.v.) innervating the motor nuclei of the cranial nerves in the brain stem.

CORTICOSPINAL TRACT—Pyramidal tract (q.v.).

CRANIAL NERVES–Nerves that innervate the head and some of the viscera. With the exception of the olfactory and optic nerves, they emerge from the brain stem where their nuclei of origin are located. Sensory cranial nerves have their cells of origin in extracerebral ganglia. There are 12 pairs of cranial nerves.

CT or COMPUTERIZED TRANSAXIAL TOMOGRAPHY SCANNING (also known as CAT or EMI SCAN)—An X-ray method that, with the use of computers, enables one to produce images of the brain where structural details as small as a few millimeters can be visualized. It is very useful for detecting brain anomalies, tumors, blood clots, swelling, atrophy, etc.

DECUSSATION—Crossing of a fiber tract from one side of the brain or spinal cord to the other.

DEMENTIA—Loss of cognitive skills because of an acquired brain lesion or dysfunction. If the underlying condition is progressive, the dementia will be progressive.

DENDRITES—Often multiple and extensively branched receptor processes of neurons. They are studded with synaptic sites, some of which form specialized areas called dendritic spines. The postsynaptic membranes of dendrites generate excitatory or inhibitory postsynaptic potentials that are graded potentials. These are continuously integrated and their sum (together with the generally inhibitory postsynaptic potentials generated in postsynaptic receptors on the shaft of the dendrite and cell body) will determine whether or not the neuron fires. Through its dendritic tree, each neuron receives thousands of inputs from potentially hundreds of thousands of other neurons.

DENERVATION—Loss of innervation, of afferent inputs.

DERMATOGLYPHICS—The pattern of creases and ridges on the palms of the hands and fingers and the soles of the feet and toes. These are highly individualized and do not change from their formation in early pregnancy throughout life. The patterns may be altered by pathology occurring during the first trimester of pregnancy. Characteristic patterns are seen in some chromosomal anomalies and other genetic and malformation syndromes, therefore, dermatoglyphics may be helpful to diagnosis in some developmental disorders of childhood.

DESYNCHRONIZATION—A term frequently applied to the EEG when it loses its rhythmicity. Desynchronization usually implies arousal of the cortex by the reticular formation in response to a stimulus that has alerting properties. Desynchronization usually denotes activation.

DEVELOPMENTAL LANGUAGE DISABILITY (DYSPHASIA)—Impaired development of language for communicative use in children who are not deaf, have adequate intelligence, and social environment. Several types of language disability depend on whether reception or expression are primarily affected and whether phonology, syntax, semantics, and/or pragmatics are implicated. The nosology of dysphasia is still tentative. In some children genetic factors may be at fault, in others, brain maldevelopment or adventitious dysfunction are likely etiologies. Some dysphasic children have associated signs of brain dysfunction such as delayed motor milestones, oromotor dysfunction, seizures, or autistic behavior. Prognosis is variable but children are at risk for later learning disabilities. In toddlers, the differential diagnosis between delayed language development and pathologically deviant language development is often difficult.

DIAZEPAM (VALIUM®)—An anxiolytic drug that also has anticonvulsant effects. It is a drug of choice, used intravenously, in patients with status epilepticus. It may be helpful against infantile spasms and some forms of myoclonus.

DICHOTIC STIMULATION—Presentation of competing messages simultaneously to the two ears. Verbal messages (e.g., digits, letters) are reported preferentially and more reliably when they are presented to the ear contralateral to the hemisphere dominant for language than when presented to the other ear. The reverse is true for some nonverbal sounds such as melodies. This test is one of those used to study cerebral dominance for language.

DIENCEPHALON—Deep midline area of the brain that contains such structures as the thalamus; hypothalamus; mammillary bodies; subthalamic nuclei; pineal gland; third ventricle; and various fiber tracts, in particular, some belonging to the limbic system.

DIPARESIS—Weakness affecting both legs because of a symmetrical lesion of both cerebral hemispheres involving the corticospinal fibers to both legs. The hands may be involved but less severely than the legs. Such lesions are typically parasagittal or located high in the white matter. If the legs are paralyzed, one may speak of a spastic diplegia.

DOMINANT HEMISPHERE—Hemisphere specialized for language and skilled movements of the preferred hand. The left hemisphere is dominant in 99% of right-handed normal persons and in 65% of left-handed persons. Other left-handed persons are either right-brained or do not have strongly lateralized language function.

DOPAMINE—A catecholamine neurotransmitter or biogenic amine in the brain. One of its precursors is L-DOPA and it is the immediate precursor of norepinephrine. There are dopaminergic neurons in the hypothalamus that inhibit the release of prolactin by the pituitary, and in the substantia nigra where they give rise to the well-known nigrostriatal tract that projects to the caudate and putamen, and in the tegmentum of the mesencephalon, projecting to the nucleus accubens via the mesolimbic tract. Dopaminergic pathways can be traced by fluorescence-microscopy. The action of dopamine is generally inhibitory. Dopamine pathways are involved in motor control and are presumed to be involved in many other brain functions.

DYSARTHRIA—Nonlinguistic (i.e., motor) deficit of speech articulation resulting from lesions of the corticobulbar pathway, of "lower motor neurons" to the muscles of articulation, from weakness of these muscles, or from pathology in extrapyramidal or cerebellar circuits.

DYSESTHESIA—Abnormal, disagreeable cutaneous sensation.

DYSGRAPHIA—Inadequate acquisition of writing skills not accounted for by a motor deficit, mental deficiency, lack of motivation, or inadequate educational opportunity. Dysgraphia implies dysorthographia. It may be associated with graphomotor inadequacy.

DYSLEXIA—Failure to develop competence for reading despite normal vision and hearing, adequate intelligence and motivation, and average educational exposure. Several syndromes of dyslexia have been delineated based on an analysis of neuropsychologic deficits and the type of reading problems in individual children. Dyslexia may be caused by either genetic or acquired brain dysfunction or both. Etiology appears to cut across the various syndromes.

DYSMETRIA—Goal directed movement that lacks smoothness, that is decomposed.

DYSPHASIA—Developmental language disability (q.v.).

DYSPLASIA—Developmental abnormality or malformation.

DYSTONIA—Movement disorder with phasic alterations in tone resulting in grotesque postures. It is presumed to result from dysfunction in the basal ganglia although its pathology and chemical basis are still unknown.

ECHOLALIA—The verbatim repetition of what was heard. Characteristic of verbal autistic children and of some hydrocephalic children and children with frontal lobe syndromes. Echolalia is often associated with pronominal reversal (I-you confusion) and with the child referring to himself by his name or in the third person. Echolalia may be immediate or it may be delayed, in the latter case the children will often recite "canned" phrases or stock sentences. Echolia strongly suggests inadequate comprehension.

ECHOPRAXIA—The repetition of gestures a person has just seen. Characteristic of some patients with frontal lobe syndromes.

ELECTROENCEPHALOGRAM (EEG)—The recording of the electrical activity of the brain from surface electrodes pasted to the scalp. The EEG reflects electrical activity of the underlying cortex, which varies with age, alertness, sleep phase, and with a variety of disease states. The EEG is especially useful for the diagnosis of convulsive disorders.

EFFERENT—Output of a neuron or neuronal system.

ENCEPHALITIS—Inflammation of the brain, most often because of a viral infection.

ENCEPHALOPATHY—Damage or dysfunction of the brain, etiology unspecified.

EPILEPSY—A chronic convulsive disorder. A single seizure and seizures in the course of an acute illness or encephalopathy do not necessarily imply that the patient is an epileptic. Epilepsy has many causes (see Chapter 4).

EPINEPHRINE (ADRENALIN)—A hormone produced by the adrenal medulla that is a catecholamine that may be utilized as a neurotransmitter by some brain stem cells. Its immediate precursor is norepinephrine (q.v.).

ESTROGEN—A female sex hormone.

ETHOSUXIMIDE (ZARONTIN®)—An anticonvulsant drug especially useful against petit mal absences. It produces gastric discomfort in some children and, rarely, bone marrow toxicity.

ETIOLOGY—The specific cause for an illness, for instance, infection with a particular organism, genetic enzymatic deficit, trauma, etc. Etiology is often confused with pathogenesis (q.v.).

EVOKED POTENTIALS OR EVOKED RESPONSES—Cerebral electrical activity usually evoked by repeated auditory, visual, or somatosensory stimulation and recorded, with the help of computers, from the scalp EEG. Some originate in the cerebral cortex (cortical evoked responses), others in the brain stem (brain stem evoked responses). They reflect physiologic activity in the living brain.

EXTRAOCULAR MUSCLES—Muscles that move the eye in the orbit.

EXTRAPYRAMIDAL SYSTEM—This term refers to all descending pathways to motor neurons and interneurons that do not travel in the pyramidal tract. Vestibulo-, rubro-, tecto-, and reticulospinal tracts are extrapyramidal, as are the interconnections of the basal ganglia, thalamus, mesencephalic and pontine nuclei.

FASCICULATION—Spontaneous contraction of a motor unit (q.v.). Fasciculations can be seen with the naked eye and are often a sign of denervation of muscle.

FOCAL MOTOR SEIZURE—A motor seizure limited to a part of the body on one side. Most focal motor seizures denote a focal lesion in the contralateral hemisphere. Any focal motor seizure may be the prelude to a generalized seizure. *Jacksonian seizures* are characterized by slow spread of clonic movements from one part of the body to another (for example, from the thumb to the hand, the arm, the face and the leg on the same side).

FOCAL SEIZURE—Any seizure discharge involving, for a time at least, a limited part of the brain. Focal seizures may be motor, sensory, visual, auditory, complex partial, etc. Sensory or psychical experiences as part of a focal seizure are often called auras.

FOLIUM—A convolution of the cerebellum.

FORNIX—A pathway linking the hippocampal formation of the temporal lobe with various diencephalic structures. An important limbic pathway (q.v.).

FOVEA—The region of the retina which has the sharpest visual acuity.

FRONTAL LOBE—The most anterior portion of the cerebral hemispheres, comprising their largest cortical area. Except for the motor cortex, premotor cortex, and supplementary motor area, the frontal cortex is an association area. It has strong connections with other cortical areas, with the neostriatum, anterior parts of the thalamus, and limbic system. The posterior orbital surface of the frontal lobe is considered a part of the limbic system. The frontal lobe is concerned, *inter alia*, with programming of behavior and with decision making. On the dominant side it is concerned with the programming of speech.

GABA—Gamma amino butyric acid (q.v.). Gabergic cells release GABA as neurotransmitter. Gabergic receptors bind GABA.

GAMMA AMINO BUTYRIC ACID (GABA)— An inhibitory neurotransmitter of the brain.

GAMMA LOOP—A spinal motor control system that involves muscle spindles (q.v.). These specialized fibers are arranged in parallel to striated motor fibers. The gamma loop is concerned with the regulation of muscle tone.

GANGLIA—Aggregate of neuronal cell bodies, either in the periphery (e.g., dorsal root ganglia) or within the brain (e.g., the basal ganglia). Groups of interconnected neurons within the brain are usually called nuclei.

GENERALIZED SEIZURE—Tonic-clonic seizure affecting all parts of the body, with loss of consciousness (see GRAND MAL SEIZURE).

GLIA or GLIAL CELLS—Supporting cells in the central nervous system. Glial cells are of three types, astrocytes, oligodendroglia, and microglia. The oligodendroglia make the myelin sheaths of axons.

GLOBUS PALLIDUS (PALEOSTRIATUM)—Part of the basal ganglia (q.v.).

GLUTAMATE (GLUTAMIC ACID)—An amino acid acting as an excitatory neurotransmitter.

GLYCINE—An inhibitory neurotransmitter, notably of the Renshaw cell that inhibits alpha motor neurons (anterior horn cells) of the spinal cord.

GRAND MAL SEIZURE—Strictly speaking, a generalized seizure with loss of consciousness from the onset and falling, with tonic contraction of all the muscles of the body followed by clonic or jerking contractions, followed by post ictal depression and sleep. In practice, any generalized seizure tends to be loosely referred to as a grand mal seizure even if it has a focal onset.

GRAY MATTER—Portions of the nervous system that look gray to the naked eye and contain nerve cell bodies and their dendrites. The cerebral cortex, basal ganglia, thalamus and many other nuclei, and the core of the spinal cord, belong to the gray matter.

GYRUS—A convolution of the cerebral cortex.

HABITUATION—Progressive loss of response to and of arousal by a repetitive stimulus.

HALLUCINATIONS—Vivid sensory experiences (usually visual or auditory, but also olfactory, gustatory, cutaneous, etc.) that result from endogenous excitation of the corresponding sensory pathways or cortical projection areas. They may occur as part of a seizure, be the result of drug ingestion, metabolic illness, psychosis, and occur under other circumstances such as prolonged sensory deprivation.

HAPTIC—Perceived by active palpation with the hand.

HEMIANOPSIA—Blindness for one side of visual space. Hemianopsias denote a defect in the central visual pathway from the level of the optic chiasm back to the visual cortex. When both eyes are blind for the same side of space, the hemianopsia is homonymous and the lesion retrochiasmatic on the contralateral side of the brain. Chiasmatic lesions almost always produce blindness for the temporal side of space seen with the nasal retina of each eye (bitemporal hemianopsia) because they involve the crossing fibers selectively (see also OPTIC CHIASM).

HEMIPARESIS—Spastic weakness affecting one side of the body, including the lower part of the face, resulting from a cerebral lesion on the contralateral side. If the hemiparesis is caused by a lesion in the cerebral hemisphere the hand is usually more affected than the leg. Hemiparetic patients can walk, albeit with a limp. The hemiparesis may be associated with a hemisensory loss and with a homonymous hemianopsia. The pattern of weakness and associated findings help in localizing the level of the lesion along the pyramidal tract.

HEMIPLEGIA—A severe hemiparesis (q.v.) with complete paralysis of the hand. Chronically hemiplegic patients usually can walk with a limp but may require a brace because of weakness of dorsiflexors of the foot resulting in a foot drop.

HIPPOCAMPUS—Part of the limbic cortex situated in the mesial temporal lobe. Comprises the hippocampus proper, hippocampal gyrus, and several other structures. The hippocampus plays a key role in learning and the retrieval of long-term memories.

HOLOPROSENCEPHALY—A rare severe malformation of the brain arising early in the first trimester of gestation in which the brain does not divide into two hemispheres. Children with holoprosencephaly are severely mentally defective and spastic and may have seizures. In some children, the cause of this malformation is a trisomy (extra chromosome 13), and in such cases other malformations, of the face and eyes especially, are usually present.

HOMONYMOUS HEMIANOPSIA—Inability to see one side of visual space with each of the eyes. The blind hemifield is contralateral to a lesion in the optic tract, lateral geniculate body, optic radiations, or visual cortex.

HOMUNCULUS—Representation of the body surface and muscles in the sensorimotor cortex.

HORMONES—Biologically active substances released by the endocrine glands into the blood stream that exert their effects at a distance. There are many hormones produced by many endocrine glands widely scattered in the body. Insulin, thyroid hormones, adrenal hormones, sex hormones, pituitary hormones are but a few typical ones.

HUNTINGTON'S CHOREA—A dominantly inherited chronic disease that usually presents in adult life with a movement disorder and dementia. It may present in childhood when rigidity and seizures accompany the dementia. It is invariably fatal after a course of several years. It affects the neostriatum and cortex predominantly.

HYDRANENCEPHALY—Congenital anomaly in which virtually the entire cerebral hemispheres are replaced by cerebrospinal fluid. Hydranencephaly is usually the result of intrauterine infarction of the cerebral hemispheres or of extreme hydrocephalus. The size of the skull may be normal or enlarged, less often microcephalic. The children are usually severely to profoundly retarded and spastic and do not undergo meaningful development, except in a few cases with extreme hydrocephalus treated with shunting at birth.

HYDROCEPHALUS—An accumulation of cerebrospinal fluid in the cerebral ventricles that have become enlarged as a result. There are several types and causes of hydrocephalus, the severity of which varies. In general, hydrocephalus produces more destruction of the white matter (and of the tracts contained therein) than of the gray matter. For unclear reasons, hydrocephalus in children is often more severe in the occipital than the frontal horns.

HYPERACTIVITY, HYPERKINETIC SYNDROME (See ATTENTION DEFICIT DISORDER)— Excessive motor activity, motor restlessness. Hyperkinetic children often have sleep problems, are distractible, and have been hyperactive since infancy. In some children, hyperkinesis is associated with motor clumsiness or with a learning disability, but these are associated symptoms rather than consequences of the hyperkinesis. Some hyperkinetic children respond favorably to stimulants like methylphenidate (Ritalin®) or amphetamine (Dexedrine®).

HYPOTHALAMUS—Portion of the diencephalon situated below the thalamus and above the optic chiasm. It is considered to be part of the limbic system. It controls the autonomic nervous system (parasympathetic and sympathetic) and endocrine system. It contains many nuclei, some of which release neuropeptides that control the anterior pituitary gland, others that act as posterior pituitary hormones (vasopressin and oxytocin). The hypothalamus is concerned with temperature control, eating and drinking, sexual activity, and attack and defense behavior. It is affected by olfaction, taste, vision, audition, and many visceral sensations such as hunger, thirst, sexual stimulation, gastrointestinal inputs, blood pressure, temperature, and pain. The hypothalamus is directly involved in the control of body homeostasis, drives, and motivated behavior. It participates in the control of mood and affect.

HYPOTONIA—Decreased muscle tone. Hypotonia usually suggests a cerebellar deficit, dysfunction of the "lower motor neuron" (anterior horn cell and peripheral nerve), or of muscle. The causes of "central" hypotonia are not well defined and may involve vestibular or other brain stem mechanisms.

HYPSARRHYTHMIA—An EEG pattern with high voltage slow waves and multifocal spikes seen in infants who have infantile spasms (q.v.). This condition, which has many etiologies, is usually the prelude to severe mental deficiency. The EEG pattern rarely persists into childhood but is replaced by other abnormalities, notably slow spike-and-waves.

IDEOGRAM—A single graphic symbol standing for a whole word. Chinese writing is ideographic. Japanese uses a combination of ideograms, borrowed from the Chinese, called kanji, and of a phonetic notation, called kana.

INDOLE AMINES—A group of compounds with indole groups that affect behavior. Serotonin (5-hydroxytryptamine) is the principal one. It exerts its effects by acting as a neurotransmitter. Interference with serotonin affects sleep. Serotonin blocking agents like LSD and mescaline produce florid hallucinations and other behavioral effects.

INFANTILE SPASMS—Myoclonic jerks with flexion of the body and dropping of the head (salaam seizures) or other brief motor seizures occurring in runs in infancy. The EEG usually shows a hypsarrhythmic pattern (q.v.). This condition has multiple etiologies but is usually the prelude to severe mental deficiency. It is sometimes referred to as Best's syndrome.

INSULA or ISLAND of REIL—A portion of the neocortex that is folded into the Sylvian fissure.

INTERICTAL INTERVAL—A period of time of any duration separating two epileptic seizures.

INTERNEURON—A neuron, often with a short axon, that is interposed between two neurons in a circuit. It may be inhibitory or play the role of a comparator or integrator.

JACKSONIAN SEIZURE—A spreading focal motor seizure (q.v.). The spread of the seizure is often called a march and reflects show spread of unbridled excitation in the motor cortex contralateral to the affected side of the body.

KINDLING—Development of self-sustaining epileptic activity as a result of intermittent stimulation at subconvulsive intensity. Kindling can be produced in the laboratory; some believe it may account for the late development of clinical seizures in some patients many months or even years after they sustained a brain insult. It is also thought by some to be responsible for the development of epileptic activity (mirror focus) in the hemisphere contralateral to the one originally containing an epileptic focus. Kindling seems to occur with particular ease in the amygdala and hippocampus of the temporal lobe.

KLÜVER-BUCY SYNDROME—A syndrome produced in monkeys by bilateral temporal resection that has been attributed to ablation of the amygdala. Visual identification of objects is deficient, the animals mouth edible and inedible objects unselectively, are hypersexual, and inappropriately tame.

KORSAKOFF SYNDROME—A permanent anterograde amnesic state often caused by chronic alcoholic encephalopathy and associated with pathology in the mammillary bodies and dorsal medial nucleus of the thalamus.

LABYRINTH (VESTIBULE, q.v.)—Part of the inner ear concerned with balance.

LEARNING—The cascade of overlapping processes that enable one to store items in long-term memory and to retrieve them therefrom.

LEARNING DISABILITY—A general term referring to scholastic failure that cannot be ascribed to general cognitive incompetence, lack of motivation, or lack of educational opportunity. The child may have dyslexia with or without dysgraphia, dyscalculia, or all three. Learning disability is thought to reflect neocortical dysfunction limited to particular systems. The children may have associated deficits such as a language disorder, visual-perceptual deficits, graphomotor dyscoordination, sequencing deficits, memory problems, or an attention deficit disorder. Neuropsychologic testing shows uneven subtest scores with at least (by definition) some scores in the average range while others may be defective. Management consists of special education tailored to the child's particular deficits, taking advantage of areas of adequate skill in order to circumvent deficiencies.

LEMNISCAL PATHWAYS—Sensory pathways with few synapses carrying modality-specific information reliably to distant targets (as opposed to multisynaptic diffuse pathways). The medial lemniscus carries somatosensory information (not pain) and the lateral lemniscus carries auditory information, both from the brain stem to the thalamus.

LEPTOMENINGES—The arachnoid and pial membranes (cf. meninges).

LEXICON—Repository of word meanings, long-term memory for words.

LIMBIC SYSTEM (RHINENCEPHALON, VISCERAL BRAIN)—A phylogenetically old portion of the brain with extremely complex connections. Many portions of the limbic system are arranged in a roughly circular region of the mesial aspect of the hemispheres surrounding the third ventricle. The limbic system extends from the upper midbrain through the hypothalamus and parts of the thalamus to the septum and posterior orbital surface of the frontal lobes. Some other parts of the limbic system are: the hypothalamus, the hippocampus (situated in the temporal lobe), cingulate gyrus (a gyrus curving above the corpus callosum), fornix (a pathway between the hippocampus and diencephalon, situated below the corpus callosum), amygdala (a nucleus in the anterior temporal lobe), mammillary bodies (two paired nuclei projecting from the posterior hypothalamus). The limbic system has to do with the control of motivated behavior, sexual behavior, fighting, fleeing, mood and affect, and learning. It is involved in decision making when behavioral alternatives have to be weighed. It is concerned with overall organismic and species-specific behaviors.

LOCUS COERULEUS—Paired nuclei in the pons which are rich in noradrenergic neurons that send widespread projections to the Purkinje cells of the cerebellum and to the neocortex, limbic system, and hypothalamus.

LONG-TERM MEMORY—Repository of consolidated memories. Items in long-term memory are organized in such a way that items are activated together with their features and can be accessed via a variety of these. Items in long-term storage are cross-linked and organized meaningfully. Storage and retrieval are strongly influenced by attentional and affective variables and engage activity of the hippocampus and other limbic and brain stem circuits.

LONG TRACTS—Pathways containing the axons of neurons that interconnect distant areas of the nervous system, notably the cortex and spinal cord, spinal cord and cerebellum, etc.

"LOWER MOTOR NEURONS" (MOTOR NEURONS)—Pyramidal cells of the anterior horn of the spinal cord and of the cranial nerve motor nuclei innervating striated muscles. Pathology in "lower motor neurons" is characteristically associated with weakness, wasting, hypotonia, and loss of tendon stretch reflexes.

MAINSTREAMING—Placing a handicapped child in school in a class with his normal peers for as many hours a day as is compatible with his particular specialized educational needs.

MBD—Minimal brain dysfunction (or damage) (q.v.).

MEDIAL FOREBRAIN BUNDLE—An important diencephalic pathway linking various structures of the midbrain, hypothalamus, and septal area.

MEDULLA—The caudal portion of the brain stem, continuous with the cervical portion of the spinal cord. It contains many fiber tracts, the nuclei of many cranial nerves, notably the vagus (parasympathetic), the acoustic and vestibular nuclei, the inferior olive—a large relay nucleus projecting to the cerebellum, descending reticular formation, respiratory center, and other autonomic nuclei. The medulla (and pons) form the floor of the fourth ventricle. The cerebellum lies dorsally to the medulla (and pons).

MENINGES—Membranes enveloping the brain and spinal cord.
The *dura*, the outermost one, is a tough connective tissue sac.
The *arachnoid*, the middle one, contains the spinal fluid pathways.
The *pia*, the innermost one, is adherent to the brain and spinal cord surface.
Blood vessels to the brain and cord travel in the pia-arachnoid.

MENTAL DEFICIENCY—Overall cognitive incompetence resulting in consistently maladaptive behaviors. Mental deficiency reflects diffuse or multifocal brain dysfunction. This term is used interchangeably with mental retardation (q.v.). For some, but not all workers, mental deficiency implies organic factors more strongly than mental retardation.

MENTAL RETARDATION (MR)—Overall cognitive incompetence resulting in consistently maladaptive behaviors. This term is often used interchangeably with mental deficiency. Failure to achieve one's cognitive potential because of genetic factors or social environmental deprivation has been called "simple," "mild," or "endogenous" MR, while MR caused by gross brain damage was called "exogenous" MR. "Retardation" does not imply that MR is due to a maturational lag or that catch-up will occur. A definition of MR based on IQ levels is useful in practice but fraught with many possibilities for error, especially among patients with focal brain dysfunction. The upper limit of MR is conventionally set at IQ 70.

MESENCEPHALON—Midbrain (q.v.).

MESIAL—Located on the inner surface of the cerebral hemisphere, adjacent to the interhemispheric fissure.

METHYLPHENIDATE (RITALIN®)—A stimulant drug prescribed for some children with Attention Deficit Disorder.

MICRENCEPHALY—Small brain. Developmental anomaly with many causes, the result of either maldevelopment or severe brain damage incurred *in utero* or in infancy. Usually associated with mental deficiency of varying severity.

MICROCEPHALY—Small head. Often reflects micrencephaly (q.v.).

MIDBRAIN (MESENCEPHALON)—Rostral part of the brain stem. It contains the aqueduct of Sylvius, a canal linking the third and fourth ventricles, many fiber tracts, the nuclei of oculomotor nerves, pupilloconstrictor neurons, the substantia nigra (part of the basal ganglia), the red nucleus (a motor pathway waystation). It also comprises the superior colliculus (a subcortical nucleus concerned with oculomotor control), inferior colliculus (a waystation of the central auditory pathway), the reticular activating system, raphé nuclei, and some nuclei of the limbic system. Some periaqueductal neurons are rich in opioid receptors and are involved in pain perception.

MINIMAL BRAIN DYSFUNCTION or DAMAGE (MBD)—A vague term describing children who are clumsy, who have a learning deficit or an attention deficit disorder (ADD). The term says little or nothing about the severity or kind of deficit the child has, its location, or pathogenesis. It does imply that the child does not have severe deficits like cerebral palsy, mental deficiency, or psychotic behavior, and that the problem is static rather than progressive. It does not imply that the child "will grow out of it" though some symptoms may improve or change with age.

MORPHOLOGY—Subsystem of language which includes words and inflectional endings.

MONOSYNAPTIC—A two neuron pathway with but one synapse.

MOTOR CORTEX (MOTOR STRIP)—Situated in the ascending frontal gyrus, immediately in front of the central sulcus that separates the frontal from the parietal lobe. The motor homunculus is upside down, with the leg area in the mesial aspect of the gyrus, adjacent to the interhemispheric fissure. Each half of the body receives inputs predominantly from the contralateral hemisphere, with the lower face and hand areas being most strongly lateralized and occupying the largest cortical area.

MOTOR NEURON (ALPHA MOTOR NEURON)—"Lower motor neuron" (q.v.).

MOTOR UNIT—Muscle fibers innervated by one motor neuron.

MUCOPOLYSACCHARIDOSES—A class of genetic-metabolic diseases in which complex molecules cannot be broken down because of the lack of degradative enzymes. Some affect both connective tissue and the nervous system and thus have widespread effects. Their prototype is gargoylism or Hurler disease.

MUSCLE SPINDLES—Specialized muscle fibers with sensory receptors found in striated muscle that provide proprioceptive information about muscle length and tension (stretch) and play an important role in the control of muscle tone. Muscle spindles are under the control of gamma loops, a reflex feedback pathway activated during muscle contraction.

MYELIN—A complex proteolipid membrane sheath that surrounds axons and serves as an insulator between adjacent axons and as a facilitator for the propagation of nerve impulses in axons. In the central nervous system myelin is derived from extensions of the cytoplasm of glial cells, called oligodendroglia, wrapped around axons. In peripheral nerves myelin is derived from extensions of the cytoplasm of Schwann cells wrapped around axons. Not all axons are myelinated.

MYOCLONUS—Sudden, brief, jerky, abnormal involuntary movement that may involve a single muscle, a part of a limb, or occasionally the whole limb or body. Myoclonus precipitated by movement is called intention myoclonus. Myoclonus is a form of seizure that may have either a cortical or subcortical origin. It does not impair consciousness.

NARCOLEPSY—A sleep disorder, rarely seen in children, in which REM sleep occurs at the onset of sleep. It is characterized by frequent brief sleeps during the day, cataplexy or sudden falls with laughter or strong emotion, sleep paralysis or inability to move for a brief period on awakening, and hypnagogic hallucinations or vivid visual hallucinations during drowsiness. These symptoms can be explained by muscle atonia and by the occurrence of the visual hallucinations of dreams dissociated from the sleeping state.

NEOCEREBELLUM—Largest portion of the cerebellar hemispheres having to do with the control of skilled movement (as opposed to the archicerebellum having to do with vestibular function, and to the anterior lobe or paleocerebellum having effects on motor tone and posture).

NEOCORTEX—Major portion of the cerebral cortex concerned with sensorimotor processing and with many higher order processes like language, planning, conscious awareness, etc.

NEOPLASM—Tumor.

NEOSTRIATUM—Caudate nucleus and putamen. Part of the basal ganglia (q.v.). Loss of small striatal neurons results in chorea.

NEURAL CREST—An embryonic structure from which spinal ganglia, autonomic ganglia, cells of the adrenal medulla, melanoblasts (pigment forming cells), peptidergic cells (peptide producing cells), and other specialized cells originate.

NEUROFIBROMATOSIS—(von RECKLINGHAUSEN'S DISEASE)—A common autosomal dominant trait resulting in a variety of skin lesions, in particular light brown spots called café au lait spots, tumors in many organs including peripheral nerves, brain, and spinal cord, and various malformations. Only a minority of patients who carry the trait have neurologic problems but these may be life threatening.

NEUROHORMONES—Substances produced by neurons that have endocrine effects. The hypothalamic releasing factors and the hormones synthesized in the hypothalamus and released by the posterior pituitary (the neurohypophyseal hormones oxytocin and vasopressin or antidiuretic hormone) are neurohormones.

NEUROHUMOR—General term referring to neurotransmitters, neuromodulators, and neurohormones.

NEUROMODULATORS—Class of molecules, usually peptides, that influence neural activity transsynaptically but that have more prolonged excitatory or inhibitory effects than neurotransmitters.

NEUROPEPTIDES—Polypeptides with stimulating or inhibitory effects on endocrine cells and on gastrointestinal glands. They are also found in the brain where at least some are produced and thought to act as neuromodulators with a more prolonged action than neurotransmitters. Some of the better known neuropeptides are hormone releasing factors (thyrotropin releasing factor, gonadotropin releasing factor, etc.), the growth hormone inhibitory factor somatostatin, substance P, neurotensin, bradykinin, cholecystokinin, gastrin, and others.

NEUROPSYCHOLOGY—A branch of psychology that attempts to relate particular behaviors to specific brain structures and functions. Neuropsychology is based on the study of the behavioral effects of focal lesions in man and in experimental animals, and on the recording of neuronal activity during behavior in man and animals. Clinical neuropsychologists attempt to make hypotheses concerning brain dysfunction by analyzing the performance of patients on standardized test batteries and specialized tests.

NEUROSECRETION—Secretion of peptides into the blood stream by neurons that play an endocrine as well as a neuronal role. Neurosecretion was first recognized in hypothalamic neurons that send their axons into the posterior lobe of the pituitary gland where they release oxytocin and vasopressin or antidiuretic hormone into the blood stream. Many other neurons of the hyopthalamus are now known to release their products into the portal circulation of the pituitary, thus stimulating or inhibiting the release of pituitary hormones. Neurosecretion may be an even more widespread phenomenon.

NEUROTRANSMITTERS—Chemicals released by presynaptic nerve endings that alter the excitability of postsynaptic neuronal receptors. Neurotransmitters are often stored in presynaptic vesicles. Neurotransmitters may have excitatory (depolarizing) or inhibitory (hyperpolarizing) effects. Most neurons release one neurotransmitter but are sensitive to several. Some of the better known neurotransmitters are acetylcholine, norepinephrine (noradrenalin), dopamine (the latter two called catecholamines), serotonin (5-hydroxytryptamine), and amino acids such as gamma-aminobutyric acid (GABA), glutamic acid, aspartic acid, and others. Pathways containing particular neurotransmitters, notably the catecholamines and serotonin, can be traced by fluorescence microscopy.

NONDOMINANT HEMISPHERE—The hemisphere specialized for visual-spatial processing, some other nonlinguistic skills, and perhaps emotion. The right hemisphere is nondominant in over 95% of right-handed persons and in some 65% of left-handed persons.

NONSPECIFIC THALAMIC NUCLEI—Nuclei that project to widespread areas of the neocortex and to the striatum and that receive inputs from the reticular activating system. They are part of a system concerned with the maintenance of vigilance and with generalized cortical activation.

NORADRENALIN—Norepinephrine (q.v.).

NOREPINEPHRINE (NORADRENALIN)—A neurotransmitter, one of the catecholamines or biogenic amines. The locus coeruleus of the pons contains most of the noradrenergic neurons in the brain; these send their processes to the Purkinje cells of the cerebellum and have extensively branched projections to the neocortex and limbic system. Norepinephrine seems to control mood and vigilance. Norepinephrine is also the neurotransmitter produced by postganglionic fibers of the sympathetic nervous system. The action of norepinephrine is mostly inhibitory. Its immediate precursor is dopamine (q.v.).

NUCLEI—*1*. Nucleus of a cell, containing its DNA. *2*. Group of interconnected neurons within the brain, acting as an integrated system or relay (e.g., the nuclei of the thalamus, hypothalamus, or cranial nerves).

NUCLEUS ACCUMBENS SEPTI—A large nucleus in the septal area that receives dopaminergic fibers from the mesencephalon (mesolimbic pathway).

OCCIPITAL LOBE—The portion of neocortex situated at the back of the head. It is particularly concerned with the processing of visual information. The primary visual area (calcarine cortex) is situated in the mesial aspect of the occipital lobe, adjacent to the interhemispheric fissure. Macular vision is projected to an area near the occipital pole.

OLIVES—Certain paired nuclei of the brain stem.
The *superior olive* is a relay in the central auditory pathway.
The *inferior olive* is a large relay nucleus in the medulla that receives fibers from subcortical motor relays, oculomotor nuclei, and superior colliculus and projects to the cerebellum.

OPERCULUM—(Literaly, cover). These parts of frontal, parietal, and temporal cortex that cover the insula (q.v.).

OPSOCLONUS—Chaotic involuntary movements of the eyes denoting brain stem or cerebellar dysfunction.

OPTIC CHIASM—Crossing of optic fibers originating from the nasal half of each retina to join the fibers originating from the temporal half of the retina of the contralateral eye. As a result of the optic chiasm and of inversion of retinal images by the lens, the right hemisphere sees objects in the left half of visual space and vice versa. The optic chiasm is located in the midline under the diencephalon and hypothalamus and above the pituitary gland.

OROMOTOR APRAXIA—Apraxia for movements of the buccolingual musculature.

PALEOSTRIATUM (GLOBUS PALLIDUS)—Part of the basal ganglia (q.v.).

PARADOXICAL SLEEP—REM sleep (q.v.).

PARAPARESIS, PARAPLEGIA—Weakness of both legs, usually because of cauda equina or spinal cord dysfunction. Paraparesis of cerebral origin (parasagittal lesion) is usually called diplegia.

PARAPHASIA—Substitution in speech.

Phonemic (literal) paraphasias result from substitution of one phoneme or syllable for another.

Semantic paraphasias result from substitution of one word or expression for another, often one that is semantically related.

PARASAGITTAL—Adjacent to the interhemispheric fissure, to the midline plane of the brain.

PARESIS—Weakness.

PARIETAL LOBE—A portion of the neocortex surrounded by the frontal lobe anteriorly, occipital lobe posteriorly, and temporal lobe inferiorly. It receives somatosensory and vestibular projections. Its posterior inferior region (inferior parietal lobule), at the junction of parietal, occipital, and temporal lobes, is an area of association cortex where spatial (somatosensory and visual) and auditory information is integrated. This area myelinates very late and in the dominant hemisphere is concerned with high order linguistic processing.

PARKINSON'S DISEASE (PARKINSONISM)—A chronic disease of unknown etiology which is most common in late adult life and is characterized pathologically by the loss of pigmented neurons in the substantia nigra. This causes loss of dopaminergic innervation to the neostriatum. Parkinsonism also occurred as a sequella of encephalitis lethargica (von Economo's disease) after World War I. Its main signs are a resting tremor, rigidity, and akinesia. It can be ameliorated, at least for a time, by the administration of the precursor of dopamine L-DOPA.

PARTIAL COMPLEX (PSYCHOMOTOR, TEMPORAL LOBE) SEIZURES— Complex partial seizures (q.v.).

PATHOGENESIS—Mechanism giving rise to a given symptom. Pathogenesis and etiology (specific cause of an illness) are often confused. For example, the etiology of reading disability may be a genetic disorder in one child and brain damage as the result of perinatal asphyxia in another, but in both the children, the pathogenesis of dyslexia may be a language disorder.

PEPTIDES—Molecules made up of a chain of amino acids. Some hormones like insulin, ACTH, vasopressin, and growth hormone are peptides; many endocrine releasing or inhibitory factors like thyroid hormone releasing factor, luteinizing hormone releasing factor, and somatostatin are also peptides, as are the endorphins and enkephalins. Many peptides are thought to act as neuromodulators or neurotransmitters in the brain.

PERIPHERAL NERVES—Nerves to the body. They are divided into the cranial nerves (q.v.) and spinal nerves, the latter having their origin in the spinal cord. Sensory fibers in peripheral nerves have their cells of origin in ganglia outside of the brain stem and spinal cord, called the cranial nerve ganglia and the dorsal root ganglia. Motor fibers have their cells of origin in the motor cranial nerve nuclei of the brain stem and in the anterior horns of the spinal cord. There is one pair of spinal nerves for each segment of the spinal cord.

PETIT MAL SEIZURE—Brief absence, usually lasting less than 15 sec, that may be accompanied by minor automatisms such as eye fluttering, rarely by more complex ones. The sine qua non for the diagnosis of petit mal is an EEG showing 3 to 3½ Hz spike-and-wave activity occurring synchronously in all leads against a normal background EEG.

PETIT MAL VARIANT—see SPIKE-AND-WAVE DISCHARGE.

PHENOBARBITAL—A barbiturate drug widely used as an anticonvulsant in children because of its safety and wide therapeutic range. It is most helpful for generalized, focal, and complex partial (psychomotor) seizures. It is generally ineffective against petit mal absences. In high doses, it may produce drowsiness and ataxia. In some children, it worsens attention deficit disorders and hyperactivity.

PHENOTHIAZINES—A group of potent antipsychotic drugs or major tranquilizers that include chlorpromazine (Thorazine®), thioridazine (Mellaril®) and others. They are thought to exert at least some of their effects by suppressing catecholamine, notably dopamine, activity in the brain. They also exert effects on indolamine metabolism.

PHENYLKETONURIA (PKU)—A recessively inherited disorder of amino acid metabolism resulting in severe mental retardation if untreated. All infants are now tested for it at birth since the effects of the disease on the brain can be avoided by providing a diet low in phenylalanine.

PHENYTOIN (DILANTIN®, DIPHENYLHYDANTOIN)—An anticonvulsant drug that is widely used in children and adults against major motor, focal, and complex partial (psychomotor) seizures. It is generally ineffective against febrile seizures, petit mal absence seizures, and myoclonus. It produces ataxia in toxic dose. Prolonged administration produces gum hypertrophy and hirsutism in some children. Occasional individuals are allergic to this drug and will develop a generalized rash, usually within 8 days to a few weeks of its introduction.

PHONOLOGY—The subsystem of language dealing with the sounds used in speech, how they are produced, and how they are decoded.

PLANUM TEMPORALE—Horizontal or superior surface of the temporal lobe which is tucked into the Sylvian fissure and where the primary auditory projection area or gyrus of Heschl is located, as well as auditory association cortex which is located just behind it. This is an area of the brain which is considerably larger on the left than on the right in about 65% of brains. This finding is thought to be correlated with dominance for language.

PLASTICITY—Modification of structure or function as a result of injury or altered environment. Plasticity in the brain implies reorganization in order to preserve behavioral competence; it probably takes many forms, from altered synaptic connections, development of new functional pathways, changes in excitability, to the adoption of alternate behavioral strategies.

POLYSYNAPTIC—A pathway in which the nerve impulse has to traverse two or more synapses from input to output.

PONS—Midportion of the brain stem containing many longitudinal fiber tracts, and a very large transverse fiber tract linking the pontine nuclei with the cerebellum. It comprises many cranial nerve nuclei, parts of the reticular formation, raphé nucleus, and locus coeruleus (the main noradrenergic nucleus in the brain). The pons (and medulla) form the floor of the fourth ventricle. The cerebellum is located behind (dorsally) to the pons and forms the roof of the fourth ventricle.

PORENCEPHALY—Focal loss of brain substance, usually as the result of an intrauterine vascular occlusion (stroke) or other destructive lesion.

POSITRON EMISSION TOMOGRAPHY (PET)—A computer assisted imaging technique using short-lived stable isotopes that enables one to record metabolic changes in particular brain areas. Thus far, it has been most useful in patients with epileptic seizure foci, vascular accidents, and other brain lesions. It has been used experimentally to show metabolic changes related to specific behaviors such as vision.

PRAGMATICS—The communicative use of language. It comprises such aspects of communication as asking and answering questions, making comments, giving orders, taking turns, looking at the person one is speaking to, gestures, nods, tone of voice, as well as choosing the appropriate verbal utterance.

PREFRONTAL CORTEX—The major part of the frontal lobe, situated anteriorly to the premotor cortex. It is by far the largest association area of the neocortex. It has extensive cortico-cortical, thalamic, and limbic connections and strong projections to the caudate nucleus.

PREMOTOR CORTEX—Area of the frontal cortex anterior to the motor strip that appears concerned with motor programming. It receives a strong input from the cerebellum and basal ganglia via the thalamus and has strong projections to the striatum. One area, known as Area 8, is concerned with the voluntary turning of the eyes to the contralateral side. Broca's area, in the foot of the third frontal convolution, is concerned with speech production.

PRIMARY BILATERAL SYNCHRONY—An epileptic EEG pattern in which the entire cortex fires bilaterally synchronously; it is presumed to be driven by a subcortical pacemaker, perhaps in the upper brain stem or thalamus. When the pattern consists of 3 to 3½ Hz spike-and-waves, it is usually indicative of petit mal (q.v.).

PRIMIDONE (MYSOLINE®)—An anticonvulsant drug effective against major motor, focal and complex partial (psychomotor) seizures. It is generally ineffective against petit mal absences and myoclonic seizures. It is degraded in part to phenobarbital. In toxic doses it produces ataxia, drowsiness and, occasionally, mental changes. It is tolerated best if introduced in slowly increasing dosage.

PROPRIOCEPTION—Input from mechanoreceptors providing information about active and passive muscle stretch, joint position, movement, pressure. This information is largely processed subcortically. Proprioception plays a major role in the control of posture and movement.

PROSODY—The melody or suprasegmental features of speech; it includes pitch, stress, and juncture (spaces between words and inside words). Prosody enables one, for example, to distinguish between questions, statements, and commands, and to convey such emotional features as sarcasm and anger. There is evidence to suggest prosody may be processed, in part at least, in the nondominant temporal lobe.

PROSOPAGNOSIA—Inability to recognize familiar faces, usually because of dysfunction in the nondominant mesial temporo-occipital cortex.

PSEUDOATHETOSIS—Inability to maintain the fingers immobile, especially when the eyes are closed, usually because of proprioceptive loss or of a lesion in the contralateral parietal lobe.

PSEUDOBULBAR PALSY—Spasticity and lack of motor control of the muscles of articulation and swallowing because of bilateral dysfunction of "upper motor neurons." It is characteristically associated with increased oral reflexes such as the jaw jerk. Adult patients with pseudobulbar palsy due to subcortical pathology often have forced crying and laughter (emotional incontinence).

PSYCHOMOTOR SEIZURE—Complex partial seizures (q.v.).

PSYCHOSIS—A severe psychiatric illness affecting thought processes, affect, and behavior. The major types of psychoses include the schizophrenias, manic-depressive psychosis, several types of psychotic depression, and paranoid states. In contrast to the neuroses, whose pathogenesis is thought to be predominantly environmental, the psychoses are viewed as multidetermined illnesses where endogenous genetic-metabolic factors play a predominant role and environmental factors a facilitatory or triggering role. Current theories suggest that the psychoses may reflect disorders of neurotransmitter or neuromodulator metabolism. Infantile autism and "childhood onset pervasive developmental disorder" are considered by many to represent psychotic disorders of early childhood. These two disorders encompass several previously used labels such as atypical children, symbiotic psychosis, early childhood schizophrenia, and childhood psychosis.

PULVINAR—Large caudal nucleus of the thalamus, concerned in part with visual perception and, on the dominant side, with language.

PURKINJE CELLS—Large neurons of the cerebellar cortex which have a very large and complex dendritic tree. They are the output cells of the cerebellar cortex and project to the deep cerebellar nuclei.

PUTAMEN—Part of the basal ganglia (q.v.).

PYRAMIDAL CELLS—Neurons with a pyramidal shape. They have extensively branched dendrites and a single basal axon which is often very long, usually with recurrent axon collaterals. Pyramidal cells are output cells. The largest pyramidal neurons are the Betz cells of layer V of the motor cortex that send their axons all the way to the spinal cord. Anterior horn cells of the spinal cord are also pyramidal neurons. Pyramidal neurons are found in many other places, including layer III of the neocortex, in the hippocampus, and also elsewhere.

PYRAMIDAL TRACT (CORTICOSPINAL TRACT)—Tract originating in the motor cortex and ending on anterior horn cells of the contralateral side of the spinal

cord. (In fact, there is both a crossed and a smaller uncrossed corticospinal tract).
Part of the corticospinal tract, called *corticobulbar tract*, innervates the motor
nuclei of the cranial nerves in the brain stem. The corticospinal tract sends axon
collaterals to the sensory cortex, and to brain stem relays such as the red nucleus,
reticular formation, and to other subcortical way stations.

QUADRIPLEGIA, QUADRIPARESIS—Weakness affecting all four limbs.

RAPHÉ NUCLEI—Pontomesencephalic nucleus that is very rich in serotonin (5-
hydroxytryptamine). It is concerned, in particular, with sleep onset and pain.

RECURRENT AXON COLLATERALS—Branches of an axon that leave the main
axon close to its origin and that are distributed to often inhibitory interneurons
in the vicinity of the cell soma. Axon collaterals provide local feedback concerning neuronal output (corollary discharges, q.v.).

QUADRANTANOPSIA—Loss of vision in a single quadrant of the visual field.

QUADRIGEMINAL BODIES—Superior and inferior colliculi of the midbrain (see
COLLICULI).

RELEASING FACTORS—Hypothalamic peptides that regulate the release of pituitary hormones by direct action on the anterior pituitary gland to which they
are transported by a specialized system of vessels called portal vessels. There
are at least 9 releasing factors; some of them, for example, prolactin, are inhibitory.
Corticotropin releasing factor (CRF) stimulates the secretion of ACTH.
Luteinizing hormone releasing hormone (LHRH) or (LRF) stimulates the secretion of gonadal stimulating hormones.
Thyrotropin releasing factor (TRF) stimulates the secretion of thyroid stimulating
hormone.

RAPID EYE MOVEMENT (REM) OR PARADOXICAL SLEEP—A stage of sleep
during which the EEG is low voltage and fast, there are rapid eye movements
and occipital spikes in the EEG, and atonia of the muscles. Dreams are particularly
likely to occur during REM sleep.

RENSHAW CELLS—Inhibitory interneurons in the anterior horn of the spinal cord
that receive recurrent axon collaterals from alpha motor neurons. They are thus
interneurons in an inhibitory feedback loop.

RESERPINE—A major tranquilizer and antipsychotic drug thought to exert its
effects by depleting the brain of catecholamines (dopamine and norepinephrine)
and indolamines. It is not used very much any more because of its lowering
effects on the blood pressure and because it produces parkinsonian side effects
if given in high dose. It is the antipsychotic drug whose effect has been known
the longest.

RETICULAR FORMATION (RETICULAR ACTIVATING SYSTEM)—A series
of deep nuclei extending from the medulla to the midbrain. In general, the reticular
formation receives and integrates inputs from widespread areas (spinal cord,
cerebellum, cranial nerve nuclei, limbic system, cortex). The lower part of the
reticular formation projects downward to the spinal cord. The rostral part of the
reticular formation projects upwards toward the nonspecific thalamic nuclei, basal

ganglia, limbic system, and cortex. The descending reticular formation has a major influence on motor tone. The ascending reticular formation mediates arousal. Reticular neurons are rich in neurotransmitters, in particular, catecholamines. The reticular formation has many other effects, not totally understood, but it is known that alerting through sensory or cortical inputs is mediated through their effects on the reticular formation.

RETROGRADE AMNESIA—See AMNESIA.

RIGIDITY—Increased tone in the muscles whose intensity remains constant throughout the range of a passively imparted movement. Rigidity suggests pathology in the basal ganglia (e.g., parkinsonism) and other brain stem circuits.

SACCADIC MOVEMENTS—Rapid, preprogrammed movements.

SCANNING SPEECH—Disorder of the rhythm of speech seen in patients with cerebellar pathology.

SCHWANN CELLS—Supporting cells in peripheral nerves that make the myelin sheaths of axons.

SCOLIOSIS—Curvature of the spine.

SECONDARY BILATERAL SYNCHRONY—An epileptic EEG pattern, often consisting of spikes-and-waves, in which a subcortical epileptic generator is thought to be fired by a cortical epileptic focus, often in the temporal lobe. Firing of the subcortical generator then fires the entire cortex. Secondary bilateral synchrony can be distinguished from primary bilateral synchrony by the presence of a spike focus in the resting EEG or by the focal onset of the spike and wave discharge. Recent data suggest that commissural fibers play an essential role in the genesis of secondary bilateral synchrony.

SEGMENTAL—Affecting a single segment of the spinal cord and its nerves and circuits.

SEIZURE—Uncontrolled discharge of neurons producing a variety of symptoms and seizure types (see Table 3, p. 41). Repetitive seizures imply a chronic convulsive disorder or epilepsy in most patients. There are multiple causes for seizures (see Chapter 4).

SEMANTICS—Rules for attaching meaning to words in the repository of word meanings or lexicon and for extracting the idea or message in a sentence or longer utterance.

SENSORIMOTOR CORTEX—The motor (ascending frontal gyrus) and somatosensory (ascending parietal gyrus) areas of the neocortex considered as an integrated system controlling movement.

SEPTUM—A part of the limbic system situated in the most rostral part of the diencephalon, beneath the genu of the corpus callosum and above the anterior commissure. It contains many important nuclei, some of them concerned with olfaction. It has strong connections with the hippocampus, hypothalamus, mesencephalon, and other areas.

SEROTONIN (5-HYDROXYTRYPTAMINE)—A neurotransmitter in the brain with generally inhibitory actions. The raphé nuclei of the brain stem are rich in serotonergic neurons that send processes to widespread areas of the brain and spinal cord. It appears to play a role in the control of slow-wave sleep. Serotonergic blocking drugs such as LSD produce vivid visual hallucinations.

SHORT-TERM MEMORY—A process that enables one to register stimuli while they are recognized by cross-checking with the items in long-term storage they have activated, determining their relevance, and deciding whether to act upon them or let them decay. Short-term memory has a large capacity and is sensory modality-specific. Its span is strongly dependent upon focused attention; it does not exceed a few seconds unless rehearsal takes place.

SLOW-WAVE SLEEP—A stage of sleep during which the EEG shows high voltage slow waves and, at times, characteristic sleep spindles and vertex waves. It is rarely associated with dreaming except for night terrors but may be associated with sleep walking, and, in young children, with bed wetting (enuresis).

SOMA—Body. Used with reference to the human body and with reference to cell bodies.

SOMATOSENSORY—Sensation arising from excitation of cutaneous, soft tissue, bone, and joint receptors. Somatosensory information includes pain, temperature, light touch, pressure, vibration, movement. Vestibular information is often considered together with somatosensory information since it informs about position and acceleration of the head.

SOMATOSENSORY CORTEX—Situated in the ascending parietal gyrus, immediately behind the central sulcus that separates the frontal from the parietal lobes. The sensory homunculus is upside-down, with the leg area in the mesial aspect of the gyrus, adjacent to the interhemispheric fissure. Each half of the body projects predominantly to the contralateral hemisphere, with the lower face and hand areas being most strongly lateralized and having the largest surface of representation. Each of the primary sensory modalities has a discrete representation.

SPASTICITY—Phasic increase in tone denoting loss of "upper motor neuron" innervation (pyramidal tract involvement q.v.). Resistance to passive stretch yields suddenly (clasp-knife phenomenon), tendon stretch reflexes are hyperactive, often with clonus, and stroking of the lateral aspect of the sole of the foot results in dorsiflexion of the big toe and fanning out of the other toes (Babinski reflex).

SPHINGOLIPIDOSES (SPHINGOLIPID STORAGE DISEASES)—A class of genetic-metabolic diseases of the nervous system where neurons store complex glycolipids that they cannot break down because of the lack of a degradative enzyme. The prototype is Tay-Sachs disease.

SPIKE-AND-WAVE DISCHARGE—An epileptic EEG pattern in which each spike is followed by a slow wave. This pattern, at a frequency of 3 to 3½ Hz, occurring diffusely and bilaterally sychronously for brief periods against a normal background, is indicative of petit mal (q.v.). Slow spike-and-wave at a frequency of 2 Hz is called petit mal variant; it occurs most often in preschool children with minor motor seizures (drop attacks); this latter syndrome is called the Lennox-Gastaut syndrome.

SPLIT-BRAIN—A person (or animal) who has had the commissures between the two cerebral hemispheres severed. As a result there is no direct interhemispheric communication, and processing occurs in isolation in each hemisphere.

STEREOGNOSIS—Perception of shape and recognition of objects by palpation.

STEREOTAXIC SURGERY—The placement of a small lesion in a specified target in the brain through a burr hole in the skull using thin wires or cannulas directed by X-ray determination of the target's coordinates. The lesion may be produced by electrical currents, freezing, the injection of small amounts of chemicals, radiowaves, etc.

STORAGE DISEASES—A group of genetic-metabolic diseases where a particular chemical substrate accumulates in particular tissues because of a block in its metabolism, usually because of the lack of a degradative enzyme. Typical storage diseases affecting the brain include the sphingolipidoses (Tay-Sachs disease and many others), mucopolysaccharidoses (Hurler's disease or gargoylism and many others), etc.

STRABISMUS (SQUINT)—Disconjugate position and movement of the eyes because of functional imbalance in one or more of the extraocular muscles.

STRIATE CORTEX—Visual or calcarine (q.v.) cortex of the occipital lobe.

STRIATUM—Part of the basal ganglia (q.v.).

SUBACUTE SCLEROSING PANENCEPHALITIS (SSPE)—A chronic encephalitis caused by the measles virus that produces a progressive and usually fatal dementia in children.

SUBSTANCE P—Peptide that appears to play a role as sensory neurotransmitter, notably in pain pathways. It is found in the dorsal (sensory) horns of the spinal cord, in the substantia nigra, limbic system, and elsewhere. It is often found in areas rich in enkephalins, which mediate analgesia.

SUBSTANTIA NIGRA—Paired large pigmented nuclei in the midbrain, considered part of the basal ganglia (q.v.). Loss of dopaminergic neurons in the substantia nigra projecting to the neostriatum produces the symptoms of parkinsonism (akinesia, rigidity, resting tremor).

SUBTHALAMIC NUCLEUS—Part of the basal ganglia (q.v.). A lesion in the subthalamic nucleus on one side produces contralateral ballismus (q.v.).

SUPPLEMENTARY MOTOR AREA—A region of the mesial frontal lobe, immediately anterior to the leg area of the motor cortex. It is concerned with speech production and, it seems, with the programming of some automatized motor acts. It may not be as strongly lateralized as other areas concerned with speech production, judging from the data provided by cerebral blood flow studies.

SUPRAMARGINAL GYRUS—Gyrus at the posterior end of the Sylvian fissure, at the junction of parietal, temporal, and occipital cortex. Involved in cross-modal and linguistic processing operations, *inter alia*.

SYLVIAN FISSURE—A deep hemispheric fissure separating the frontal and parietal lobes from the temporal lobe, and in the depth of which the insular cortex is hidden. Perisylvian areas of the dominant hemisphere are concerned with linguistic processing.

SYNAPSE—Specialized area of neurons where an axon terminal with its presynaptic membrane makes contact with the postsynaptic membrane of an adjacent neuron. Pre- and postsynaptic membranes are separated by a narrow space called the synaptic cleft that is traversed by the neurotransmitter released by the presynaptic membrane. Classical synapses are axodendritic or axosomatic. Dendrodendritic or axoaxonal synapses also exist.

SYNKINESIS—Involuntary movements of one part of the body that occur when another part is moved. For example, mirror movements are the spillover to the opposite hand of movements supposed to be performed with one hand only. Synkinesis denotes lack of inhibition (or, rarely, atypical decussation of the pyramidal tract).

SYNTAX—Set of rules for arranging words and constructions relative to each other in order to generate meaningful sentences.

TECTUM—Portion of the brain stem, situated dorsally to the aqueduct of Sylvius. Its most important constituents are the superior and inferior colliculi (quadrigeminal bodies).

TEGMENTUM—Portion of the brain stem, just ventral to the aqueduct and fourth ventricle.

TEMPORAL LOBE—A lobe of the brain situated in the middle fossa of the skull, below the parietal lobe, behind the frontal lobe, and in front of the occipital lobe. The superior surface of the temporal lobe, tucked into the Sylvian fissure, contains the primary and secondary auditory projection areas. The mesial aspect of the temporal lobe contains the hippocampus and other limbic structures. The amygdala, a relay nucleus of the limbic system, is located in the temporal lobe. The temporal lobe is particularly concerned with auditory processing, and, on the dominant side, with the comprehension of speech.

THALAMUS—Paired deep nuclear masses of the diencephalon comprising many nuclei. Major way station for (a) ascending sensory systems (somatosensory—ventroposterolateral nucleus, auditory—medial geniculate body, visual—lateral geniculate body), with projections to the primary sensory cortical areas for each modality; (b) motor control systems (neocerebellar and basalganglia outputs converge on and are integrated in the ventrolateral and ventroanterior nuclei with projections to the sensorimotor and premotor cortex; (c) the brain stem reticular activating system (nonspecific thalamic nuclei) with widespread cortical and neostriatal projections; (d) the limbic system with inputs from the amygdala, mammillary bodies, and other limbic nuclei and projections to the limbic cortical areas (from the anterior nucleus of the thalamus in particular); (e) language systems with reciprocal connections of the large posterior nucleus or pulvinar to the temporoparietal cortex (dominant hemisphere); (f) the visual system with connections between secondary and tertiary visual cortical areas, pulvinar, and superior colliculus.

TIC—Sudden repetitive involuntary movements of small amplitude, involving the face or upper limbs most commonly. May be associated with respiratory tics, involuntary noises, or speech (Tourette syndrome q.v.).

TITUBATION—Inability to maintain the stability of the head and trunk in the erect posture. Titubation suggests cerebellar dysfunction, especially of the vermis. It is of course common in alcohol and other intoxications.

TONIC MUSCLE CONTRACTION—Sustained contraction (as opposed to phasic or intermittent voluntary contraction or to clonic or jerking involuntary contraction). Tonic contraction is usually involuntary as it is governed by subcortical, brain stem, or spinal circuits; it also occurs during the initial phase of a generalized seizure and reflects massive cortical and subcortical discharge.

TONIC NECK REFLEX—Extension of the arm and leg on the side of the face and flexion of the limbs on the side of the occiput upon forceful turning of the head to one side. A spontaneous tonic neck position is normal in infancy but is always abnormal if obligatory. It then denotes spasticity or athetosis.

TOTAL COMMUNICATION—The deliberate use of all possible channels to convey linguistic meaning; specifically, the combination of speech with sign language. Signed Exact English is a form of Total Communication which provides a manual sign for each word and signs for word endings to indicate the past, plurals, etc. Signed Exact English is not the language of the deaf community, called American Sign Language or Ameslan for short; Ameslan has a totally different syntax and word order than English.

TOURETTE SYNDROME—Syndrome characterized by multiple changing tics associated with vocal tics (throat clearing, snorts, involuntary swearing or coprolalia). May have a genetic origin and be associated with a learning disability. Responds to dopamine receptor blocking agent like haloperidol. Does not lead to dementia or neurologic deterioration.

TRANQUILIZERS—Drugs whose calming effects are not primarily due to sedation. *Major tranquilizers* have antipsychotic effects and include the phenothiazines, butyrophenones, reserpine, lithium, and others. They are thought to exert their effects by altering catechol- or indolamine metabolism.
Minor tranquilizers have anxiolytic effects and include the benzodiazepines e.g., diazepam (Valium®) and chlordiazepoxide (Librium®), meprobamate (Equanil®), hydroxyzine (Atarax®), and others. Some of them are thought to exert their effects by stimulating GABA receptors.

TREMOR—Trembling or shaking. A tremor at rest that improves during movement suggests nigrostriatal dysfunction (parkinsonism). A tremor that appears during movement and gets worse as movement approaches its goal (intention tremor) suggests neocerebellar dysfunction. Tremor is frequent in many intoxications, including alcohol. It may be the sign of benign familial tremor.

TRIMETHADIONE (TRIDIONE®)—An anticonvulsant drug with selective effect against petit mal absences. It is not used very much today because of possible bone marrow and kidney toxicity.

TUBEROUS SCLEROSIS—A common autosomal dominant genetic trait in which patients may have skin lesions (depigmented spots, raised macules on the face—adenoma sebaceum, and others), seizures, intracranial calcifications, mental deficiency, and other symptoms.

"UPPER MOTOR NEURON"—Pyramidal cell of the motor cortex innervating "lower motor neurons" in the cranial nerve nuclei and anterior horns of the spinal cord. Dysfunction of "upper motor neurons" are characteristically associated with weakness, loss of voluntary control, spasticity, increased stretch reflexes, and pathologic reflexes like upgoing toes (Babinski reflex).

VALPROIC ACID (DEPAKENE®, SODIUM VALPROATE)—An anticonvulsant especially useful against petit mal absences, but which also is effective against febrile seizures and, to some degree, against other major seizures. It produces troublesome gastrointestinal side effects in some children and has significant liver and bone marrow toxicity, so that careful monitoring of its use is required.

VASOPRESSIN (ANTIDIURETIC HORMONE)—A peptide produced in the brain, notably in the hypothalamus and in extrahypothalamic sites. It appears to act as a neuromodulator in the brain where it may foster learning, as well as being released by the posterior pituitary gland into the blood where it acts as a hormone.

VENTRICLES—Cavities within the brain filled with cerebrospinal fluid. Each hemisphere contains a lateral ventricle that is a curved structure with a frontal horn, body, occipital horn, and temporal horn. The two lateral ventricles communicate via the foramen of Monro with the third ventricle, located in the diencephalon. The third ventricle opens via the aqueduct of Sylvius, in the core of the midbrain, into the fourth ventricle situated between the pons and medulla ventrally and the cerebellum dorsally. CSF is formed by the choroid plexus in each of the ventricles and escapes through the foramina of the fourth ventricle into the subarachnoid spaces surrounding the spinal cord and brain where it is reabsorbed into the blood stream. Dilatation of the cerebral ventricles with accumulation of cerebrospinal fluid is called hydrocephalus (q.v.).

VERBRAL AUDITORY AGNOSIA (WORD DEAFNESS)—Selective inability to decode language presented acoustically. It is usually caused by bilateral pathology affecting auditory association areas. In young children, it produces mutism and total inability to understand speech with preserved ability to interpret gestures.

VERMIS—Midline portion of the cerebellum.

VESTIBULE (LABYRINTH)—Portion of the inner ear consisting of the semicircular canals, the utricle, and saccule that provides information about movement of the head in space and about its position relative to gravity. The vestibule projects to vestibular nuclei in the brain stem that have extensive connections with the cerebellum, oculomotor nuclei, superior colliculus, spinal cord, etc.

VISUAL CORTEX (STRIATE CORTEX)—Situated along the calcarine fissure in the mesial surface of the occipital lobe, adjacent to the interhemispheric fissure. The upper half of the visual field is represented below the fissure, the lower half of the visual field above the fissure. This inversion of the image of space corresponds to its inversion on the retina by the lens of the eye. Because of the optic chiasm, the left side of visual space projects to the right hemisphere and the right side of the left hemisphere.

WERNICKE'S (FLUENT) APHASIA—An acquired aphasia produced by a posterior (temporoparietal) lesion of the dominant hemisphere. The patient's spontaneous speech is fluent or even verbose. It has communicative intent; prosody, phonology, and syntax are spared. Its content is grossly deficient; it contains many clichés and empty phrases. The patient often makes semantic paraphasic errors. His comprehension of oral and written language is grossly impaired. He usually cannot write.

WHITE MATTER—Portions of the nervous system that look white to the naked eye because they contain myelinated fiber tracts (bundles of axons or neuronal processes).

X-LINKED RECESSIVE TRAIT—A trait due to a gene located on the X chromosome (females carry two X chromosomes, males one X and one Y). X-linked recessive disease usually is manifested by males who inherit the disease from their healthy but carrier mother (healthy because she is heterozygous for the trait, the abnormal recessive gene on one of her X chromosomes being masked by the corresponding healthy dominant gene on her other X chromosome). Affected males, if they reproduce, do not have affected children but all their daughters will be carriers and capable of transmitting the trait to half of their sons. The sons of an affected male are unaffected and do not transmit the trait to their descendents. A number of neurologic diseases are transmitted in this way, for example Duchenne muscular dystrophy.

References

1. Abrams, H. L., and McNeil, B. J. (1978): Medical implications of computed tomography ("cat scanning"). *N. Engl. J. Med.*, 298:255–261, 310–318.
2. Adams, J., Kenny, T. J., Peterson, R. A., and Canter, A. (1975): Age effects and revised scoring of the Canter BIP for identifying children with cerebral dysfunction. *J. Consult. Clin. Phychol.*, 43:117–118.
3. Agranoff, B. W. (1976): Learning and memory: Approaches to correlating behavioral and bio-chemical events. In: *Basic Neurochemistry, 2nd Ed.*, edited by G. J. Siegel, R. W. Albers, R. Katzman, and B. W. Agranoff, pp. 765–784. Little Brown, Boston.
4. Aicardi, J., and Chevrie, J. J. (1971): Convulsive status epilepticus in infants and children: A study of 239 cases. *Epilepsia*, 11:187–197.
5. Ajuriaguerra, J. de, and Auzias, M. (1975): Preconditions for the development of writing in the child. In: *Foundations of Language Development, Vol. 2*, edited by E. H. Lenneberg, and E. Lenneberg, pp. 311–328. Academic Press, New York.
6. Ajuriaguerra, J. de, Jaeggi, A., Guignard, F., Kocher, F., Maquard, M., Roth, S., and Schmid, E. (1976): The development and prognosis of dysphasia in children. In: *Normal and Deficient Child Language*, edited by D. M. Morehead, and A. E. Morehead, pp. 345–385. University Park Press, Baltimore.
7. Akil, H., Richardson, D. E., Hughes, J., and Barchas, J. D. (1978): Enkephalin-like material elevated in ventricular cerebrospinal fluid of pain patients after analgetic focal stimulation. *Science*, 201:463–465.
8. Alajouanine, T., and Lhermitte, F. (1965): Acquired aphasia in children. *Brain*, 88:653–662.
9. Albert, M. L. (1978): Subcortical dementia. In: *Alzheimer's Disease: Senile Dementia and Related Disorders*, edited by R. Katzman, R. D. Terry, and K. L. Bick, pp. 173–180. Raven Press, New York.
10. Albert, M. L., Soffer, D., Silverberg, R., and Reches, A. (1979): The anatomic basis of visual agnosia. *Neurology*, 29:876–879.
11. Allen, D. A., and Rapin, I. (1980): Language disorders in preschool children: Predictors of outcome—A preliminary report. *Brain Dev.*, 2:73–80.
12. Aman, M. G. (1978): Drugs, learning, and the psychotherapies. In: *Pediatric Psychopharmacology: The Use of Behavior Modifying Drugs in Children*, edited by J. S. Werry, pp. 79–108. Brunner/Mazel, New York.
13. Ameli, N. O. (1980): Hemispherectomy for the treatment of epilepsy and behavior disturbance. *Can. J. Neurol. Sci.*, 7:33–38.
14. Andermann, F., and Robb, M. P. (1972): Absence status. *Epilepsia*, 13:177–187.
15. Annett, M. (1973): Laterality of childhood hemiplegia and the growth of speech and intelligence. *Cortex*, 9:4–29.
16. Antelman, S. M., and Caggiula, A. R. (1977): Norepinephrine-dopamine interactions and behavior. *Science*, 195:646–653.
17. Aram, D. M., and Nation, J. E. (1975): Patterns of language behavior in children with developmental language disorders. *J. Speech Hear. Res.*, 18:229–241.

18. Aram, D. M., and Nation, J. E. (1980): Preschool language disorders and subsequent language and academic difficulties. *J. Commun. Dis.*, 13:159–170.
19. Armstrong, D. M. (1978): The mammalian cerebellum and its contribution to movement control. *Int. Rev. Physiol.*, 17:239–294.
20. Aron, A. M., Freeman, J. M., and Carter, S. (1965): The natural history of Sydenham's chorea. *Am. J. Med.*, 38:83–95.
21. Averbach, E., and Coriell, A. S. (1961): Short-term memory in vision. *Bell System Technical J.*, 40:309–328.
22. Axelrod, J. (1974): The pineal gland: A neurochemical transducer. Chemical signals from nerves regulate synthesis of melatonin and convey information about internal clocks. *Science*, 184:1341–1348.
23. Baird, H. W., John, E. R., Ahn, H., and Maisel, E. (1980): Neurometric evaluation of epileptic children who do well and poorly in school. *Electroencephalogr. Clin. Neurophysiol.*, 48:683–693.
24. Bakker, D. J. (1979): Hemispheric differences and reading strategies: Two dyslexias. *Bull. Orton Soc.*, 29:84–100.
25. Balazs, R. (1972): Effects of hormones and nutrition on brain development. In: *Human Development and the Thyroid Gland: Relation to Endemic Cretinism*, edited by J. B. Stanbury, pp. 385–415. Plenum Press, New York.
26. Baltaxe, C. A. M., and Simmons, J. Q., III (1975): Language in childhood psychosis. A review. *J. Speech Hear. Dis.*, 40:439–458.
27. Barbizet, J. (1970): *Human Memory and its Pathology.* W. H. Freeman. San Francisco.
28. Barchas, J. D., Akil, H., Elliott, G. R., Holman, R. B., and Watson, S. J. (1978): Behavioral neurochemistry: Neuroregulators and behavioral states. *Science*, 200:964–973.
29. Barkley, R. A. (1977): A review of stimulant drug research with hyperactive children. *J. Child Psychol. Psychiatry*, 18:137–165.
30. Barondes, S. H. (1970): Cerebral protein synthesis inhibitors block long-term memory. *Int. Rev. Neurobiol.*, 12:177–205.
31. Basser, L. S. (1962): Hemiplegia of early onset and the faculty of speech with special reference to the effects of hemispherectomy. *Brain*, 85:427–460.
32. Bateson, M. C. (1975): Mother-infant exchanges: The epigenesis of conversational interaction. *Ann. N.Y. Acad. Sci.*, 263:101–113.
33. Bax, M., and MacKeith, R., editors (1963): *Minimal Cerebral Dysfunction, Little Club Clinics in Developmental Medicine*, No. 10. William Heinemann Medical Books, London.
34. Bayley, N. (1969): *Bayley Scales of Infant Development*. Psychological Corp., New York.
35. Bear, D. M. (1979): The temporal lobes: An approach to the study of organic behavioral changes. In: *Handbook of Behavioral Neurobiology, Vol. 2: Neuropsychology*, edited by M. S. Gazzaniga, pp. 75–95. Plenum Press, New York.
36. Beery, K. F., and Buktenica, N. A. (1967): *Developmental Test of Visual Motor Integration*. Follet Educational Corporation, Chicago.
37. Bellak, L. (1977): Psychiatric states in adults with minimal brain dysfunction. *Psychiatr. Ann.*, 7:575–589.
38. Benbow, C. P., and Stanley, J. C. (1980): Sex differences in mathematical ability: Fact or artifact? *Science*, 210:1262–1264.
39. Bennett, E. L., Diamond, M. C., Krech, D., and Rosenzweig, M. R. (1964): Chemical and anatomical plasticity of brain. *Science*, 146:610–619.
40. Bennett, H. S., Selman, J. E., Rapin, I., and Rose, A. (1982): Nonconvulsive epileptiform activity appearing as ataxia. *Am. J. Dis. Child.*, 136:30–32.
41. Bensman, A. S., and Szegho, M. (1978): Cerebellar electrical stimulation: A critique. *Arch. Phys. Med. Rehab.*, 59:485–487.
42. Benton, A. L. (1959): *Right-Left Discrimination and Finger Localization: Development and Pathology*. Paul B. Hoeber, New York.
43. Benton, A. L. (1975): Developmental dyslexia: Neurological aspects. In: *Advances in Neurology, Vol. 7*, edited by W. J. Friedlander, pp. 1–47. Raven Press, New York.
44. Benton, A. (1975): Neuropsychological assessment. In: *The Nervous System, Vol. 2.: The Clinical Neurosciences*, edited by D. B. Tower, pp. 67–74. Raven Press, New York.
45. Benton, A. (1979): Body scheme disturbances: Finger agnosia and right-left disorientation. In: *Clinical Neuropsychology*, edited by K. M. Heilman, and E. Valenstein, pp. 140–158. Oxford University Press, New York.

46. Benton, A. (1979): Visuoperceptive, visuospatial, and visuoconstructive disorders. In: *Clinical Neuropsychology*, edited by K. M. Heilman, and E. Valenstein, pp. 186–232. Oxford University Press, New York.

47. Benton, A. L., and Pearl, D., editors (1978): *Dyslexia: An Appraisal of Current Knowledge.* Oxford University Press, New York.

48. Benton, A. L., and Spreen, O. (1969): *Embedded Figures Test.* Neuropsychology Laboratory, Department of Psychology, University of Victoria, Victoria, B.C.

49. Benton, A. L., and Spreen, O. (1969): *Right-Left Orientation Test.* Neuropsychology Laboratory, Department of Psychology, University of Victoria, Victoria, B.C.

50. Berges, J., and Lezine, I. (1965): *The Imitation of Gestures. Clin. Dev. Med.*, No. 18. William Heinemann Medical Books, London.

51. Berkeley, M. (1978): Vision: Geniculocortical system. In: *Handbook of Behavioral Biology. Vol. 1: Sensory Integration*, edited by R. B. Masterton, pp. 165–207. Plenum Press, New York.

52. Berlin, C. I., and Lowe, S. S. (1972): Temporal and dichotic factors in central auditory testing. In: *Handbook of Clinical Audiology*, edited by J. Katz, pp. 280–312. Williams and Wilkins, Baltimore.

53. Berridge, M. J. (1979): Modulation of nervous activity by cyclic nucleotides and calcium. In: *The Neurosciences: Fourth Study Program*, edited by F. O. Schmitt, and F. G. Worden, pp. 873–889. MIT Press, Cambridge, Mass.

54. Bever, T. G., and Chiarello, R. J. (1974): Cerebral dominance in musicians and nonmusicians. *Science*, 185:537–539.

55. Binnie, L. D., Rowan, A. J., Overweg, J., Meinardi, H., Wisman, T., Kamp, A., and Lopes de Silva, F. (1981): Telemetric EEG and video monitoring in epilepsy. *Neurology*, 31:298–303.

56. Birch, H. G., editor (1964): *Brain Damage in Children: The Biological and Social Aspects.* Williams and Wilkins, Baltimore.

57. Birch, H. G., and Lefford, A. (1963): Intersensory development in children. *Monogr. Soc. Res. Child Dev.*, 28:1–47.

58. Bird, E. D., and Iversen, L. L. (1974): Huntington's chorea: Post-mortem measurement of glutamic acid decarboxylase, choline acetyltransferase, and dopamine in basal ganglia. *Brain*, 97:457–472.

59. Bishop, D. V. M., Jancey, C., and Steel, A. McP. (1979): Orthoptic status and reading disability. *Cortex*, 15:659–666.

60. Blank, M. (1975): Mastering the intangible through language. *Ann. N.Y. Acad. Sci.*, 263:44–58.

61. Blom, S., Heijbel, J., and Bergfors, P. G. (1972): Benign epilepsy of children with centrotemporal EEG foci. Prevalence and follow-up study of 40 patients. *Epilepsia*, 13:609–619.

62. Bloom, F., Segal, D., Ling, N., and Guillemin, R. (1976): Endorphins: Profound behavioral effects in rats suggest new etiological factors in mental illness. *Science*, 194:630–632.

63. Bloom, L., and Lahey, M. (1978): *Language Development and Language Disorders.* John Wiley & Sons, New York.

64. Bobath, K. (1980): A Neurophysiological Basis for the Treatment of Cerebral Palsy. In: *Clin. Dev. Med. No. 75:* pp. 1–98. J. B. Lippincott, Philadelphia.

65. Boder, E. (1973): Developmental dyslexia: A diagnostic approach based on three atypical reading-spelling patterns. *Dev. Med. Child Neurol.*, 15:663–687.

66. Boller, F., and Dennis, M. (1979): *Auditory Comprehension: Clinical and Experimental Studies with the Token Test.* Academic Press, New York.

67. Bortner, M., editor (1968): *Evaluation and Education of Children with Brain Damage.* Charles C. Thomas, Springfield, Ill.

68. Bossom, J. (1974): Movement without proprioception. *Brain Res.*, 71:285–296.

69. Boyar, R. M. (1978): Sleep related endocrine rhythms. In: *Res. Publ. Assoc. Res. Nerv. Ment. Dis.*, Vol. 56, *The Hypothalamus*, edited by S. Reichlin, R. J. Baldessarini, and J. B. Martin, pp. 373–386. Williams and Wilkins, Baltimore.

70. Bradley, C. (1937): The behavior of children receiving benzedrine. *Am. J. Psychiatry*, 94:577–585.

71. Bradley, L. (1981): The organization of motor patterns for spelling: An effective remedial strategy for backward readers. *Dev. Med. Child Neurol.*, 23:83–91.

72. Brazelton, T. B. (1973): *Neonatal Behavioral Assessment Scale*, In: *Clin. Dev. Med., No. 50.* pp. 1–66. J. B. Lippincott, Philadelphia.

73. Brazier, M. A. B., editor (1979): *Brain Mechanisms in Memory and Learning: From the Single Neuron to Man.* Raven Press, New York.

74. Bremer, F. (1954): The neurophysiological problem of sleep. In: *Brain Mechanisms and Consciousness*, edited by J. F. Delafresnaye, pp. 137–158. Charles C. Thomas, Springfield, Ill.
75. Brett, E. M. (1966): Minor epileptic status. *J. Neurol. Sci.*, 3:52–75.
76. Brinkman, J., and Kuypers, H. G. J. M. (1973): Cerebral control of contralateral and ipsilateral hand and finger movements in the split-brain rhesus monkey. *Brain*, 96:653–674.
77. Brodmann, K. (1909): *Vergleischende Lokalisationslehre der Grosshirnrinde in ihren prinzipien dargestelt auf Grund des Zellenbaues*. J. A. Barth, Leipzig.
78. Broman, S. H., Nichols, P. L., and Kennedy, W. A. (1975): *Preschool IQ*, Erlbaum, Hillsdale, N.J.
79. Brooks, V. B. (1975): Role of cerebellum and basal ganglia in initiation and control of movements. *Can. J. Neurol. Sci.*, 2:265–277.
80. Brown, J. K. (1977): Migraine and migraine equivalents in children. *Dev. Med. Child Neurol.*, 19:683–692.
81. Brown, J. W. (1972): *Aphasia, Apraxia, and Agnosia: Clinical and Theoretical Aspects*. Charles C. Thomas, Springfield, Ill.
82. Brown, J. W. (1979): Thalamic mechanisms in language. In: *Neuropsychology*, edited by M. S. Gazzaniga, pp. 215–238. Plenum Press, New York.
83. Brown, R., and McNeill, D. (1966): The "tip of the tongue" phenomenon. *J. Verb. Learn. Verb. Behav.*, 5:325–337.
84. Buchwald, N. A., Hull, C. D., and Levine, M. S. (1979): Neuronal activity of the basal ganglia related to the development of "behavioral sets." In: *Brain Mechanisms in Memory and Learning: From the Single Neuron to Man*, edited by M. A. B. Brazier, pp. 93–103. Raven Press, New York.
85. Burkland, C. W., and Smith, A. (1977): Language and the cerebral hemispheres: Observation of verbal and nonverbal responses during 18 months following left ("dominant") hemispherectomy. *Neurology*, 27:627–633.
86. Buschke, H. (1974): Spontaneous remembering after recall failure. *Science*, 184:579–581.
87. Buschke, H. (1976): Learning is organized by chunking. *J. Verb. Learn. Verb. Behav.*, 15:313–324.
88. Buschke, H., and Schaier, A. H. (1979): Memory units, ideas, and propostions in semantic remembering. *J. Verb. Learn. Verb. Behav.*, 18:549–563.
89. Butters, N. (1979): Amnesic disorders. In: *Clinical Neuropsychology*, edited by K. M. Heilman, and E. Valenstein, pp. 439–474. Oxford University Press, New York.
90. Calloway, E., Tueting, P., and Koslow, S. H., editors (1978): *Event-related Potentials in Man.*, Academic Press, New York.
91. Campbell, M. (1978): Use of drug treatment in infantile autism and childhood schizophrenia. A review. In: *Psychopharmacology: A Generation of Progress*, edited by M. A. Lipton, A. DiMascio, and K. F. Killam, pp. 1451–1461. Raven Press, New York.
92. Carr, E. G. (1979): Teaching autistic children to use sign language: Some research issues. *J. Autism Devel. Dis.*, 9:345–359.
93. Carroll, B. J. (1978): Neuroendocrine function in psychiatric disorders. In: *Psychopharmacology: A Generation of Progress*, edited by M. A. Lipton, A. DiMascio, and K. F. Killam, pp. 487–497. Raven Press, New York.
94. Carrow, E. (1973): *Test for Auditory Comprehension of Language*. Learning Concepts, Austin, Tx.
95. Casey, K. L. (1978): Neural mechanisms of pain. In: *Handbook of Perception, Vol. 6B: Feeling and Hurting*, edited by E. C. Carterette, and M. P. Friedman, pp. 183–230. Academic Press, New York.
96. Casey, L. O. (1978): Development of communication behavior in autistic children: A parent program using manual signs. *J. Autism Child. Schizo.*, 8:45–59.
97. Chalfant, J. C., and Schefflin, M. A. (1969): *Central Processing Dysfunctions in Children*, N.I.N.D.S. Monograph No. 9. U.S. Department of Health, Education, and Welfare, Washington, D.C.
98. Chall, J. S., and Mirsky, A. F., editors (1978): *Education and the Brain*. University of Chicago Press, Chicago.
99. Chao, D., Carter, S., and Gold, A. P. (1977): Paroxysmal disorders. In: *Pediatrics, 16th Ed.*, edited by A. M. Rudolph, pp. 1838–1855. Appleton-Century-Crofts, New York.
100. Chapanis, N. P. (1981): The patterning method: A critique. In: *Brain Dysfunction in Children: Etiology, Diagnosis, and Management*, edited by P. Black, pp. 265–280. Raven Press, New York.

101. Chapman, R. M., McCrary, J. W., and Chapman, J. A. (1978): Short-term memory: The "storage" component of human brain responses predicts recall. *Science*, 202:1211–1213.

102. Charles, D. C. (1953): Ability and accomplishment of persons earlier judged mentally deficient. *Genet. Psychol. Monogr.*, 47:3–71.

103. Charlton, M. H., and Yahr, M. D. (1967): Long-term follow-up of patients with petit mal. *Arch. Neurol.*, 16:595–598.

104. Chase, J. B. (1968): *Retrolental Fibroplasia and Autistic Symptomatology*. American Foundation for the Blind, New York.

105. Chase, T. N. (1975): Extrapyramidal disorders induced by drugs. In: *The Nervous System, Vol. 2: The Clinical Neurosciences*, edited by D. B. Tower, pp. 331–335. Raven Press, New York.

105a. Chatrian, G. E., and Petersen, M. C. (1960): The convulsive patterns provoked by indoklon, metrazol and electroshock: Some depth electrographic observations in human patients. *Electroenceph. Clin. Neurophysiol.*, 12:715–725.

106. Chess, S. (1960): Diagnosis and treatment of the hyperactive child. *N.Y. State J. Med.*, 60:2379–2385.

107. Chess, S., Korn, S. J., and Fernandez, P. B. (1971): *Psychiatric Disorders of Children with Congenital Rubella*. Brunner/Mazel, New York.

108. Chevrie, J. J., and Aicardi, J. (1972): Childhood epileptic encephalopathy with slow spike-wave. A statistical study of 80 cases. *Epilepsia*, 13:259–271.

109. Childers, A. T. (1935): Hyperactivity in children having behavior disorders. *Amer. J. Orthopsychiatry*, 5:227–243.

110. Chomsky, N., and Walker, E. (1978): Introduction: The linguistic and psycholinguistic background. In: *Explorations in the Biology of Language*, edited by E. Walker, pp. 15–26. Bradford Books, Montgomery, Vermont.

111. Cioffi, J., and Kandel, G. L. (1979): Laterality of stereognostic accuracy of children for words, shapes, and bigrams: A sex difference for bigrams. *Science*, 204:1432–1434.

112. Clark, D. L., Kreutzberg, J. R., and Chee, F. K. W. (1977): Vestibular stimulation influence on motor development in infants. *Science*, 196:1228–1229.

113. Clarke, A. M., and Clarke, A. D. B., editors (1965): *Mental Deficiency: The Changing Outlook (Rev. Ed.)*. The Free Press, New York.

114. Clements, S. D., editor (1966): *Minimal Brain Dysfunction in Children*, N.I.N.D.S. Monograph No. 3. US Department of Health, Education, and Welfare, Washington, D.C.

115. Clopton, B. M., and Silverman, M. S. (1977): Plasticity of binaural interaction. II. Critical period and changes in midline response. *J. Neurophysiol.*, 40:1275–1280.

116. Cogan, D. G. (1956): *Neurology of the Ocular Muscles*. Charles C. Thomas, Springfield, Ill.

117. Cohen, H. J., and Kligler, D., editors (1980): *Urban Community Care for the Developmentally Disabled*. Charles C. Thomas, Springfield, Ill.

118. Cohen, H. J., Taft, L. T., Mahadeviah, M. S., and Birch, H. G. (1967): Developmental changes in overflow in normal and aberrantly functioning children. *J. Pediatr.*, 71:39–47.

119. Cohen, M. M., and Rapin, I. (1978): Evoked potential audiometry in neurologically impaired children. In: *Evoked Electrical Activity in the Auditory Nervous System*, edited by R. F. Naunton, and C. Fernandez, pp. 551–572. Academic Press, New York.

120. Cohen, N. J., and Squire, L. R. (1980): Preserved learning and retention of pattern-analyzing skill in amnesia: Dissociation of knowing how and knowing that. *Science*, 210:207–210.

121. Coleman, M. (1979): Studies of the autistic syndrome. In: *Res. Publ. Assoc. Res. Nerv. Ment Dis. Vol. 57: Congenital and Acquired Cognitive Disorders*, edited by R. Katzman, pp. 265–267. Raven Press, New York.

122. Coleman, M., Steinberg, G., Tippet, J., Bhagavan, H. N., Coursin, D. B., Gross, M., Lewis, C., and DeVeau, L. (1979): A preliminary study of the effect of pyridoxine administration in a subgroup of hyperkinetic children: A double-blind crossover comparison with methylphenidate. *Biol. Psychiatry*, 14:741–751.

123. Commission on Classification and Terminology of the International League Against Epilepsy (1981): Proposal for revised clinical and electroencephalographic classification of epileptic seizures. *Epilepsia*, 22:489–501.

124. Connolly, A. J., Nachtman, W., and Pritcheff, E. M. (1976): *The Key Math Diagnostic Arithmetic Test. 2nd Ed.*, American Guidance Service, Circle Pines, Minn.

125. Conrad, R. (1972): Speech and Reading. In: *Language by Ear and by Eye*, edited by J. F. Kavanagh, and I. G. Mattingly, pp. 205–240. MIT Press, Cambridge, Mass.

126. Conrad, R. (1979): *The School Age Deaf Child*. Harper & Row, London.
127. Cooper, I. S. (1969): *Involuntary Movement Disorders*. Hoeber, New York.
128. Cooper, I. S., Amin, I., Upton, A., Ricklan, M., Watkins, S., and McLellan, L. (1977/78): Safety and efficacy of chronic cerebellar stimulation. *Appl. Neurophysiol.*, 40:124–134.
129. Coss, R. G., and Globus, A. (1978): Spine stems on tectal interneurons in jewel fish are shortened by social stimulation. *Science*, 200:787–790.
130. Cott, A. (1977): *The Orthomolecular Approach to Learning Disabilities*. Academic Therapy, Novato, Ca.
131. Cotzias, G. O., Papavasilliou, P. S., Ginos, J. Z., and Tolosa, E. S. (1975): Treatment of Parkinson's disease and allied conditions. In: *The Nervous System, Vol. 2: The Clinical Neurosciences*, edited by D. B. Tower, pp. 323–329. Raven Press, New York.
132. Critchley, M. (1953): *The Parietal Lobes*. Edward Arnold, London.
133. Critchley, M. (1970): *The Dyslexic Child*. William Heinemann Medical Books, London.
134. Critchley, M., and Henson, R. A., editors (1977): *Music and the Brain: Studies in the Neurology of Music*. William Heinemann Medical Books, London.
135. Cromer, R. F. (1976): The cognitive hypothesis of language acquisition and its implications for child language deficiency. In: *Normal and Deficient Child Language*, edited by D. M. Morehead, and A. E. Morehead, pp. 283–333. University Park Press, Baltimore.
136. Cronbach, L. J., and Meehl, P. E. (1955): Construct validity in psychological tests. *Psychol. Bull.*, 52:281–302.
137. Crothers, B., and Paine, R. S. (1959): *The Natural History of Cerebral Palsy*. Harvard University Press, Cambridge, Mass.
138. Crowder, R. G. (1972): Visual and auditory memory. In: *Language by Ear and by Eye*, edited by J. F. Kavanagh, and I. G. Mattingly, pp. 251–275. MIT Press, Cambridge, Mass.
139. Cytryn, L., McKnew, D. H., Jr., and Bunney, W. E., Jr. (1980): Diagnosis of depression in children: A reassessment. *Am. J. Psychiatry*, 137:22–25.
140. Damasio, A. (1979): The frontal lobes. In: *Clinical Neuropsychology*, edited by K. M. Heilman, and E. Valenstein, pp. 159–185. Oxford University Press, New York.
141. Damasio, A. R., and Maurer, R. G. (1978): A neurological model for childhood autism. *Arch. Neurol.*, 35:777–786.
142. Damasio, H., Maurer, R. G., Damasio, A. R., and Chui, H. C. (1980): Computerized tomographic scan findings in patients with autistic behavior. *Arch. Neurol.*, 37:504–510.
143. Darlington, R. B., Royce, J. M., Snipper, A. S., Murray, H. W., and Lazar, I. (1980): Preschool programs and later school competence of children from low-income families. *Science*, 208:202–204.
144. Daube, J. R. (1966): Sensory precipitated seizures: A review. *J. Nerv. Ment. Dis.*, 141:524–539.
145. Davis, K. L., Mohs, R. C., Tinklenberg, J. R., Pfefferbaum, A., Hollister, L. E., and Kopell, B. S. (1978): Physostigmine: Improvement of long-term memory processes in normal humans. *Science*, 201:272–274.
146. DeFrancesca, S. (1972): *Academic Achievement Test Results of a National Testing Program for Hearing Impaired Students—United States: Spring 1971*. Gallaudet College, Office of Demographic Studies, Washington, D.C.
147. Delacato, C. H. (1963): *The Diagnosis and Treatment of Speech and Reading Problems*. Charles C. Thomas, Springfield, Ill.
148. de la Fuente, J. R., and Rosenbaum, A. H. (1979): Psychoendocrinology. *Mayo Clin. Proc.*, 54:109–118.
149. Delgado-Escueta, A. V., Mattson, R. H., King, L., Goldensohn, E. S., Spiegel, H., Madsen, J., Crandall, P., Dreifuss, F., and Porter, R. J. (1981): The nature of aggression during epileptic seizures. *N. Engl. J. Med.*, 305:711–716.
150. DeLong, G. R. (1978): A neuropsychologic interpretation of infantile autism. In: *Autism: A Reappraisal of Concepts and Treatment*, edited by M. Rutter, and E. Schopler, pp. 207–218. Plenum Press, New York.
151. DeLong, M. R., and Strick, P. L. (1974): Relation of basal ganglia, cerebellum, and motor cortex units to ramp and ballistic limb movements. *Brain Res.*, 71:327–335.
152. Dement, W., Holman, R. B., and Guilleminault, C. (1976): Neurochemical and neuropharmacological foundations of the sleep disorders. *Psychopharmacol. Comm.*, 2:77–90.
153. DeMyer, M. K., Barton, S., DeMyer, W. E., Norton, J. A., Allen, J., and Steele, R. (1973): Prognosis in autism: A follow-up study. *J. Autism Child. Schizophr.*, 3:199–246.

154. Denckla, M. B. (1973): Development of speed in repetition and successive finger movements in normal children. *Dev. Med. Child Neurol.*, 15:635–645.

155. Denckla, M. B. (1974): Development of coordination in normal children. *Dev. Med. Child Neurol.*, 16:729–741.

156. Denckla, M. B. (1977): Minimal brain dysfunction and dyslexia: Beyond diagnosis by exclusion. In: *Topics in Child Neurology*, edited by M. E. Blaw, I. Rapin, and M. Kinsbourne, pp. 243–262. Spectrum, New York.

157. Denckla, M. B. (1979): Childhood learning disabilities. In: *Clinical Neuropsychology*, edited by K. M. Heilman, and E. Valenstein, pp. 535–573. Oxford University Press, New York.

158. Denckla, M. B., and Heilman, K. M. (1979): The syndrome of hyperactivity. In: *Clinical Neuropsychology*, edited by K. M. Heilman, and E. Valenstein, pp. 574–597. Oxford University Press, New York.

159. Denny-Brown, D., and Chambers, R. A. (1976): Physiological aspects of visual perception. I. Functional aspects of visual cortex. *Arch. Neurol.*, 33:219–227.

160. Desmedt, J. E. (1977): Active touch exploration of extrapersonal space elicits specific electrogenesis in the right cerebral hemisphere of intact right-handed man. *Proc. Natl. Acad. Sci. U.S.A.*, 74:4037–4040.

161. Desmedt, J. E. (1981): Scalp-recorded cerebral event-related potentials in man as point of entry into the analysis of cognitive processing. In: *The Organization of Cerebral Cortex*, edited by F. O. Schmitt, F. G. Worden, G. Adelman, and S. G. Dennis, pp. 440–473. MIT Press, Cambridge, Mass.

162. DeWied, D., and Versteeg, D. H. G. (1979): Neurohypophyseal principles and memory. *Fed. Proc.*, 38:2348–2354.

163. Diaz, J., and Schain, R. J. (1978): Phenobarbital: Effects of long-term administration on behavior and brain of artificially reared rats. *Science*, 199:90–91.

164. Dimond, S. J., and Beaumont, J. G., editors (1974): *Hemisphere Function in the Human Brain*. John Wiley & Sons, New York.

165. Dimond, S. J., and Blizard, D. A., editors (1977): *Evolution and Lateralization of the Brain. Ann. N.Y. Acad. Sci.*, 299.

166. DiSimoni, F. (1978): *The Token Test for Children*. Teaching Resources Corp, Hingham, Mass.

167. Doll, E. A. (1946): *Oseretsky Tests of Motor Proficiency*. American Guidance Service, Circle Pines, Minn.

168. Drachman, D. A. (1978): Memory, dementia, and the cholinergic system. In: *Alzheimer's Disease: Senile Dementia and Related Disorders*, edited by R. Katzman, R. D. Terry, and K. L. Bick, pp. 141–148. Raven Press, New York.

169. Drillien, C. M. (1963): Obstetric hazard, mental retardation, and behaviour disturbances in primary school. *Dev. Med. Child Neurol.*, 5:3–13.

170. Drillien, C. M., and Drummond, M. B. (1977): *Neurodevelopmental Problems in Early Childhood: Assessment and Management*. Blackwell Scientific Publications, Oxford.

171. *D.S.M. III. Diagnostic and Statistical Manual of Mental Disorders, 3rd Ed.* (1980): American Psychiatric Association, Washington, D. C.

172. Dublin, W. B. (1976): *Fundamentals of Sensorineural Auditory Pathology*. Charles C. Thomas, Springfield, Ill.

173. Duffy, F. H., Burchfiel, J. L., and Lombroso, C. T. (1979): Brain electrical activity mapping (BEAM): A method for extending the clinical utility of EEG and evoked potential data. *Ann. Neurol.*, 5:309–321.

174. Duffy, F. H., Denckla, M. B., Bartels, P. H., and Sandini, G. (1980): Dyslexia: Regional differences in brain electrical activity by topographic mapping. *Ann. Neurol.*, 7:412–420.

175. Dunn, L. M. (1965): *Peabody Picture Vocabulary Test*. American Guidance Service, Circle Pines, Minn.

176. Economo, C., von (1929): *The Cytoarchitectonics of the Human Cerebral Cortex* (translated by S. Parker). London, Humphrey Milford, Oxford University Press.

177. Ehrhardt, A. A. (1978): Behavioral sequellae of prenatal hormonal exposure in animals and man. In: *Psychopharmacology: A Generation of Progress*, edited by M. A. Lipton, A. DiMascio, and K. F. Killam, pp. 531–539. Raven Press, New York.

178. Ehrhardt, A. A., and Meyer-Bahlburg, H. F. L. (1981): Effects of prenatal sex hormones on gender-related behavior. *Science*, 211:1312–1318.

179. Eimas, P. D. (1979): On the processing of speech: Some implications for language development. In: *The Neurological Bases of Language Disorders in Children: Methods and Directions for*

Research, edited by C. L. Ludlow, and M. E. Doran-Quine, pp. 159–171. N.I.N.C.D.S. Monograph No. 22, Bethesda, Md.

180. Eisenberg, L. (1977): Psychiatry and society: A sociobiologic synthesis. *N. Engl. J. Med.*, 296:903–910.

181. Eisenson, J. (1972): *Aphasia in Children*. Harper & Row, New York.

182. Emerson, R., D'Souza, B. J., Vining, E. P., Holden, K. R., Mellits, E. D., and Freeman, J. M. (1981): Stopping medication in children with epilepsy: Predictors of outcome. *N. Engl. J. Med.*, 304:1125–1129.

183. Erenberg, G. (1972): Drug therapy in minimal brain dysfunction: A commentary. *J. Pediatr.*, 81:359–365.

184. Ervin, F. R., and Anders, T. R. (1970): Normal and pathological memory: Data and a conceptual scheme. In: *The Neurosciences: Second Study Program*, edited by F. O. Schmitt, pp. 163–176. Rockefeller University Press, New York.

185. Falck, B., Hillarp, N. -A., Thieme, G., and Tarp, A. (1962): Fluorescence of catecholamines and related compounds condensed with formaldehyde. *J. Histochem. Cytochem.*, 10:348–354.

186. Falconer, M. A. (1973): Reversibility by temporal-lobe resection of the behavioral abnormalities of temporal-lobe epilepsy. *N. Engl. J. Med.*, 289:451–455.

187. Falconer, M. A. (1974): Mesial temporal (Ammon's horn) sclerosis as a common cause of epilepsy. *Lancet*, 2:767–770.

188. Fedio, P. and van Buren, J. (1975): Memory and perceptual deficits during electrical stimulation in the left and right thalamus and parietal subcortex. *Brain Lang.*, 2:78–100.

189. Feingold, B. F. (1975): *Why Your Child is Hyperactive*. Random House, New York.

190. Feldman, A. S., and Wilber, L. A., editors (1976): *Acoustic Impedance and Admittance: The Measurement of Middle Ear Function*. Williams and Wilkins, Baltimore.

191. Ferry, P. C., Hall, S. M., and Hicks, J. L. (1975): 'Dilapidated' speech: Developmental verbal dyspraxia. *Dev. Med. Child Neurol.*, 17:749–756.

192. Finger, S., editor (1978): *Recovery from Brain Damage. Research and Theory*. Plenum Press, New York.

193. Firkowska, A., Ostrowska, A., Sokolowska, M., Stein, Z., Susser, M., and Wald, I. (1978): Cognitive development and social policy: The contribution of parental occupation and education to mental performance in 11-year-olds in Warsaw. *Science*, 200:1357–1362.

194. Fish, B. (1971): The "one child, one drug" myth of stimulants in hyperkinesis. *Arch. Gen. Psychiatry*, 25:193–203.

195. Fisk, J. L., and Rourke, B. P. (1979): Identification of subtypes of learning-disabled children at three age levels: A neuropsychological, multivariate approach. *J. Clin. Neuropsychol.*, 1:289–310.

196. Fletcher, C. M., and Oldham, P. D. (1959): Diagnosis in group research. In: *Medical Surveys and Clinical Trials*, edited by L. J. Witts, pp. 23–38. Oxford University Press, London.

197. Fog, R. (1972): On stereotypy and catalepsy: Studies on the effects of amphetamine and neuroleptics in rats. *Acta. Neurol. Scand.*, 48:(Suppl. 50),1–66.

198. Forster, F. M. (1977): *Reflex Epilepsy, Behavioral Therapy, and Conditional Reflexes*. Charles C. Thomas, Springfield, Ill.

199. Frankenburg, W. K., and Dodds, J. B. (1966): *Denver Developmental Screening Test*. University of Colorado Medical Center, Denver.

200. Frederickson, J. M., Kornhuber, H. H., and Schwarz, D. W. F. (1974): Cortical projections of the vestibular nerve. In: *Vestibular System, Part 1: Basic Mechanisms*, edited by H. H. Kornhuber, pp. 565–582. Springer-Verlag, Berlin.

201. Frederickson, R. C. A., Burgis, V., Harrell, C. E., and Edwards, J. D. (1978): Dual actions of substance P on nociception. Possible role of endogenous opioids. *Science*, 199:1359–1361.

202. French, J. (1964): *Pictorial Test of Intelligence*. Houghton Mifflin, Boston.

203. Frumkin, B., and Rapin, I. (1980): Perception of vowels and consonant-vowels of varying duration in language impaired children. *Neuropsychologia*, 18:443–454.

204. Fuxe, K., Hökfelt, T., Aguati, L. F., Johannson, O., Goldstein, M., Perez de la Mora, M., Possani, L., Tapia, R., Teran, L., and Palacios, R. (1978): Mapping out central catecholamine neurons: Immunohistochemical studies on catecholamine-synthesizing enzymes. In: *Psychopharmacology. A Generation of Progress*, edited by M. A. Lipton, A. DiMascio, and K. F. Killam, pp. 67–94. Raven Press, New York.

205. Galaburda, A. M., and Kemper, T. L. (1978): Cytoarchitectonic abnormalities in developmental dyslexia: A case study. *Ann. Neurol.*, 6:94–100.

206. Galaburda, A. M., LeMay, M., Kemper, T. L., and Geschwind, N. (1978): Right-left asymmetries in the human brain. *Science*, 199:852–856.

207. Galambos, R. (1959): Electrical correlates of conditioned learning. In: *Conference on The Central Nervous System and Behavior*, edited by M. A. B. Brazier, pp. 375–415. Josiah Macy Jr. Foundation, New York.

208. Galin, D. (1979): EEG studies of lateralization of verbal processes. In: *The Neurological Bases of Language Disorders in Children: Methods and Directions for Research*, edited by C. L. Ludlow, and M. E. Doran-Quine, pp. 129–141. N.I.N.C.D.S. Monograph No. 22, Bethesda, Md.

209. Gardner, R. A. (1978): *Purdue Pegboard: Normative Data (Revised). Examiner Manual for the Purdue Pegboard Test.* Science Research Associates, Chicago.

210. Gardner, W. I. (1978): *Children with Learning and Behavior Problems: A Behavior Management Approach, 2nd Ed.* Allyn and Bacon, Boston.

211. Garfinkel, B. D., Webster, C. D., and Sloman, L. (1975): Methylphenidate and caffeine in the treatment of children with minimal brain dysfunction. *Am. J. Psychiatry*, 132:723–728.

212. Garrettson, L. K., Perel, J. M., and Dayton, P. G. (1969): Methylphenidate interaction with both anticonvulsants and ethyl biscoumacetate. *J.A.M.A.*, 207:2053–2056.

213. Gascon, G. G., and Lombroso, C. T. (1971): Epileptic (gelastic) laughter. *Epilepsia*, 12:63–76.

214. Gazzaniga, M. S. (1970): *The Bisected Brain.* Appleton-Century-Crofts, New York.

215. Gazzaniga, M. S., editor (1979): *Handbook of Behavioral Neurobiology, Vol. 2: Neuropsychology.* Plenum Press, New York.

216. Gazzaniga, M. S., and LeDoux, J. E. (1978): *The Integrated Mind.* Plenum Press, New York.

217. Gelman, R., and Gallistel, C. R. (1978): *The Child's Understanding of Number.* Harvard University Press, Cambridge, Mass.

218. Geschwind, N. (1965): Disconnexion syndromes in animals and man. *Brain*, 88:237–294, 585–644.

219. Geschwind, N. (1974): The apraxias. In: *Selected Papers on Language and the Brain*, pp. 314–323. D. Reidel, Boston, Mass.

220. Geschwind, N. (1974): Disorders of higher cortical function in children. In: *Selected Papers on Language and the Brain*, pp. 467–481. D. Reidel, Boston, Mass.

221. Geschwind, N. (1979): Anatomical foundations of language and dominance. In: *The Neurological Bases of Language Disorders in Children: Methods and Directions for Research*, edited by C. L. Ludlow, and M. E. Doran-Quine, pp. 145–157. N.I.N.C.D.S. Monograph No. 22, Bethesda, Md.

222. Geschwind, N., and Fusillo, M. (1966): Color naming defects in association with alexia. *Arch. Neurol.*, 15:137–146.

223. Geschwind, N., and Levitsky, W. (1968): Human brain: Left-right asymmetries in temporal speech region. *Science*, 161:186–187.

223a. Gibbs, F. A., and Gibbs, E. L. (1952): *Atlas of Electroencephalography. Volume 2: Epilepsy.* Addison-Wesley Press, Cambridge, Mass.

224. Gibson, J. J. (1966): *The Senses Considered as Perceptual Systems.* Houghton Mifflin, Boston, Mass.

225. Gilman, S. (1975): Primate models of postural disorders. In: *Advances in Neurology, Vol. 10*, edited by B. S. Meldrum and C. D. Marsden, pp. 55–76. Raven Press, New York.

226. Gittelman-Klein, R. (1978): Psychopharmacological treatment of anxiety disorders, mood disorders, and Tourette's disorder in children. In: *Psychopharmacology: A Generation of Progress*, edited by M. A. Lipton, A. DiMascio, and K. F. Killam, pp. 1471–1480. Raven Press, New York.

227. Gittelman-Klein, R., Klein, D. F., Abikoff, H., Katz, S., Gloisten, A. C., and Kates, W. (1976): Relative efficacy of methylphenidate and behavior modification in hyperkinetic children: An interim report. *J. Abnorm. Child Psychol.*, 4:361–379.

228. Gloor, P. (1978): Inputs and outputs of the amygdala: What the amygdala is trying to tell the rest of the brain. In: *Limbic Mechanisms*, edited by K. L. Livingston, and O. Hornykiewicz, pp. 189–209. Plenum Press, New York.

229. Goff, W. R., Allison, T., and Vaughan, H. G., Jr. (1978): The functional neuroanatomy of event-related potentials. In: *Event-Related Brain Potentials in Man*, edited by E. Callaway, P. Tueting, and S. H. Koslow, pp. 1–79. Academic Press, New York.

230. Goldberg, M. E., and Robinson, D. L. (1978): Visual system: Superior colliculus. In: *Handbook of Behavioral Neurobiology, Vol. 1: Sensory Integration*, edited by R. B. Masterton, pp. 119–164. Plenum Press, New York.

231. Goldberger, M. E. (1974): Recovery of movement after CNS lesions in monkeys. In: *Plasticity and Recovery of Function in the Central Nervous System*, edited by D. G. Stein, J. J. Rosen, and N. Butters, pp. 265–337. Academic Press, New York.

232. Golden, G. S. (1974): Gilles de la Tourette's syndrome following methylphenidate administration. *Dev. Med. Child Neurol.*, 16:76–78.

233. Goldensohn, E. S., and Gold, A. P. (1960): Prolonged behavioral disturbances as ictal phenomena. *Neurology*, 10:1–9.

234. Goldensohn, E. S., and Koehle, R. (1981): *EEG Interpretation: Problems of Over-reading and Under-reading*. Futura Publishing, Mt. Kisco, N. Y.

235. Goldensohn, E. S., and Ward, A. A., Jr. (1975): Pathogenesis of epileptic seizures. In: *The Nervous System, Vol. 2: The Clinical Neurosciences*, edited by D. B. Tower, pp. 249–260. Raven Press, New York.

236. Goldman, R., Fristoe, M., and Woodcock, R. W. (1970): *Goldman-Fristoe-Woodcock Test of Auditory Discrimination*. American Guidance Service, Circle Pines, Minn.

237. Goldman-Rakic, P. S. (1981): Development and plasticity of primate frontal association cortex. In: *The Organization of the Cerebral Cortex*, edited by F. O. Schmitt, F. G. Worden, G. Adelman, and S. G. Dennis, pp. 69–97. MIT Press, Cambridge, Mass.

238. Goldstein, K. (1939): *The Organism: A Holistic Approach to Biology Derived from Pathological Data in Man*. American Book, New York.

239. Gomez, M. R., editor (1979): *Tuberous Sclerosis*. Raven Press, New York.

240. Goslin, D. A. (1968): Standardized ability tests and testing. *Science*, 159:851–855.

241. Gotman, J. (1981): Interhemispheric relations during bilateral spike-and-wave activity. *Epilepsia*, 22:453–466.

242. Grastyan, E., Lissak, K., Mandarasz, I., and Donhoffer, H. (1959): Hippocampal electrical activity during the development of conditioned reflexes. *Electroencephalogr. Clin. Neurophysiol.*, 11:409–430.

243. Gray, W. S. (1967): *Gray Oral Reading Test*. Bobbs-Merrill, New York.

244. Graziani, L. J., Mason, J. C., and Cracco, J. (1981): Neurological aspects and early recognition of brain dysfunction in children: Diagnostic and prognostic significance of gestational, perinatal, and postnatal factors. In: *Brain Dysfunction in Children: Etiology, Diagnosis, and Management*, edited by P. Black, pp. 131–169. Raven Press, New York.

245. Griffith, J. F., and Dodge, P. R. (1968): Transient blindness following head injury in children. *N. Engl. J. Med.*, 278:648–651.

246. Gros, C., Frerebeam, P., Perez-Dominguez, E., Bazin, M., and Privat, J. M. (1976): Long-term results of stereotaxic surgery for infantile dystonia and dyskinesia. *Neurochirurgia*, 19:171–178.

247. Gubbay, S. S. (1975): *The Clumsy Child: A Study of Developmental Apraxic and Agnosic Ataxia*. W.B. Saunders, Philadelphia.

248. Guillemin, R. (1978): Peptides in the brain: The new endocrinology of the neuron. *Science*, 202:390–402.

249. Guilleminault, C., and Dement, W. C., editors (1978): *Sleep Apnea Syndromes*. Liss, New York.

250. Gupta, P. C., Rapin, I., Houroupian, D. S., Roy, S., Llena, J. F., and Tandon, P. N. (1982): Smoldering encephalitis causing intractable seizures and chronic neurologic deterioration in children.

251. Hagberg, B., Sanner, G., and Steen, M. (1972): *The Dysequilibrium Syndrome in Cerebral Palsy*. *Acta. Paediatr. Scand. Suppl. 226*.

252. Haith, M. M., Bergman, T., and Moore, M. J. (1977): Eye contact and face scanning in early infancy. *Science*, 198:853–855.

253. Hall, J. G. (1964): The cochlea and the cochlear nuclei in neonatal asphyxia: A histological study. *Acta. Otolaryngol.*, (Suppl. 194), pp. 1–93.

254. Hallgren, B. (1950): Specific dyslexia ("congenital word blindness"): A clinical and genetic study. *Acta. Psychiatry Neurol.* (Suppl. 65), 1–287.

255. Halliday, A. M. (1974): The neurophysiology of myoclonic jerking: A reappraisal. In: *Myoclonic Seizures*, edited by M. H. Charlton, pp. 1–32. Excerpta Medica, Amsterdam.

256. Harlan, R. E., Gordon, J. H., and Gorski, R. A. (1979): Sexual differentiation of the brain: Implications for neuroscience. In: *Reviews of Neuroscience, Vol. 4*, edited by D. M. Schneider, pp. 31–71. Raven Press, New York.

257. Harper, P. S. (1978): Benign hereditary chorea: Clinical and genetic aspects. *Clin. Genet.*, 13:85–95.

258. Harris, L. J. (1978): Sex differences in spatial ability: Possible environmental, genetic, and neurological factors. In: *Asymmetrical Function of the Brain*, edited by M. Kinsbourne, pp. 405–522. Cambridge University Press, Cambridge.

259. Harrison, J. M. (1978): Functional properties of the auditory system of the brain stem. In: *Handbook of Behavioral Neurobiology, Vol. 1: Sensory Integration*, edited by R. B. Masterton, pp. 409–458. Plenum Press, New York.

260. Hauser, S. L., de Long, G. R., and Rosman, N. P. (1975): Pneumographic findings in the infantile autism syndrome: A correlation with temporal lobe disease. *Brain*, 98:667–688.

261. Haywood, H. C., editor (1968): *Brain Damage in School Children*. Council for Exceptional Children, Washington, D.C.

262. Heath, R. G., and Mickle, W. A. (1960): Evaluation of seven years' experience with depth electrode studies in human patients. In: *Electrical Studies on the Unanesthetized Brain: A Symposium*, edited by E. R. Ramey, and D. S. O'Doherty, pp. 214–247. Paul B. Hoeber, New York.

263. Hebb, D. O. (1949): *The Organization of Behavior: A Neuropsychological Theory*. John Wiley & Sons, New York.

264. Hécaen, H. (1976): Acquired aphasia in children and the ontogenesis of hemispheric functional specialization. *Brain Lang.*, 3:114–134.

265. Hécaen, H. (1979): Aphasias. In: *Handbook of Behavioral Neurobiology, Vol. 2, Neuropsychology*, edited by M. S. Gazzaniga, pp. 239–292. Plenum Press, New York.

266. Hécaen, H., and Kremin, H. (1976): Neurolinguistic research on reading disorders resulting from left hemisphere lesions: Aphasic and "pure" alexias. In: *Studies in Neurolinguistics, Vol. 2*, edited by H. Whitaker, and H. A. Whitaker, pp. 269–329. Academic Press, New York.

267. Hécaen, H., and Sauguet, J. (1971): Cerebral dominance in left-handed subjects. *Cortex*, 7:19–48.

268. Heilman, K. M. (1979): Apraxia. In: *Clinical Neuropsychology*, edited by K. M. Heilman, and E. Valenstein, pp. 159–185. Oxford University Press, New York.

269. Heilman, K. M. (1979): Neglect and related disorders. In: *Clinical Neuropsychology*, edited by K. M. Heilman, and E. Valenstein, pp. 268–307. Oxford University Press, New York.

270. Heilman, K. M., and Abell, T. van den (1980): Right hemisphere dominance for attention: The mechanism underlying hemispheric asymmetries of inattention (neglect). *Neurology*, 30:327–330.

271. Heilman, K. M., and Valenstein, E., editors (1979): *Clinical Neuropsychology*. Oxford University Press, New York.

272. Hein, A. (1970): Recovering spatial motor coordination after visual cortex lesions. In: *Res. Publ. Assoc. Res. Nerv. Ment. Dis., Vol. 48: Perception and its Disorders*, edited by D. A. Hamburg, K. H. Pribram and A. J. Stunkard, pp. 163–175. Williams and Wilkins, Baltimore.

273. Held, R., and Bauer, J. A., Jr. (1974): Development of sensorially-guided reaching in infant monkey. *Brain Res.*, 71:265–271.

274. Hermelin, B., and O'Connor, N. (1971): Functional asymmetry in the reading of braille. *Neuropsychologia*, 9:431–435.

275. Hernández-Péon, R., and Donoso, M. (1957): Influence of attention and suggestion upon subcortical evoked electrical activity in the human brain. *Proceedings of the First International Congress of Neurologic Sciences, Vol. 3*, pp. 385–396. Pergamon Press, Brussels.

276. Hess, W. R. (1954): *Diencephalon: Autonomic and Extrapyramidal Functions*. In: *Monographs in Biology and Medicine, Vol. 3*. Grune & Stratton, New York.

277. Hier, D. B., LeMay, M., and Rosenberger, P. B. (1978): Autism: Association with reversed cerebral asymmetry. *Neurology*, 28:348–349.

278. Hillyard, S. A., Picton, T. W., and Regan, D. (1978): Sensation, perception, and attention: Analysis using ERPs. In: *Event-related Potentials in Man*, edited by E. Calloway, P. Tueting, and S. H. Koslow, pp. 223–321. Academic Press, New York.

278a. Hirano, A., Iwata, M., Llena, J. F., and Matsui, T. (1980): Color Atlas of the Pathology of the Nervous System. Igaku-Shoin, Tokyo, New York.

279. Hiskey, M. S. (1955): *The Hiskey-Nebraska Test of Learning Aptitude (Rev. Ed.)*. University of Nebraska, Lincoln.

280. Hofstadter, D. R. (1979): *Gödel, Escher, Bach: An Eternal Golden Braid*. Basic Books, New York.

281. Hökfelt, T., Elde, R., Johansson, O., et al. (1978): Distribution of peptide-containing neurons. In: *Psychopharmacology: A Generation of Progress*, edited by M. A. Lipton, A. DiMascio, and K. F. Killam, pp. 39–66. Raven Press, New York.

282. Hollenbeck, G. P., and Kaufman, A. S. (1973): Factor analysis of the Wechsler Preschool and Primary Scale of Intelligence (WPPSI). *J. Clin. Psychol.*, 29:41–45.

283. Hosobuchi, Y., Rossier, J., Bloom, F. E., and Guillemin, R. (1979): Stimulation of human periaqueductal gray for pain relief increases immunoreactive β-endorphin in ventricular fluid. *Science*, 203:279–281.

284. Hubel, D. H., and Wiesel, T. N. (1977): Functional architecture of macaque monkey cortex. *Proc. R. Soc. Lond.* B198:1–59.

285. Humphreys, L. G. (1976): A factor model for research in intelligence and problem solving. In: *The Nature of Intelligence*, edited by L. Resnick, pp. 329–340. Lawrence Erlbaum Associates, Hillsdale, N.J.

286. Hunt, J. McV. (1976): Environmental programming to foster competence and prevent mental retardation in infancy. In: *Environments as Therapy for Brain Dysfunction*, edited by R. N. Walsh, and W. T. Greenough, pp. 201–255. Plenum Press, New York.

287. Huppert, F. A., and Piercey, M. (1979): Normal and abnormal forgetting in organic amnesia: Effect of locus of lesion. *Cortex*, 15:385–390.

288. Hutchison, J. B., editor (1978): *Biological Determinants of Sexual Behavior*. Wiley-Interscience, New York.

289. Huttenlocher, P. R., and Huttenlocher, J. (1973): A study of children with hyperlexia. *Neurology*, 23:1107–1116.

290. Huttenlocher, P. R, Wilbourn, A. J., and Signore, J. M. (1971): Medium-chain triglycerides as a therapy for intractable childhood epilepsy. *Neurology*, 21:1097–1103.

291. Ingram, D. (1975): Cerebral speech lateralization in young children. *Neuropsychologia*, 13:103–105.

292. Ingram, T. T. S. (1975): Speech disorders in childhood. In: *Foundations of Language Development*, *Vol. 2*, edited by E. H. Lenneberg, and E. Lenneberg, pp. 195–261. Academic Press, New York.

293. Inhelder, B. (1976): Observations on the operational and figurative aspects of thought in dysphasic children. In: *Normal and Deficient Child Language*, edited by D. M. Morehead, and A. E. Morehead, pp. 335–343. University Park Press, Baltimore.

294. Isaacson, R. L. (1975): The myth of recovery from early brain damage. In: *Aberrant Development in Infancy*, edited by N. R. Ellis. John Ellis & Sons, New York.

295. Isaacson, R. L., and Pribram, K. H., editors (1975): *The Hippocampus, (Vol. 1 & 2)*. Plenum Press, New York.

295a. Iversen, L. L. (1979): The chemistry of the brain. *Sci. Am.*, 241, No. 3:134–149.

296. Ives, J. R., Thompson, C. J., and Gloor, P. (1976): Seizure monitoring: A new tool in electroencephalography. *Electroencephalogr. Clin. Neurophysiol.*, 41:422–427.

297. Jabbour, J. T., Ramey, D. R., and Roach, S. (1977): *Atlas of Computerized Tomography Scans in Pediatric Neurology*. Medical Examination Publishing Co., Flushing, N.Y.

298. Jastak, J., and Jastak, S. (1976): *Wide Range Achievement Test*. Guidance Associates, Wilmington, Delaware.

299. Jeavons, P. M., and Bower, B. D. (1974): Infantile Spasms. In: *Handbook of Clinical Neurology, Vol. 5: The Epilepsies*, edited by O. Magnus, and A. M. Lorentz de Haas, pp. 219–234. North Holland Publishing Co., Amsterdam.

300. Jeavons, P. M., and Harding, G. F. A. (1975): *Photosensitive Epilepsy. A Review of the Literature and a Study of 460 Patients. Clinics in Develop. Med. No. 56.* W. Heinemann Medical Books, London.

301. Jones, E. G. (1981): Anatomy of cerebral cortex: Columnar input-output organization. In: *The Organization of Cerebral Cortex*, edited by F. O. Schmitt, F. G. Worden, G. Adelman, and S. G. Dennis, pp. 203–235. MIT Press, Cambridge, Mass.

302. Jones, M. H. (1960): Management of hemiplegic children with peripheral sensory loss. *Pediatr. Clin. North Am.*, 7:765–775.

303. Joschko, M. (1979): Bilateral prefrontal leucotomy: An ex post facto archival study of a complete hospital sample. *J. Clin. Neuropsychol.*, 1:167–182.

304. Jouvet, M. (1972): The role of monoamines and acetylcholine-containing neurons in the regulation of the sleep-waking cycle. *Ergeb. Physiol.*, 64:166–307.

305. Kaas, J. H., Nelson, R. J., Sur, M., and Merzenich, M. M. (1981): Organization of somatosensory complex in primates. In: *The Organization of the Cerebral Cortex*, edited by F. O. Schmitt, F. G. Worden, G. Adelman, and S. G. Dennis, pp. 237–261. MIT Press, Cambridge, Mass.

306. Kagan, J. (1970): The distribution of attention in infancy. In: *Res. Publ. Assoc. Res. Nerv. Ment. Dis.*, Vol. 48: pp. 214–237. Williams and Wilkins, Baltimore.

307. Karczmar, A. G., and Dun, N. J. (1978): Cholinergic synapses: Physiological, pharmacological, and behavioral considerations. In: *Psychopharmacology: A Generation of Progress*, edited by M. A. Lipton, A. DiMascio, and K. F. Killam, pp. 293–305. Raven Press, New York.
308. Kaufman, A. S. (1979): Cerebral specialization and intelligence testing. *J. Res. Dev. Educ.*, 12:96–107.
309. Kavanagh, J. F., and Mattingly, I. G., editors (1972): *Language by Ear and by Eye*. The MIT Press, Cambridge, Mass.
310. Keele, S. W., and Neill, W. T. (1978): Mechanisms of attention. In: *Handbook of Perception, Vol. 9: Perceptual Processing*, edited by E. C. Carterette, and M. P. Friedman, pp. 3–47. Academic Press, New York.
311. Kelly, P. H., Seviour, P. W., and Iversen, S. D. (1975): Amphetamine and apomorphine responses in the rat following 6-OHDA lesions of the nucleus accumbens septi and corpus striatum. *Brain Res.*, 94:507–522.
312. Kimura, D. (1977): Acquisition of a motor skill after left-hemisphere damage. *Brain*, 100:527–542.
313. Kinsbourne, M. (1971): The minor hemisphere as a source of aphasic speech. *Arch. Neurol.*, 25:302–306.
314. Kinsbourne, M. (1973): Minimal brain dysfunction as a neurodevelopmental lag. *Ann. N.Y. Acad. Sci.*, 205:268–273.
315. Kinsbourne, M. (1973): School problems. *Pediatrics*, 52:697–710.
316. Kinsbourne, M. (1977): The mechanism of hyperactivity. In: *Topics in Child Neurology*, edited by M. E. Blaw, I. Rapin, and M. Kinsbourne, pp. 289–306. Spectrum, New York.
317. Kinsbourne, M., and Hiscock, M. (1977): Does cerebral dominance develop? In: *Language Development and Neurological Theory*, edited by S. J. Segalowitz, and F. A. Gruber, pp. 171–191. Academic Press, New York.
318. Kinsbourne, M., and Smith, W. L., editors (1974): *Hemispheric Disconnection and Cerebral Function*. Charles C. Thomas, Springfield, Ill.
319. Kinsbourne, M., and Warrington, E. K. (1962): A disorder of simultaneous form perception. *Brain*, 85:461–486.
320. Kinsbourne, M., and Warrington, E. K. (1963): Developmental factors in reading and writing backwardness. *Br. J. Psychol.*, 54:145–156.
321. Kinsbourne, M., and Warrington, E. K. (1963): The developmental Gerstmann syndrome. *Arch. Neurol.*, 8:490–501.
322. Kirk, S. A., McCarthy, J. J., and Kirk, W. R. (1968): *Illinois Test of Psycholinguistic Abilities*. University of Illinois Press, Urbana.
323. Klawans, H. L., and Weiner, W. J. (1976): The pharmacology of choreatic movement disorders. *Prog. Neurobiol.*, 6:49–80.
324. Klemm, W. R. (1976): Hippocampal EEG and information processing: A special role for theta rhythm. *Prog. Neurobiol.*, 7:197–214.
325. Klüver, H., and Bucy, P. C. (1939): Preliminary analysis of function of the temporal lobe in monkeys. *Arch. Neurol. Psychiatry*, 42:979–1000.
326. Knights, R. M., and Bakker, D. J., editors (1976): *The Neuropsychology of Learning Disorders: Theoretical Approaches*. University Park Press, Baltimore.
327. Knobloch, H., and Pasamanick, B. (1959): Syndrome of minimal cerebral damage in infancy. *J.A.M.A.*, 170:1384–1387.
328. Knobloch, H., and Pasamanick, B. (1974): *Developmental Diagnosis (3rd Rev Edition)*. Psychological Corp., New York.
329. Knox, C., and Kimura, D. (1970): Cerebral processing of nonverbal sounds in boys and girls. *Neuropsychologia*, 8:227–237.
330. Kools, J. A., Williams, A. F., Vickers, M. J., and Caell, A. (1971): Oral and limb apraxia in mentally retarded children with deviant articulation. *Cortex*, 7:387–400.
331. Koppitz, E. M. (1963): *The Bender Gestalt Test for Young Children*. Grune and Stratton, New York.
332. Kornhuber, H. H. (1974): Cerebral cortex, cerebellum, and basal ganglia: An introduction to their motor functions. In: *The Neurosciences, Third Study Program*, edited by F. O. Schmitt, and F. G. Worden, pp. 267–280. MIT Press, Cambridge, Mass.
333. Krasner, L., and Ullmann, L. P., editors (1965): *Research in Behavior Modification: New Developments and Implications*. Holt, Rinehart and Winston, New York.

334. Krieger, D. T., and Liotta, A. S. (1979): Pituitary hormones in brain: When, how, and why? *Science*, 205:366–372.
335. Krieger, D. T., and Martin, J. B. (1981): Brain peptides. *New Engl. J. Med.*, 304:876–885, 944–951.
336. Kuhl, D. E., Engel, J. Jr., Phelps, M. E., and Selin, D. (1980): Epileptic patterns of local cerebral metabolism and perfusion in humans determined by emission computed tomography of ¹⁸FDG and ¹³NH₃. *Ann. Neurol.*, 8:348–360.
337. Lafferman, J. A., and Silbergeld, E. K. (1979): Erythrosin B inhibits dopamine transport in rat caudate synaptosomes. *Science*, 205:410–412.
338. Lagos, J. L. (1974): *Seizures, Epilepsy, and Your Child.* Harper & Row, New York.
339. Lahey, B. B., editor (1978): *Behavior Therapy with Hyperactive and Learning Disabled Children.* Oxford University Press, New York.
340. Landau, W. M., Goldstein, R., and Kleffner, F. R. (1960): Congenital aphasia: A clinicopathologic study. *Neurology*, 10:915–921.
341. Landau, W. M., and Kleffner, F. R. (1957): Syndrome of acquired aphasia with convulsive disorder in children. *Neurology*, 7:523–530.
342. Largo, R., and Howard, J. (1979): Developmental progression in play behavior of children between nine and thirty months. I. Spontaneous play and imitation. *Dev. Med. Child Neurol.*, 21:299–310.
343. Larsen, B., Skinhøj, E., and Lassen, N. A. (1978): Variations in regional cortical blood flow in the right and left hemisphere during automatic speech. *Brain*, 101:193–209.
344. Larsen, E. J. (1931): A neurologic-etiologic study on 1,000 mental defectives. *Acta Psychiatr. Neurol.*, 6:37–54.
345. Lasley, K. S. (1929): *Brain Mechanisms and Intelligence: A Quantitative Study of Injuries to the Brain.* University of Chicago Press, Chicago.
346. Lassen, N. A., Ingvar, D. H., and Skinhøj, E. (1978): Brain function and blood flow. *Sci. Am.*, 239, No. 4:62–71.
347. Laufer, M. W., and Denhoff, E. (1957): Hyperkinetic behavior syndrome in children. *J. Pediatr.*, 50:463–474.
348. Lawrence, D. G., and Hopkins, D. A. (1976): The development of motor control in the rhesus monkey. Evidence concerning the role of corticomotoneuronal connections. *Brain*, 99:235–254.
348a. LeDoux, J. E., Wilson, D. H., and Gazzaniga, M. S. (1979): Beyond commisurotomy: Clues to consciousness. In: *Handbook of Behavioral Neurobiology, Vol. 2: Neuropsychology*, edited by M. S. Gazzaniga, pp. 543–554. Plenum Press, New York.
349. Leiter, R. (1948): *The Leiter International Performance Scale.* Stoelting, Chicago.
350. Lenneberg, E. H. (1967): *Biological Foundations of Language.* John Wiley & Sons, New York.
351. Lennerstrand, G., and Bach-y-Rita, P. (1975): *Basic Mechanisms of Ocular Motility and Their Clinical Implications.* Pergamon Press, Oxford.
352. Lennox-Buchthal, M. A. (1973): Febrile convulsions: A reappraisal. *Electroencephalogr. Clin. Neurophysiol. (Suppl. 32)*, 1–138.
353. Lerman, P., and Kivity, S. (1975): Benign focal epilepsy of childhood. A follow-up study of 100 recovered patients. *Arch. Neurol.*, 32:261–264.
354. Leshner, A. I. (1978): *An Introduction to Behavioral Endocrinology.* Oxford University Press, New York.
355. Levy, J., and Trevarthen, C. (1977): Perceptual, semantic, and phonetic aspects of elementary language processes in split-brain patients. *Brain*, 100:105–118.
356. Levy, J., Trevarthen, C., and Sperry, R. W. (1972): Perception of bilateral chimeric figures following hemispheric disconnexion. *Brain*, 95:61–78.
357. Lewis, M., and McGurk, H. (1972): Evaluation of infant intelligence: Infant intelligence scores—true or false? *Science*, 178:1174–1177.
358. Ley, R. G., and Bryden, M. P. (1979): Hemispheric differences in processing emotions and faces. *Brain Lang.*, 7:127–138.
359. Liberman, A. M., Cooper, F. S., Shankweiler, D. P., and Studdert-Kennedy, M. (1967): Perception of the speech code. *Psychol. Rev.*, 74:431–461.
360. Lindenberg, R. (1955): Compression of brain arteries as pathogenetic factor for tissue necroses and their areas of predilection. *J. Neuropathol. Exp. Neurol.*, 14:223–243.
361. Linksz, A. (1973): *On Writing, Reading, and Dyslexia.* Grune and Stratton, New York.
362. Lipman, R. S., DiMascio, A., Reatig, N., and Kirson, T. (1978): Psychotropic drugs and mentally retarded children. In: *Psychopharmacology: A Generation of Progress*, edited by M. A. Lipton, A. DiMascio, and K. F. Killam, pp. 1437–1449. Raven Press, New York.

363. Lipton, M. A., DiMascio, A., and Killam, K. F., editors (1978): *Psychopharmacology: A Generation of Progress*. Raven Press, New York.
364. Livingston, K. E., and Hornykiewicz, O., editors (1978): *Limbic Mechanisms*. Plenum Press, New York.
365. Livingston, S. (1972): *Comprehensive Management of Epilepsy in Infancy, Childhood, and Adolescence*. Charles C. Thomas, Springfield, Ill.
366. Llinás, R. (1975): The cerebellar cortex. In: *The Nervous System, Vol. 1: The Basic Neurosciences*, edited by D. B. Tower, pp. 235–244. Raven Press, New York.
367. Lockman, L. A., Swaiman, K. F., Drage, J. S., Nelson, K. B., and Marsden, A. M. editors (1979): *Workshop on the Neurobiological Basis of Autism*. N.I.H. Publication 79-1855, Bethesda, Md.
368. Loehlin, J. C., Lindzey, G., and Spuhler, J. N. (1975): *Race Differences in Intelligence*. Freeman, San Francisco.
369. Loftus, G. R., and Loftus, E. F. (1976): *Human Memory: The Processing of Information*. Lawrence Erlbaum Associates, Hillsdale, N.J.
370. Logan, W. J., and Freeman, J. M. (1969): Pseudodegenerative disease due to diphenylhydantoin intoxication. *Arch. Neurol.*, 21:631–637.
371. Lomas, J., and Kimura, D. (1976): Interhemispheric interaction between speaking and sequential manual activity. *Neuropsychologia*, 14:23–33.
372. Lou, H. C., Brandt, S., and Bruhn, P. (1977): Progressive aphasia and epilepsy with a self-limited course. In: *Epilepsy, the Eighth International Symposium*, edited by J. K. Penry, pp. 295–303. Raven Press, New York.
373. Louick, D., and Boland, T. B. (1978): Psychologic tests: A guide for pediatricians. *Pediatr. Ann.*, 7:86–101.
374. Lucas, A. R. (1981): Toward an understanding of anorexia nervosa as a disease entity. *Mayo Clin. Proc.*, 56:254–264.
375. Lucas, A. R., Kauffman, P. E., and Morris, E. M. (1967): Gilles de la Tourette's disease: A clinical study of 15 cases. *J. Am. Acad. Child Psychiatry*, 6:700–722.
376. Ludlow, C. L. (1980): Children's language disorders: Recent research advances. *Ann. Neurol.*, 7:497–507.
377. Ludlow, C. L., and Doran-Quine, M. E. (1979): *The Neurological Basis of Language Disorders in Children: Methods and Directions for Research*. N.I.N.C.D.S. Monograph No. 22, Bethesda, Md.
378. Luria, A. R. (1966): *Higher Cortical Functions in Man*. Basic Books, New York.
379. Lynch, G., Deadwyler, S., and Cotman, C. W. (1973): Postlesional axonal growth produces permanent functional connections. *Science*, 180:1364–1366.
380. Lynn, G. E., and Gilroy, J. (1972): Neuro-audiological abnormalities in patients with temporal lobe tumors. *J. Neurol. Sci.*, 17:167–184.
381. Mailman, R. B., Ferris, R. M., Tang, F. L. M., Vogel, R. A., Kilts, C. D., Lipton, M. A., Smith, D. A., Mueller, R. A., and Breese, G. R. (1980): Erythrosin (red no. 3) and its nonspecific biochemical actions: What relation to behavioral changes? *Science*, 207:535–537.
382. Mantovani, J. F., and Landau, W. M. (1980): Acquired aphasia with convulsive disorder: Course and prognosis. *Neurology*, 30:524–529.
383. Marcus, E. M. (1972): Experimental models of petit mal epilepsy. In: *Experimental Models of Epilepsy-A Manual for the Laboratory Worker*, edited by D. P. Purpura, J. K. Penry, D. B. Tower, D. M. Woodbury, and R. D. Walter, pp. 114–146. Raven Press, New York.
384. Markham, C. H., and Knox, J. W. (1965): Observations on Huntington's chorea in childhood. *J. Pediatr.*, 67:46–57.
385. Marsden, C. D., Foley, T. H., Owen, D. A. L., and McAllister, R. G. (1967): Peripheral beta-adrenergic receptors concerned with tremor. *Clin. Sci.*, 33:53–65.
386. Marx, J. L. (1980): NMR opens a new window into the body. *Science*, 210:302–305.
387. Masterton, R. B., editor (1978): *Handbook of Behavioral Neurobiology, Vol. 1: Sensory Integration*. Plenum Press, New York.
388. Matsumoto, A., Watanabe, K., Negoro, T., Sugiura, M., Iwase, K., Hara, K., and Miyazaki, S. (1981): Long-term prognosis after infantile spasms: A statistical study of prognostic factors in 200 cases. *Dev. Med. Child Neurol.*, 23:51–65.
389. Mattis, S. (1978): Dyslexia syndromes: A working hypothesis that works. In: *Dyslexia: An Appraisal of Current Knowledge*, edited by A. L. Benton, and D. Pearl, pp. 45–58. Oxford University Press, New York.

390. Mattis, S. (1981): Dyslexia syndromes in children: Toward the development of syndrome-specific treatment programs. In: *Neuropsychological and Cognitive Processes in Reading*, edited by F. J. Pirozzolo, and M. C. Wittrock, pp. 93–107. Academic Press, New York.
391. Mattis, S., French, J. H., and Rapin, I. (1975): Dyslexia in children and young adults: Three independent neuropsychological syndromes. *Dev. Med. Child Neurol.*, 17:150–163.
392. Maulsby, R., and Kellaway, P. (1964): Transient hypoxic crises in children. In: *Neurological and Electroencephalographic Correlative Studies in Infancy*, edited by P. Kellaway, and I. Petersen, pp. 349–360. Grune & Stratton, New York.
393. Maurer, D., and Salapatek, P. (1976): Developmental changes in the scanning of faces by young infants. *Child Dev.*, 47:523–527.
394. Maurer, R. G., and Damasio, A. R. (1979): Vestibular dysfunction in autistic children. *Dev. Med. Child Neurol.*, 21:656–659.
395. McCall, R. B. (1970): Intelligence quotient pattern over age: Comparisons among siblings and parent-child pairs. *Science*, 170:644–648.
396. McCall, R. B. (1977): Childhood IQ's as predictors of adult educational and occupational status. *Science*, 197:482–483.
397. McCarley, R. W. (1980): Mechanisms and models of behavioral state control. In: *The Reticular Formation Revisited*, edited by J. A. Hobson, and M. A. B. Brazier, pp. 375–403. Raven Press, New York.
398. McCarthy, D. (1972): *McCarthy Scales of Children's Abilities*. Psychological Corporation, New York.
398a. McCleary, R. A., and Moore, R. Y. (1965): *Subcortical Mechanisms of Behavior: The Psychological Functions of Primitive Parts of the Brain*, Basic Books, New York.
399. McCloskey, D. I. (1978): Kinesthetic sensibility. *Physiol. Rev.*, 58:763–820.
400. McKusick, V. A. (1978): *Mendelian Inheritance in Man. Catalogs of Autosomal Dominant, Autosomal Recessive, and X-linked Phenotypes, 5th Ed*. The Johns Hopkins University Press, Baltimore.
401. McKusick, V. A., and Ruddle, F. H. (1977): The status of the gene map of the human chromosomes. *Science*, 196:390–405.
402. McLaughlin, J. F., and Kriegsmann, E. (1980): Developmental dyspraxia in a family with X-linked mental retardation (Rennpenning syndrome). *Dev. Med. Child Neurol.*, 22:84–92.
403. McNamara, J. O., Byrne, M. C., Dasheiff, R. M., and Fitz, J. G. (1980): The kindling model of epilepsy: A review. *Prog. Neurobiol.*, 15:139–159.
404. Meadows, J. C. (1974): The anatomical basis of prosopagnosia. *J. Neurol. Neurosurg. Psychiatry*, 37:489–501.
405. Meadows, J. C. (1974): Disturbed perception of colors associated with localized cerebral lesions. *Brain*, 97:615–632.
406. Meehl, P. E. (1954): *Clinical Versus Statistical Prediction: A Theoretical Analysis and a Review of the Evidence*. University of Minnesota Press, Minneapolis.
407. Mehegan, C. C., and Dreifuss, F. E. (1972): Hyperlexia: Exceptional reading ability in brain-damaged children. *Neurology*, 22:1105–1111.
408. Meichenbaum, D., and Goodman, S. (1977): The nature and modification of impulsivity. In: *Topics in Child Neurology*, edited by M. E. Blaw, I. Rapin, and M. Kinsbourne, pp. 263–278. Spectrum, New York.
409. Meldrum, B. (1978): Physiological changes during prolonged seizures and epileptic brain damage. *Neuropaediatrie*, 9:203–212.
410. Melzack, R., and Wall, P. D. (1965): Pain mechanisms: A new theory. *Science*, 150:971–979.
411. Menyuk, P. (1969): *Sentences Children Use*. MIT Press, Cambridge, Mass.
412. Metrakos, K., and Metrakos, J. D. (1961): Genetics of convulsive disorders. II. Genetic and electroencephalographic studies in centrencephalic epilepsy. *Neurology*, 11:474–483.
413. Metrakos, K., and Metrakos, J. D. (1974): Genetics of epilepsy. In: *Handbook of Clinical Neurology, Vol. 15: The Epilepsies*, edited by P. J. Vinken, and G. W. Bruyn, pp. 429–439. North Holland, Amsterdam.
414. Miceli, G., and Gainotti, G. (1979): Selective impairment of perception of articulatory place in a case of cortical auditory disorder. *Exp. Brain Res., (Suppl. 2)* 2:358–364.
415. Miles, T. R. (1974): *The Dyslexic Child*. Priory Press, London.
416. Miller, G. A. (1956): The magical number seven, plus or minus two: Some limits on our capacity for processing information. *Psychol. Rev.*, 63:81–97.

417. Milner, B. (1970): Memory and the medial temporal regions of the brain. In: *Biology of Memory*, edited by K. H. Pribram, and D. E. Broadbent, pp. 29–50. Academic Press, New York.

418. Milner, B. (1974): Hemispheric specialization: Scope and limits. In: *The Neurosciences, Third Study Program*, edited by F. O. Schmitt, and F. G. Worden, pp. 75–89. MIT Press, Cambridge, Mass.

419. Milner, B., Corkin, S., and Teuber, H.-L. (1968): Further analysis of hippocampal amnesic syndrome: Fourteen year follow-up study. *Neuropsychologia*, 6:215–234.

420. Minde, K. (1977): Hyperactivity: Where do we stand? In: *Topics in Child Neurology*, edited by M. E. Blaw, I. Rapin, and M. Kinsbourne, pp. 279–287. Spectrum, New York.

421. *Minimal Brain Dysfunction in Children: Educational, Medical and Health Related Services*. Public Health Service Publication No. 2015. U.S. Department of Health, Education, and Welfare, Washington, D.C.

422. Mitchell, D. E., Freeman, R. D., Millodot, M., and Haegerstrom, G. (1973): Meridional amblyopia: Evidence for modification of human visual system by early visual experience. *Vision Res.*, 13:535–558.

423. Moe, P. G. (1971): Spike-wave stupor. Petit mal stupor. *Am. J. Dis. Child.*, 121:307–313.

424. Mohr, J. P., Pessin, M. S., Finkelstein, S., Funkenstein, H. H., Duncan, G. W., and Davis, K. R. (1978): Broca's aphasia: Pathologic and clinical. *Neurology*, 28:311–324.

425. Moore, R. Y. (1974): Visual pathways and the central neural control of diurnal rhythms. In: *The Neurosciences, Third Study Program*, edited by F. O. Schmitt, and F. G. Worden, pp. 537–542. MIT Press, Cambridge, Mass.

426. Mori, S., Nishimura, H., and Aoki, M. (1980): Brain stem activation of the spinal stepping generator. In: *The Reticular Formation Revisited*, edited by J. A. Hobson, and M. A. B. Brazier, pp. 241–259. Raven Press, New York.

427. Morrell, F. (1960): Secondary epileptogenic lesions. *Epilepsia*, 1:538–560.

428. Morrell, F. (1961): Electrophysiological contributions to the neural basis of learning. *Psychol. Rev.*, 41:443–494.

429. Morse, P. A. (1976): Speech perception in the human infant and rhesus monkey. *Ann. N.Y. Acad. Sci.*, 280:694–707.

430. Moskowitz, B. A. (1978): The acquisition of language. *Sci. Am.*, 239, No. 5:92–108.

431. Mountcastle, V. B., editor (1962): *Interhemispheric Relations and Cerebral Dominance*. The Johns Hopkins Press, Baltimore.

432. Mountcastle, V. B. (1979): An organizing principle for cerebral function: The unit module and the distributed system. In: *The Neurosciences, Fourth Study Program*, edited by F. O. Schmitt, and F. G. Worden, pp. 21–42. MIT Press, Cambridge, Mass.

433. Mountcastle, V. B., Lynch, J. C., Georgopoulos, A., Sakata, H., and Acuna, A. (1975): Posterior parietal association cortex of the monkey: Command functions for the operations within extrapersonal space. *J. Neurophysiol.*, 38:871–908.

434. Murphy, E. A. (1975): Clinical genetics: Some neglected facets. *N. Engl. J. Med.*, 292:458–462.

435. Naidu, S., and Narasimhachari, N. (1980): Syndenham's chorea: A possible presynaptic dopaminergic dysfunction initially. *Ann. Neurol.*, 8:445–446.

436. Naidu, S., Wolfson, L. I., and Sharpless, N. S. (1978): Juvenile parkinsonism: A patient with possible primary striatal dysfunction. *Ann. Neurol.*, 3:453–455.

437. Narabayashi, H. (1977): Stereotaxic amygdalotomy for epileptic hyperactivity-Long range results. In: *Topics in Child Neurology*, edited by M. Blaw, I. Rapin, and M. Kinsbourne, pp. 319–331. Spectrum Publication, New York.

438. Naunton, R. F., and Fernandez, C., editors (1978): *Evoked Electrical Activity in the Auditory Nervous System*. Academic Press, New York.

439. Nauta, W. J. H. (1971): The problem of the frontal lobe: A reinterpretation. *J. Psychiatry Res.*, 8:167–187.

440. Needleman, H. L., Gunnoe, C., Leviton, A., Reed, R., Peresie, H., Maher, C., and Barrett, P. (1979): Deficits in psychologic and classroom performance of children with elevated dentine lead levels. *N. Engl. J. Med.*, 300:689–695.

441. Nelson, K. B., and Ellenberg, J. H. (1976): Predictors of epilepsy in children who have experienced febrile seizures. *N. Engl. J. Med.*, 295:1029–1033.

442. Nelson, K. B., and Ellenberg, J. H. (1981): Apgar scores as predictors of chronic neurologic disability. *Pediatrics*, 68:36–44.

443. Nichols, P. L., and Chen, T.-C. (1981): *Minimal Brain Dysfunction: A Prospective Study*. Laurence Erlbaum Assoc., Hillsdale, N.J.

443a. Noback, C. R., and Demarest, R. J. (1981): *The Human Nervous System (Third Edition)*. McGraw Hill, New York.

444. O'Brien, J. L., Goldensohn, E. S., and Hoefer, P. (1959): Electroencephalographic abnormalities in addition to bilaterally synchronous 3/sec spike and wave activity in petit mal. *Electroencephalogr. Clin. Neurophysiol.*, 13:747–761.

445. O'Donohoe, N. V. (1979): *Epilepsies of Childhood*. Butterworth, London.

446. Öhman, A., and Lader, M. (1977): Short-term changes of the human auditory evoked potentials during repetitive stimulation. In: *Auditory Evoked Potentials in Man: Psychopharmacology Correlates of EPs, Prog. Clin. Neurophysiol. Vol. 2*, edited by J. E. Desmedt, pp. 93–118. Karger, Basel.

447. Ojemann, G. A. (1977): Asymmetric function of the thalamus in man. *Ann. N.Y. Acad. Sci.*, 299:380–396.

448. Ojemann, G., and Mateer, C. (1979): Human language cortex: Localization of memory, syntax, and sequential motor-phoneme identification systems. *Science*, 205:1401–1403.

449. Ojemann, G. A., and Whitaker, H. A. (1978): The bilingual brain. *Arch. Neurol.*, 35:409–412.

450. Olds, J. (1977): *Drives and Reinforcements: Behavioral Studies of Hypothalamic Functions*. Raven Press, New York.

451. Orgogozo, J. M., and Larsen, B. (1979): Activation of the supplementary motor area during voluntary movement in man suggests it works as a supramotor area. *Science*, 206:847–850.

452. Orton, S. T. (1937): *Reading, Writing, and Speech Problems in Children*. Chapman and Hall, London.

453. Paine, R. S. (1962): Minimal chronic brain syndromes in children. *Dev. Med. Child Neurol.*, 4:21–27.

454. Palfrey, J. S., Mervis, R. C., and Butler, J. A. (1978): New directions in the evaluation and education of handicapped children. *N. Engl. J. Med.*, 298:819–824.

455. Pappas, G. D., and Purpura, D. P., editors (1972): *The Structure and Function of Synapses*. Raven Press, New York.

456. Pasik, T., and Pasik, P. (1971): The visual world of monkeys deprived of striate cortex: Effective stimulus parameters and the importance of the accessory optic system. *Vision Res. (Suppl.)*3:419–435.

457. Pearlman, A. L., Birch, J., and Meadows, J. C. (1979): Cerebral color blindness: An acquired defect in hue discrimination. *Neurology*, 29:253–261.

458. Peiper, A. (1963): *Cerebral Function in Infancy and Childhood*. Consultants Bureau, New York.

459. Penfield, W., and Jasper, H. (1954): *Epilepsy and the Functional Anatomy of the Human Brain*. Little, Brown, Boston.

459a. Penfield, W., and Rasmussen, T. (1952): *The Cerebral Cortex of Man. A Clinical Study of Localization of Function*. Macmillan, New York.

460. Penfield, W., and Roberts, L. (1959): *Speech and Brain Mechanisms*. Princeton University Press, Princeton, N.J.

461. Penry, J. K., and Newmark, M. E. (1979): The use of antiepileptic drugs. *Ann. Intern. Med.*, 90:207–218.

462. Penry, J. K., Porter, R. J., and Dreifuss, F. E. (1975): Simultaneous recording of absence seizures with videotape and electroencephalography-A study of 374 seizures in 48 patients. *Brain*, 98:427–440.

463. Perret, C. (1976): Neural control of locomotion in the decorticate cat. In: *Neural Control of Locomotion*, edited by R. M. Herman, S. Grillner, P. S. G. Stein, and D. G. Stuart, pp. 587–615. Plenum Press, New York.

464. Peters, J. E., Romine, J. S., and Dyckman, R. A. (1975): A special neurological examination of children with learning disabilities. *Dev. Med. Child Neurol.*, 17:63–78.

465. Phelps, M. E., Hoffman, E. J., Sung-Cheng, H., and Kuhl, D. E. (1978): ECAT: A new computerized tomographic imaging system for positron-emitting radiopharmaceuticals. *J. Nucl. Med.*, 19:635–647.

466. Phillips, C. G., and Porter, R. (1977): *Corticospinal Neurons: Their Role in Movement*. Academic Press, New York.

467. Piaget, J. (1926): *The Language and Thought of the Child*. Harcourt Brace, New York.

468. Piaget, J. (1972): *The Psychology of Intelligence*. Littlefield Adams & Co., Totowa, N.J.

468a. Picton, T. W., Woods, D. L., Baribeau-Braun, J., and Healey, T. M. G. (1977): Evoked potential audiometry. *J. Otolaryngol.* 6:90–119.

469. Piercy, M., Hécaen, H., and Ajuriaguerra, J. de (1960): Constructional apraxia associated with unilateral cerebral lesions. Left and right-sided cases compared. *Brain*, 83:225–242.

470. Pincus, J. H. (1980): Can violence be a manifestation of epilepsy? *Neurology*, 30:304–307.

471. Pinel, J. P. J., and Van Oot, P. H. (1975): Generality of the kindling phenomenon: Some clinical implications. *Can. J. Neurol. Sci.*, 2:467–475.

472. Pitlyk, P. J., Miller, R. H., and Johnson, G. M. (1965): Diencephalic syndrome of infancy presenting with anorexia and emaciation: Report of a case. *Mayo Clin. Proc.*, 40:327–333.

473. Plum, F., and Posner, J. B. (1980): *The Diagnosis of Stupor and Coma, 3rd Ed.* F.A. Davis, Philadelphia.

474. Prange, A. J., Jr., Nemeroff, C. B., and Lipton, M. A. (1978): Behavioral effects of peptides: Basic and clinical studies. In: *Psychopharmacology: A Generation of Progress*, edited by M. A. Lipton, A. DiMascio, and K. F. Killam, pp. 441–458. Raven Press, New York.

475. Prechtl, H. F. R., and Stemmer, C. J. (1962): The choreiform syndrome in children. *Dev. Med. Child Neurol.*, 4:119–127.

476. Prescott, J. W., Read, M. S., and Coursin, D., editors (1975): *Brain Function and Malnutrition-Neuropsychological Methods of Assessment*. John Wiley, New York.

477. Pribram, K. H. (1971): *Languages of the Brain: Experimental Paradoxes and Principles in Neuropsychology*. Prentice Hall, Englewood Cliffs, N.J.

478. Pribram, K. H. (1974): How is it that sensing so much we can do so little? In: *The Neurosciences, Third Study Program*, edited by F. O. Schmitt, and F. G. Worden, pp. 249–261. MIT Press, Cambridge, Mass.

479. Pribram, K. H., and Broadbent, D. E., editors (1970): *Biology of Memory*. Academic Press, New York.

480. Pribram, K. H., and Luria, A. R., editors (1973): *Psychophysiology of the Frontal Lobes*. Academic Press, New York.

481. Pritchard, P. B., III, Lombroso, C. T., and McIntyre, M. (1980): Psychological complications of temporal lobe epilepsy. *Neurology*, 30:227–232.

482. Purpura, D. P. (1979): Pathobiology of cortical neurons in metabolic and unclassified amentias. In: *Res. Publ. Assoc. Res. Nerv. Ment. Dis. Vol. 57: Congenital and Acquired Cognitive Disorders* edited by R. Katzman, pp. 43–68. Raven Press, New York.

483. Pyles, M. K., Stolz, H. R., and MacFarlane, J. W. (1935): The accuracy of mother's report on birth and developmental data. *Child Dev.*, 6:165–176.

483a. Rakic, P. (1982): Geniculo-cortical connections in primates: Normal and experimentally altered development. *Prog. In Brain Res. (In press)*.

483b. Ramón y Cajal, S. (1902): *Studien über die Hirnrinde des Menschen 3. Heft: Die Hörrinde*. Barth, Leipzig.

483c. Ramón y Cajal, S. (1909): *Histologie du Système Nerveux de l'Homme et des Vertébrés*. A. Maloine, Paris.

484. Rapin, I. (1974): Hypoactive labyrinths and motor development. *Clin. Pediatr.*, 13:922–937.

485. Rapin, I. (1976): Progressive genetic-metabolic diseases of the central nervous system in children. *Pediatr. Ann.*, 5:313–349.

486. Rapin, I. (1977): Progressive genetic metabolic diseases of the central nervous system. In: *Pediatrics, 16th Ed.*, edited by A. M. Rudolph, pp. 1892–1939. Appleton-Century-Crofts, New York.

487. Rapin, I. (1979): Effects of early blindness and deafness on cognition. In: *Res. Publ. Assoc. Res. Nerv. Ment. Dis., Congenital and Acquired Cognitive Disorders*, edited by R. Katzman, Vol. 57:189–245. Raven Press, New York.

488. Rapin, I. (1982): Developmental language disorders and brain dysfunction as precursors of reading disability. In: *Topics in Child Neurology, Vol. 2.*, edited by G. A. Wise, M. E. Blaw, and P. G. Procopis. Spectrum Publications, New York. *(in press)*.

489. Rapin, I., and Allen, D. A. (1982): Developmental language disorders: Nosologic considerations. In: *Neuropsychology of Language, Reading and Spelling*, edited by U. Kirk. Academic Press, New York. *(in press)*.

490. Rapin, I., Allen, D. A. (1982): Progress toward a nosology of developmental dysphasia *(in press)*.

491. Rapin, I., Allen, D. A., and Mattis, S.: The semantic-pragmatic syndrome in two brothers *(in preparation)*.

492. Rapin, I., Mattis, S., Rowan, A. J., and Golden, G. G. (1977): Verbal auditory agnosia in children. *Dev. Med. Child Neurol.*, 19:192–207.

493. Rapin, I., Tourk, L. M., and Costa, L. D. (1966): Evaluation of the Purdue pegboard as a screening test for brain damage. *Dev. Med. Child Neurol.*, 8:45–54.

494. Rapin, I., and Wilson, B. C. (1978): Children with developmental language disability: Neurologic aspects and assessment. In: *Developmental Dysphasia*, edited by M. A. Wyke, pp. 13–41. Academic Press, London.

495. Rapoport, J. L., Buchsbaum, M. S., Zahn, T. P., Weingartner, H., Ludlow, C., and Mikkelsen, E. J. (1978): Dextroamphetamine: Cognitive and behavioral effects in normal prepubertal boys. *Science*, 199:560–563.

496. Rasmussen, T., and Milner, B. (1977): The role of early left-brain injury in determining lateralization of cerebral speech functions. *Ann. N.Y. Acad. Sci.*, 299:355–369.

497. Raven, J. C. (1956): *The Coloured Progressive Matrices*. Psychological Corporation, New York.

498. Raven, J. C. (1958): *Raven's Progressive Matrices*. Dunfries, Scotland: Crichton, Royal.

499. Ravizza, R. J., and Belmore, S. M. (1978): Auditory forebrain: Evidence from anatomical and behavioral experiments involving human and animal subjects. In: *Handbook of Behavioral Neurobiology, Vol. 1: Sensory Integration*, edited by R. B. Masterton, pp. 459–501. Plenum Press, New York.

500. Reichlin, S., Baldessarini, R. J., and Martin, J. B., editors (1978): *The Hypothalamus. Res. Publ. Assoc. Res. Nerv. Ment. Dis.*, vol 56. Raven Press, New York.

501. Reitan, R. M. (1964): *Manual for Administering and Scoring the Reitan-Indiana Neuropsychology Battery for Children (Aged 5 through 8)*. University of Indiana Medical Center, Indianapolis.

502. Reynell, J. (1977): *The Reynell Developmental Language Scales, Rev. Ed.* N.F.E.R. Publishing Co., Windsor, England.

503. Robinson, B. W. (1976): Limbic influences on human speech. *Ann. N.Y. Acad. Sci.*, 280:761–771.

504. Roscuzway, M. R., and Bennett, E. L., editors (1976): *Neuronal Mechanisms of Learning and Memory*. MIT Press, Cambridge, Mass.

505. Rose, F. C., and Symonds, C. P. (1960): Persistent memory defect following encephalitis. *Brain*, 83:195–212.

506. Rose, R. J., Harris, E. L., Christian, J. C., and Nance, W. E. (1979): Genetic variance in nonverbal intelligence: Data from the kinships of identical twins. *Science*, 205:1153–1155.

507. Rosen, J. A., and Barsoum, A. H. (1979): Failure of chronic dorsal column stimulation in multiple sclerosis. *Ann. Neurol.*, 6:66–67.

508. Rosenberg, P. E. (1966): Misdiagnosis of children with auditory problems. *J. Speech Hear. Disord.*, 31:279–283.

509. Rosenthal, J. H. (1977): *The Neuropsychopathology of Written Language*. Nelson-Hall, Chicago.

510. Rosenzweig, M. R., and Bennett, E. L., editors (1976): *Neural Mechanisms of Learning and Memory*. MIT Press, Cambridge, Mass.

511. Rosman, N. P., and Pearce, J. (1967): The brain in multiple neurofibromatosis (von Recklinghausen's disease): A suggested neuropathological basis for the associated mental defect. *Brain*, 90:829–838.

512. Ross, E. D. (1980): Sensory-specific and fractional disorders of recent memory in man. I. Isolated loss of visual recent memory. *Arch. Neurol.*, 37:193–200.

513. Ross, E. D., and Mesulam, M.-M. (1979): Dominant language functions of the right hemisphere? Prosody and emotional gesturing. *Arch. Neurol.*, 36:144–148.

514. Ross, M., Berger, P. A., and Goldstein, A. (1979): Plasma β-endorphin immunoreactivity in schizophrenia. *Science*, 205:1163–1164.

515. Roswell, F. G., and Natchez, G., editors (1977): *Reading Disability, 3rd Ed.*, Basic Books, New York.

516. Routtenberg, A. (1978): The reward system of the brain. *Sci. Am.*, 239, No. 5:154–164.

517. Ruben, R. J., Elberling, C., and Salomon, G., editors (1976): *Electrocochleography*. University Park Press, Baltimore.

518. Ruben, R. J., and Rapin, I.: Theoretical issues in the development of audition. In: *Developmental Disabilities in the Preschool Child*, edited by M. Lewis, and L. T. Taft. *(in press)*.

519. Rubens, A. B. (1979): Agnosia. In: *Clinical Neuropsychology*, edited by K. M. Heilman, and E. Valenstein, pp. 233–267. Oxford University Press, New York.

520. Ruff, R. L., and Arbit, E. (1981): Aphemia resulting from a left frontal hematoma. *Neurology*, 31:353–356.

521. Russell, I. S., and Ochs, S. (1963): Localization of a memory trace in one cortical hemisphere and transfer to the other hemisphere. *Brain*, 86:37–54.

522. Rutter, M. (1979): Language, cognition, and autism. In: *Res. Publ. Assoc. Res. Nerv. Ment. Dis., Vol. 57: Congenital and Acquired Cognitive Disorders*, edited by R. Katzman, pp. 247–264. Raven Press, New York.

523. Safer, D. J., and Allen, R. P. (1973): Factors influencing the suppressant effects of two stimulating drugs on the growth of hyperactive children. *Pediatrics*, 51:660–667.

524. Safer, D. J., and Allen, R. P. (1976): *Hyperactive Children: Diagnosis and Management*. University Park Press, Baltimore.

525. Samuels, I. (1959): Reticular mechanisms and behavior. *Psychol. Bull.*, 56:1–25.

526. Schaeffer, B. (1978): Teaching spontaneous sign language to nonverbal children: Theory and method. *Sign Language Studies*, 21:317–352.

527. Schain, R. J., Ward, J. W., and Guthrie, D. (1977): Carbamazepine as an anticonvulsant in children. *Neurology*, 27:476–480.

528. Scheibel, M. E., and Scheibel, A. B. (1967): Anatomical basis of attention mechanisms in vertebrates. In: *The Neurosciences, A Study Program*, edited by G. C. Quarton, T. Melnechuk. and F. O. Schmitt, pp. 577–602. Rockefeller University Press, New York.

529. Schif, M., Duyme, M., Dumaret, A., Stewart, J., Tomkiewicz, S., and Feingold, J. (1978): Intellectual status of working-class children adopted early into upper-middle-class families. *Science*, 200:1503–1504.

530. Schildkraut, J. J. (1978): Current status of the catecholamine hypothesis of affective disorders. In: *Psychopharmacology: A Generation of Progress*, edited by M. A. Lipton, A. DiMascio, and K. F. Killam, pp. 1223–1234. Raven Press, New York.

531. Scoville, W. B., and Milner, B. (1957): Loss of recent memory after bilateral hippocampal lesions. *J. Neurol. Neurosurg. Psychiatry*, 20:11–21.

532. Sem-Jacobsen, C. W., and Torkildsen, A. (1960): Depth recording and electrical stimulation in the human brain. In: *Electrical Studies on the Unanesthetized Brain: A Symposium*, edited by E. R. Ramey, and D. S. O'Doherty, pp. 275–290. Paul B. Hoeber, New York.

533. Semmes, J., Weinstein, S., Ghent, L., and Teuber, H.-L. (1960): *Somatosensory Changes after Penetrating Brain Wounds in Man*. Harvard University Press, Cambridge, Mass.

534. *Sex Hormones and Behavior*. (1979): CIBA Foundation Symposium No. 62. (new series). Excerpta Medica, Amsterdam.

535. Shapiro, A. K., Shapiro, E. S., Bruun, R. D., and Sweet, R. D. (1978): *Gilles de la Tourette Syndrome*. Raven Press, New York.

536. Shaywitz, D. A., Yager, R. D., and Klapper, J. H. (1976): Selective brain dopamine depletion in developing rats: An experimental model of minimal brain dysfunction. *Science*, 191:305–308.

537. Shebilske, W. L. (1976): Extraretinal information in corrective saccades and inflow versus outflow theories of visual direction constancy. *Vision Res.*, 16:621–628.

538. Sher, P. K., and Brown, S. B. (1975): A longitudinal study of head growth in pre-term infants. II. Differentiation between "catch-up" head growth and early infantile hydrocephalus. *Dev. Med. Child Neurol.*, 17:711–718.

539. Shik, M. L., and Orlovsky, G. N. (1976): Neurophysiology of locomotor automatism. *Physiol. Rev.*, 56:465–501.

540. Shlaer, R. (1971): Shift in binocular disparity causes compensatory changes in the cortical structure of kittens. *Science*, 173:638–643.

541. Shoulson, I. (1979): Huntington's disease: Overview of experimental therapeutics. In: *Advances in Neurology*, 23:751–757. Raven Press, New York.

542. Silver, L. B. (1979): The minimal brain dysfunction syndrome. In: *Basic Handbook of Child Psychiatry, Vol. 2: Disturbance of Development*, edited by J. D. Noshpitz, pp. 416–439. Basic Books, New York.

543. Simson, R., Vaughan, H. G., Jr., and Ritter, W. (1976): The scalp topography of potentials associated with missing visual or auditory stimuli. *Electroencephalogr. Clin. Neurophysiol.*, 40:33–42.

544. Skoff, B. F., Mirsky, A. F., and Turner, D. (1980): Prolonged brain stem transmission time in autism. *Psychiatry Res.*, 2:157–166.

545. Smith, D. W. (1976): *Recognizable Patterns of Human Malformations: Genetic, Embryologic, and Clinical Aspects, 2nd Ed.* W.B. Saunders, Philadelphia.

546. Smith, I. L., Walth, T. H., and Shiply, T. (1966): Cortical blindness in congenital hydrocephalus. *Am. J. Ophthalmol.* 62:251–257.

546a. Smith, S. D., Pennington, B. F., Kimberling, W. J., and Lubs, H. A. (1979): Investigation of subgroups within specific reading disability utilizing neuropsychological and linkage analysis. *Am. J. Human Genet.*, 31:83A.

547. Snead, O. C., III, and Bearden, L. J. (1980): Anticonvulsants specific for petit mal antagonize epileptogenic effect of leucine enkephalin. *Science*, 210:1031–1033.
548. Snow, J. B., Jr., Rintelmann, W. F., Miller, J. M., and Konkle, D. F. (1977): Central auditory imperception. *Laryngoscope*, 87:1451–1471.
549. Snyder, S. H. (1974): Catecholamines as mediators of drug effects in schizophrenia. In: *The Neurosciences, Third Study Program*, edited by F. O. Schmitt, and F. G. Worden, pp. 721–732. MIT Press, Cambridge, Mass.
550. Snyder, S. H. (1979): Receptors, neurotransmitters, and drug responses. *N. Engl. J. Med.*, 300:465–472.
551. Snyder, S. H. (1980): Brain peptides as neurotransmitters. *Science*, 209:976–983.
552. Snyder, S. H., and Meyerhoff, J. L. (1973): How amphetamine acts in minimal brain dysfunction. *Ann. N.Y. Acad. Sci.*, 205:310–320.
553. Spain, B. (1974): Verbal and performance ability of pre-school children with spina bifida. *Dev. Med. Child Neurol.*, 16:773–783.
554. Sperry, R. W. (1974): Lateral specialization in the surgically separated hemispheres. In: *The Neurosciences, Third Study Program*, edited by F. O. Schmitt, and F. G. Worden, pp. 5–19. MIT Press, Cambridge, Mass.
555. Sperry, R. W., Stamm, J. S., and Miner, N. (1956): Relearning tests for interocular transfer following division of optic chiasma and corpus callosum in cats. *J. Comp. Physiol. Psychol.*, 49:529–533.
556. Spreen, O., and Benton, A. L. (1977): *Neurosensory Center Comprehensive Examination for Aphasia (1977 Revision)*. Neuropsychology Laboratory, Department of Psychology, University of Victoria, Victoria, B.C.
557. Sroufe, L. A., and Stewart, M. A. (1973): Treating problem children with stimulant drugs. *N. Engl. J. Med.*, 289:407–413.
558. Stein, D. G., Rosen, J. J., and Butters, N., editors (1974): *Plasticity and Recovery of Function in the Central Nervous System*. Academic Press, New York.
559. Stein, L. (1978): Reward transmitters: Catecholamines and opioid peptides. In: *Psychopharmacology: A Generation of Progress*, edited by M. A. Lipton, A. DiMascio, and K. F. Killam, pp. 569–581. Raven Press, New York.
560. Stein, Z. A., Susser, M., Saenger, G., and Marolla, F. (1975): *Famine and Human Development: The Dutch Hunger Winter of 1944/45*, Oxford University Press, New York.
561. Stelmach, G. E., editor (1978): *Information Processing in Motor Control and Learning*. Academic Press, New York.
562. Steriade, M., Ropert, N., Kitsikis, A., and Oakson, G. (1980): Ascending activating neuronal networks in midbrain reticular core and related rostral systems. In: *The Reticular Formation Revisited*, edited by J. A. Hobson, and M. A. B. Brazier, pp. 125–167. Raven Press, New York.
563. Stevens, J. R., and Hermann, B. P. (1981): Temporal lobe epilepsy, psychopathology, and violence: The state of the evidence. *Neurology*, 31:1127–1132.
564. Strauss, A. A., and Kephart, N. C. (1955): *Psychopathology and Education of the Brain-Injured Child, Vol. 2: Progress in Theory and Clinic*. Grune and Stratton, New York.
565. Strauss, A. A., and Lehtinen, L. E. (1947): *Psychopathology and Education of the Brain-Injured Child*. Grune & Stratton, New York.
566. Streissguth, A. P., Landesman-Dwyer, S., Martin, J. C., and Smith, D. W. (1980): Teratogenic effects of alcohol in humans and laboratory animals. *Science*, 209:353–361.
567. Student, M., and Sohmer, H. (1978): Evidence from auditory nerve and brain stem evoked responses for an organic brain lesion in children with autistic traits. *J. Autism Child. Schizophr.*, 8:13–20.
568. Swanson, J. M., and Kinsbourne, M. (1980): Food dyes impair performance of hyperactive children on a laboratory learning test. *Science*, 207:1485–1487.
569. Swisher, L. P., and Pinsker, E. J. (1971): The language characteristics of hyperverbal hydrocephalic children. *Dev. Med. Child Neurol.*, 13:746–755.
570. *Symposium on Functions of the Septo-Hippocampal System, London, 1977* (1978): (CIBA Foundation Symposium No. 58-new series) Elsevier, New York.
571. Taft, L. T., and Cohen, H. J. (1971): Hypsarrythmia and infantile autism: A clinical report. *J. Autism Child. Schizophr.*, 1:327–336.
572. Tallal, P., and Piercy, M. (1978): Defects of auditory perception in children with developmental dysphasia. In: *Developmental Dysphasia*, edited by M. Wyke, pp. 63–84. Academic Press, London.

573. Tallman, J. F., Paul, S. M., Skolnick, P., and Gallagher, D. W. (1980): Receptors for the age of anxiety: Pharmacology of the benzodiazepines. *Science*, 207:274–281.

574. Tecce, J. J., and Cole, J. O. (1974): Amphetamine effects in man: Paradoxical drowsiness and lowered electrical brain activity (CNV). *Science*, 185:451–453.

575. Technical recommendations for psychological tests and diagnostic techniques (1954): *Psychol. Bull.*, 51 (suppl):201–238.

576. Terman, L. M., and Merrill, M. A. (1960): *Stanford-Binet Intelligence Scale (Third Revision)*. Houghton Mifflin, Boston.

577. Teuber, H.-L. (1978): The brain and human behavior. In: *Perception. Handbook of Sensory Physiology, Vol. 8*, edited by R. Held, H. W. Leibowitz, and H.-L. Teuber, pp. 877–920. Springer-Verlag, Berlin.

578. Teuber, H.-L., Battersby, W. S., and Bender, M. B. (1960): *Visual Field Defects after Penetrating Missile Wounds of the Brain*. Harvard University Press, Cambridge, Mass.

579. Thal, L. J., Sharpless, N. S., Wolfson, L., and Katzman, R. (1980): Treatment of myoclonus with *L*-5-hydroxytryptophan and carbidopa: Clinical, electrophysiological, and biochemical observations. *Ann. Neurol.*, 7:570–576.

580. *The Brain*. (1979): Sci. Am., 241:No. 3: pp. 45–232.

581. *The Hyperkinesis Index. A Physician's Aid to Progress Evaluation in MBD*. (1975): Abbott Laboratories Pharmaceutical Products Division, North Chicago, Ill.

582. Thomas, A., Chess, S., and Birch, H. G. (1968): *Temperament and Behavior Disorders in Children*. New York University Press, New York.

583. Thompson, R. (1981): Rapid forgetting of a spatial habit in rats with hippocampal lesions. *Science*, 212:959–960.

584. Thomson, G. (1951): *The Factorial Analysis of Human Ability, 5th Ed*. Houghton Mifflin, Boston.

585. Tibbles, J. A. R. (1980): Dominant benign neonatal seizures. *Dev. Med. Child Neurol.*, 22:664–667.

586. Tizard, J. (1958): Longitudinal and follow-up studies. In: *Mental Deficiency: The Changing Outlook*, edited by A. M. Clarke, and A. D. B. Clarke, pp. 422–449. The Free Press, Glencoe, Ill.

587. Touwen, B. C. L. (1980): *Examination of the Child with Minor Neurological Dysfunction, 2nd Ed.*, In: *Clin. Dev. Med. No. 71*, pp. 1–141. J.B. Lippincott, Philadelphia.

588. Trevarthen, C. (1974): Cerebral embryology and the split brain. In: *Hemispheric Disconnection and Cerebral Function*, edited by M. Kinsbourne, and W. L. Smith, pp. 208–236. Charles C. Thomas, Springfield, Ill.

589. Turner, G. (1975): An aetiological study of 1,000 patients with an IQ assessment below 51. *Med. J. Aust.*, 2:927–931.

590. Turner, G., Brookwell, R., Daniel, A., Selikowitz, M., and Zilibowitz, M. (1980): Heterozygous expression of X-linked mental retardation and X-chromosome marker fra (X) (q27). *N. Engl. J. Med.*, 303:662–664.

591. Usdin, E., Hamburg, D. A., and Barchas, J. D., editors (1977): *Neuroregulators and Psychiatric Disorders*. Oxford University Press, New York.

592. Valenstein, E. S. (1977): The practice of psychosurgery: A survey of the literature (1971–1976), Chapter 9: Ethical Issues. In: *Appendix: Psychosurgery. The National Commission for the Protection of Human Subjects in Biomedical and Behavioral Research*, pp. I-87–I-94, United States Department of Health Education and Welfare, DHEW Publication No. (OS)77-0002, U.S. Government Printing Office, Washington, D.C.

593. Valenstein, E., and Heilman, K. M. (1979): Emotional disorders resulting from lesions of the central nervous system. In: *Clinical Neuropsychology*, edited by K. M. Heilman, and E. Valenstein, pp. 413–438. Oxford University Press, New York.

594. Valett, R. E. (1980): *Dyslexia: A Neuropsychological Approach to Educating Children with Severe Reading Disorders*. Fearon Pitman Publishers, Belmont, Ca.

595. Valverde, F. (1967): Apical dendritic spines of the visual cortex and light deprivation in the mouse. *Exp. Brain Res.*, 3:337–352.

596. Van Buren, J. M. (1958): Some autonomic concomitants of ictal automatism. A study of temporal lobe attacks. *Brain*, 81:505–528.

597. van Praag, H. M., and Bruinvels, J., editors (1977): *Neurotransmission and Disturbed Behavior*. Bohn, Scheltema and Holkema, Utrecht.

598. Vaughan, H. G., Jr., and Ritter, W. (1973): Physiologic approaches to the analysis of attention and performance. In: *Attention and Performance IV*, edited by S. Kornblum, pp. 129–154. Academic Press, New York.

599. Vierck, C. (1978): Somatosensory system. In: *Handbook of Behavioral Neurobiology, Vol. 1: Sensory Integration*, edited by R. B. Masterton, pp. 249–309. Plenum Press, New York.

600. Volpe, J. J. (1977): Neonatal intracranial hemorrhage: Pathophysiology, neuropathology and clinical features. *Clin. Perinatol.*, 4:77–102.

601. Volpe, J. J., and Pasternak, J. F. (1977): Parasagittal cerebral injury in neonatal hypoxic-ischemic encephalopathy: Clinical and neuroradiologic features. *J. Pediatr.*, 91:472–476.

602. Wada, J. A., Clarke, R., and Hamm, A. (1975): Cerebral hemispheric asymmetry in humans: Cortical speech zones in 100 adults and 100 infant brains. *Arch. Neurol.*, 32:239–246.

603. Wada, J., and Rasmussen, T. (1960): Intracarotid injection of sodium amytal for the lateralization of cerebral speech dominance: Experimental and clinical observations. *J. Neurosurg.*, 17:266–282.

604. Walsh, K. W. (1978): *Neuropsychology: A Clinical Approach*. Churchill Livingstone, New York.

605. Walsh, R. N., and Greenough, W. T., editors (1976): *Environments as Therapy for Brain Dysfunction*. Plenum Press, New York.

606. Warburton, D. M. (1975): *Brain, Behavior, and Drugs: Introduction to the Neurochemistry of Behavior*. John Wiley & Sons, London.

607. Ward, F., and Bower, B. D. (1978): A study of certain social aspects of epilepsy in childhood. *Dev. Med. Child Neurol. (Suppl. 39)*, Vol. 20, pp. 1–63.

608. Wasterlain, C. G. (1978): Neonatal seizures and brain growth. *Neuropaediatrie*, 9:213–228.

609. Watson, R. T., Valenstein, E., and Heilman, K. M. (1981): Thalamic neglect: Possible role of the medial thalamus and nucleus reticularis in behavior. *Arch. Neurol.*, 38:501–506.

610. Webster, D. B., and Webster, M. (1977): Neonatal sound deprivation affects brain stem auditory nuclei. *Arch. Otolaryngol.*, 103:392–396.

611. Wechsler, D. (1945): *Wechsler Memory Scale*. Psychological Corporation, New York.

612. Wechsler, D. (1949): *Wechsler Intelligence Scale for Children*. Psychological Corporation, New York.

613. Wechsler, D. (1967): *Manual for Wechsler Preschool and Primary Scale of Intelligence*. Psychological Corporation, New York.

614. Weiner, W. J., Nausieda, P. A., and Klawans, H. L. (1978): Methylphenidate-induced chorea: Case report and pharmacologic implications. *Neurology*, 28:1041–1044.

615. Weingartner, H., Gold, P., Ballenger, J. C., Smallberg, S. A., Summers, R., Rubinow, D. R., Post, R. M., and Goodwin, F. K. (1981): Effects of vasopressin on human memory functions. *Science*, 211:601–603.

616. Weiskrantz, L. (1974): The interaction between occipital and temporal cortex in vision: An overview. In: *The Neurosciences, Third Study Program*, edited by F. O. Schmitt, and F. G. Worden, pp. 189–204. MIT Press, Cambridge, Mass.

617. Weiskrantz, L. (1978): A comparison of hippocampal pathology in man and other animals. In: *Symposium on Functions of the Septo-Hippocampal System, London 1977*. CIBA Foundation Symposium No. 58 (new series), pp. 373–406. Elsevier, New York.

618. Weiss, G., and Hechtman, L. (1979): The hyperactive child syndrome. *Science*, 205:1348–1354.

619. Wender, P. H. (1971): *Minimal Brain Dysfunction in Children*. Wiley Interscience, New York.

620. Wender, P. H. (1978): Minimal brain dysfunction: An overview. In: *Psychopharmacology: A Generation of Progress*, edited by M. A. Lipton, A. DiMascio, and K. F. Killam, pp. 1429–1435. Raven Press, New York.

621. Wiesel, T. N., and Hubel, D. H. (1974): Ordered arrangement of orientation columns in monkeys lacking visual experience. *J. Comp. Neurol.*, 158:307–318.

622. Wigglesworth, R. (1961): Minimal cerebral palsy. *Cereb. Palsy Bull.*, 3:293–295.

623. Willerman, L. (1979): *The Psychology of Individual and Group Differences*. Freeman, San Francisco.

624. Williams, D. (1956): The structure of emotions reflected in epileptic experiences. *Brain*, 79:28–67.

625. Wilson, B. C., Iacovillo, J. M., Wilson, J. J., and Risucci, D. (1982): Purdue pegboard performance in normal preschool children. *J. Clin. Neuropsychol., (in press)*.

626. Wilson, B. C., and Wilson, J. J. (1967): Sensory and perceptual function in the cerebral palsied. I. Pressure threshold and two-point discrimination. *J. Nerv. Ment. Dis.*, 145:53–60.

627. Wilson, B. C., and Wilson, J. J. (1967): Sensory and perceptual functions in the cerebral palsied. II. Stereognosis. *J. Nerv. Ment. Dis.*, 145:61–68.

628. Wilson, B. C., and Wilson, J. J. (1978): Language disordered children: A neuropsychologic view. In: *Developmental Disabilities of Early Childhood*, edited by B. A. Feingold, and C. L. Bank, pp. 148–171. Charles C. Thomas, Springfield, Ill.

629. Wilson, B. C., Wilson, J. J., and Davidovicz, H. M. (1982): *The Neuropsychological Assessment of the Preschool Child*. Marcel Dekker, New York, *(in press)*.

630. Wilson, D. H., Reeves, A., Gazzaniga, M., and Culver, C. (1977): Cerebral commissurotomy for control of intractable seizures. *Neurology*, 27:708–715.

631. Wilson, J. J., Rapin, I., Wilson, B. C., and Van Denburgh, F. V. (1975): Neuropsychologic function of children with severe hearing impairment. *J. Speech. Hear. Res.*, 18:634–652.

632. Wilson, M. (1978): Visual system: Pulvinar-extrastriate cortex. In: *Handbook of Behavioral Neurobiology, Vol. 1: Sensory Integration*, edited by R. B. Masterton, pp. 209–247. Plenum Press, New York.

633. Wilson, P. J. E. (1970): Cerebral hemispherectomy for infantile hemiplegia: A report of 50 cases. *Brain*, 93:147–180.

634. Wilson, R. S. (1978): Synchronies in mental development: An epigenetic perspective. *Science*, 202:939–948.

635. Windle, C. (1962): Prognosis of mental subnormals: A critical review of research. *Am. J. Ment. Defic.*, 66; monograph suppl:1–180.

636. Winick, M., and Rosso, P. (1969): Head circumference and cellular growth of the brain in normal and marasmic children. *J. Pediatr.*, 74:774–778.

637. Witelson, S. F. (1977): Early hemispheric specialization and interhemispheric plasticity. An empirical and theoretical review. In: *Language Development and Neurological Theory*, edited by S. J. Segalowitz, and F. A. Gruber, pp. 213–287. Academic Press, New York.

638. Witelson, S. F. (1977): Developmental dyslexia: Two right hemispheres and none left. *Science*, 195:309–311.

639. Witelson, S. F., and Pallie, W. (1973): Left hemisphere specialization for language in the newborn. *Brain*, 96:641–646.

640. Wittig, M. A., and Petersen, A. C., editors (1979): *Sex-Related Differences in Cognitive Functioning*. Academic Press, New York.

641. Wolff, P. H. (1977): The development of manual asymmetries in motor sequencing skills. *Ann. N.Y. Acad. Sci.*, 299:319–327.

642. Wolpaw, T. M., Nation, J. E., and Aram, D. M. (1979): Developmental language disorders: A follow-up study. *Ill. Speech Hear. J.*, 12, No. 2:14–18.

643. Wood, D. R., Reimherr, F. W., Wender, P. H., and Johnson, G. E. (1976): Diagnosis and treatment of minimal brain dysfunction in adults. *Arch. Gen. Psychiatry*, 33:1453–1461.

644. Woodcock, R. W. (1973): *The Woodcock Reading Mastery Tests*. American Guidance Service, Circle Pines, Minn.

645. Woods, B. T., and Carey, S. (1979): Language deficit after apparent clinical recovery from childhood aphasia. *Ann. Neurol.*, 6:405–409.

646. Woods, B. T., and Teuber, H.-L. (1978): Changing patterns of childhood aphasia. *Ann. Neurol.*, 3:273–280.

647. Worster-Drought, C., and Allen, I. M. (1930): Congenital auditory imperception (congenital word-deafness): and its relation to idioglossia and other speech defects. *J. Neurol. Psychopathol.*, 10:193–236.

648. Wyke, M. (1978): *Developmental Dysphasia*. Academic Press, London.

649. Yahr, M., editor (1975): *The Basal Ganglia, Res. Publ. Assoc. Res. Nerv. Ment. Dis.*, 55. Raven Press, New York.

650. Yakovlev, P., and Lecours, A. (1967): The myelogenetic cycles of regional maturation of the brain. In: *Regional Development of the Brain in Early Life*, edited by A. Minkowski, pp. 3–64. Blackwell, Oxford.

651. Young, R. R., Growdon, J. H., and Shahani, B. T. (1975): Beta-adrenergic mechanisms in action tremor. *N. Engl. J. Med.*, 293:950–953.

652. Zaidel, E. (1979): The split and half brains as models of congenital language disability. In: *The Neurological Bases of Language Disorders in Children: Methods and Directions for Research*, edited by C. L. Ludlow, and M. E. Doran-Quine, pp. 55–89. N.I.N.C.D.S. Monograph #22, US Government Printing Office, Washington, D.C.

653. Zajonc, R. B. (1976): Family configuration and intelligence: Variations in scholastic aptitude scores parallel trends in family size and the spacing of children. *Science*, 192:227–236.

654. Zee, D. S., and Robinson, D. A. (1979): A hypothetical explanation of saccadic oscilliations. *Ann. Neurol.*, 5:405–414.

655. Zee, D. S., Yee, R. D., and Singer, H. S. (1977): Congenital ocular motor apraxia. *Brain*, 100:581–599.

656. Zuckerman, M. (1969): Hallucinations, reported sensations, and images. In: *Sensory Deprivation: Fifteen Years of Research*, edited by J. P. Zubeck, pp. 85–125. Appleton-Century-Crofts, New York.

Subject Index

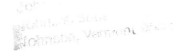

AAS-1326